Migraine and other Primary Headaches

Editor

RANDOLPH W. EVANS

NEUROLOGIC CLINICS

www.neurologic.theclinics.com

Consulting Editor
RANDOLPH W. EVANS

November 2019 • Volume 37 • Number 4

ELSEVIER

1600 John F. Kennedy Boulevard • Suite 1800 • Philadelphia, Pennsylvania, 19103-2899

http://www.theclinics.com

NEUROLOGIC CLINICS Volume 37, Number 4
November 2019 ISSN 0733-8619, ISBN-13: 978-0-323-70870-8

Editor: Stacy Eastman
Developmental Editor: Donald Mumford

Neurologic Clinics (ISSN 0733-8619) is published quarterly by Elsevier Inc., 360 Park Avenue South, New York, NY 10010–1710. Months of issue are February, May, August, and November. Periodicals postage paid at New York, NY, and additional mailing offices. Subscription prices are $323.00 per year for US individuals, $663.00 per year for US institutions, $100.00 per year for US students, $408.00 per year for Canadian individuals, $803.00 per year for Canadian institutions, $427.00 per year for international individuals, $803.00 per year for international institutions, and $210.00 for Canadian and foreign students/residents. To receive student/resident rate, orders must be accompanied by name of affiliated institution, date of term, and the *signature* of program/residency coordinator on institution letterhead. Orders will be billed at individual rate until proof of status is received. Foreign air speed delivery is included in all *Clinics* subscription prices. All prices are subject to change without notice. **POSTMASTER:** Send address changes to *Neurologic Clinics*, Elsevier Health Sciences Division, Subscription Customer Service, 3251 Riverport Lane, Maryland Heights, MO 63043. **Customer Service: Telephone: 1-800-654-2452 (U.S. and Canada); 314-447-8871 (outside U.S. and Canada). Fax: 314-447-8029. E-mail: journalscustomerservice-usa@elsevier.com (for print support); journalsonlinesupport-usa@elsevier.com (for online support).**

Reprints. For copies of 100 or more of articles in this publication, please contact the Commercial Reprints Department, Elsevier Inc., 360 Park Avenue South, New York, New York, 10010-1710; Tel.: +1-212-633-3874; Fax: +1-212-633-3820, and E-mail: reprints@elsevier.com.

Neurologic Clinics is also published in Spanish by Nueva Editorial Interamericana S.A., Mexico City, Mexico.

Neurologic Clinics is covered in *Current Contents/Clinical Medicine, MEDLINE/PubMed (Index Medicus), EMBASE/Excerpta Medica, and PsycINFO, and ISI/BIOMED.*

Contributors

CONSULTING EDITOR

RANDOLPH W. EVANS, MD
Clinical Professor, Department of Neurology, Baylor College of Medicine, Houston, Texas, USA

EDITOR

RANDOLPH W. EVANS, MD
Clinical Professor, Department of Neurology, Baylor College of Medicine, Houston, Texas, USA

AUTHORS

FRANK ANDRASIK, PhD, FAHS
Distinguished Professor and Chair, Department of Psychology, University of Memphis, Memphis, Tennessee, USA

REBECCA C. BURCH, MD
Staff Physician, John R. Graham Headache Center, Brigham and Women's Hospital, Assistant Professor of Neurology, Harvard Medical School, Boston, Massachusetts, USA

MARK J. BURISH, MD, PhD
Assistant Professor, Department of Neurosurgery, University of Texas Health Science Center at Houston, Director, Will Erwin Headache Research Center, Houston, Texas, USA

DAWN C. BUSE, PhD, FAHS
Clinical Professor, Department of Neurology, Albert Einstein College of Medicine of Yeshiva University, Assistant Professor, Clinical Health Psychology Doctoral Program, Ferkauf Graduate School of Psychology of Yeshiva University, Bronx, New York, USA

F. MICHAEL CUTRER, MD
Professor of Neurology, Mayo Clinic, Rochester, Minnesota, USA

RANDOLPH W. EVANS, MD
Clinical Professor, Department of Neurology, Baylor College of Medicine, Houston, Texas, USA

ROD FOROOZAN, MD
Associate Professor of Ophthalmology, Baylor College of Medicine, Houston, Texas, USA

BENJAMIN W. FRIEDMAN, MD, MS
Professor, Department of Emergency Medicine, Albert Einstein College of Medicine, New York, New York, USA; Montefiore Medical Center, Bronx, New York, USA

AMY A. GELFAND, MD
Department of Neurology, Director of Child & Adolescent Headache, UCSF Pediatric Headache Center, University of California, San Francisco, UCSF Benioff Children's Hospital, San Francisco, California, USA

PETER J. GOADSBY, MD, PhD
Headache Group, Basic and Clinical Neurosciences, Institute of Psychiatry, Psychology and Neuroscience, King's College, London, United Kingdom

VICENTE GONZÁLEZ-QUINTANILLA, MD, PhD
Service of Neurology, University Hospital Marqués de Valdecilla, IDIVAL, Santander, Spain

KAITLIN GREENE, MD
Department of Neurology, Pediatric Headache Fellow, UCSF Pediatric Headache Center, University of California, San Francisco, UCSF Benioff Children's Hospital, San Francisco, California, USA

PHILIP R. HOLLAND, PhD
Headache Group, Basic and Clinical Neurosciences, Institute of Psychiatry, Psychology and Neuroscience, King's College, London, United Kingdom

ANGELA HOU, MD
Thomas Jefferson University, Jefferson Headache Center, Philadelphia, Pennsylvania, USA

SAMANTHA L. IRWIN, MD, MSc, MB BCh BAO, FRCPC
Department of Neurology, Assistant Professor of Clinical Neurology, UCSF Pediatric Headache Center, University of California, San Francisco, UCSF Benioff Children's Hospital, San Francisco, California, USA

ANA MARISSA LAGMAN-BARTOLOME, MD, FRCPC
Assistant Professor, Pediatric Neurology and Headache Medicine, Women's College Hospital, Hospital for Sick Children, University of Toronto, Toronto, Ontario, Canada

CHRISTINE LAY, MD, FRCPC, FAHS
Professor, Neurology and Headache Medicine, Women's College Hospital, Hospital for Sick Children, University of Toronto, Toronto, Ontario, Canada

THOMAS LEMPERT, MD
Department of Neurology, Schlosspark-Klinik, Berlin, Germany

RICHARD B. LIPTON, MD
Edwin S. Lowe Professor and Vice Chair of Neurology, Professor of Epidemiology and Population Health, Professor of Psychiatry and Behavioral Science, Albert Einstein College of Medicine, Co-Director, Montefiore Headache Center, Bronx, New York

MICHAEL J. MARMURA, MD
Thomas Jefferson University, Jefferson Headache Center, Philadelphia, Pennsylvania, USA

ANDREA PÉREZ-MUÑOZ, BA
Graduate Student, Department of Psychology, University of Memphis, Memphis, Tennessee, USA

SIMY K. PARIKH, MD
Assistant Professor of Neurology, Jefferson Headache Center, Thomas Jefferson University Hospital, Thomas Jefferson University, Philadelphia, Pennsylvania, USA

JULIO PASCUAL, MD, PhD
Service of Neurology, University Hospital Marqués de Valdecilla, IDIVAL, Santander, Spain

TODD D. ROZEN, MD
Department of Neurology, Mayo Clinic Florida, Jacksonville, Florida, USA

STEPHEN D. SILBERSTEIN, MD
Professor of Neurology, Director, Jefferson Headache Center, Thomas Jefferson University Hospital, Thomas Jefferson University, Philadelphia, Pennsylvania, USA

STEWART J. TEPPER, MD, FAHS
Professor of Neurology, Geisel School of Medicine at Dartmouth, Hanover, New Hampshire, USA; Director, Dartmouth Headache Center, Neurology Department, Dartmouth-Hitchcock Medical Center, Lebanon, New Hampshire, USA

MICHAEL VON BREVERN, MD, PhD
Neurologisches Zentrum, Berlin, Germany

Contents

> The term vestibular migraine designates recurrent vertigo that is caused by migraine. Vestibular migraine presents with episodes of spontaneous or positional vertigo lasting seconds to days that are accompanied by migraine symptoms. Because headache is often absent during acute attacks, other migraine features have to be identified by thorough history taking. In contrast, vestibular testing serves mainly for the exclusion of other diagnoses. Treatment still lacks solid evidence. It is targeted at the underlying migraine and comprises explanation and reassurance, lifestyle modifications, and drugs.

> Most primary headaches can be diagnosed using the history and examination. Judicious use of neuroimaging and other testing, however, is indicated to distinguish primary headaches from the many secondary causes that may share similar features. This article evaluates the reasons for diagnostic testing and the use of neuroimaging, electroencephalography, lumbar puncture, and blood testing. The use of diagnostic testing in adults and children who have headaches and a normal neurologic examination, migraine, trigeminal autonomic cephalalgias, hemicrania continua, and new daily persistent headache are reviewed.

> All patients with migraine merit acute treatment, which should optimally achieve a sustained pain-free response. Maximum acute treatment is associated with reduced risk of transformation of episodic to chronic migraine. The American Headache Society published the most recent complete evidence assessment of acute migraine treatments in 2015. Noninvasive neuromodulation represents a new, Food and Drug Administration–approved nonsignificant risk alternative for acute migraine therapy. The future of acute migraine treatment includes new devices and formulations of existing medications, new classes of acute medications, and new noninvasive nonsignificant risk neuromodulation devices, with many anticipated in the next few years.

> Diagnostic testing is of limited value among patients with migraine who present to an emergency department. Various nonopioid, disease-specific treatments are available for patients who present to an emergency department with migraine headache and associated features. Emergency physicians should recognize that the acute migraine presentation is part of an underlying disorder; care should be geared to the underlying headache disorder in addition to the acute attack.

Episodic migraine is a debilitating condition. Preventive therapy is used to reduce frequency, duration, or severity of attacks. This review discusses principles of preventive treatment with a focus on preventive treatment options for people with episodic migraine. Specifically discussed is evidence and use of new migraine-specific treatment options for episodic migraine, such as calcitonin gene-related peptide monoclonal antibodies, a noninvasive transcutaneous electrical nerve stimulation device, and a single-pulse transcranial magnetic stimulator device. Also discussed are evidence-based updates from the 2012 American Academy of Neurology and the American Headache Society guidelines regarding major medication classes recommended for preventive episodic migraine treatment.

Migraine is a frequently disabling neurologic condition which can be complicated by medication overuse headache and comorbid medical disorders, including obesity, anxiety and depression. Although most migraine management takes place in outpatient clinics, inpatient treatment is indicated for migraine refractory to multiple outpatient treatments, with intractable nausea or vomiting, need for detoxification from medication overuse (such as opioids and barbiturates), and significant medical and psychiatric disease. The goals of inpatient treatment include breaking the current cycle of headache pain, reducing the frequency and/or severity of future attacks, monitored detoxification of overused medications, and reducing disability and improving quality of life.

Biobehavioral interventions for migraine incorporate both physiologic and psychological factors. This article details treatments for migraine management and prevention, ranging from traditional to newly emerging interventions. Similarly, this article reviews key person-related factors that may affect migraine prevalence and management. Aspects related to patient-physician relationships and communication are also reviewed. Research involving childhood and adolescent migraine is reviewed, and special considerations regarding this population are summarized. Clinical trials and other studies have provided evidence that these behavioral interventions, when combined with pharmacotherapy, show a marked improvement in primary treatment outcomes, such as a decrease in headache frequency and duration.

This article outlines key features of diagnosis and treatment of migraine in children and adolescents. It emphasizes techniques that can be used by clinicians to optimize history taking in this population, as well as recognition of episodic conditions that may be associated with migraine and present in childhood. Acute treatment strategies include use of over-the-counter analgesics and triptan medications that have been approved by the US Food and Drug Administration for use in children and adolescents. Preventive treatment approach includes lifestyle modifications, behavioral strategies, and consideration of preventive medications with the lowest side effect profiles.

Migraine is a lifelong condition that disproportionately affects women and, if not effectively managed, can lead to significant disability. It is important for clinicians to have a good understanding of the impact of the hormonal fluctuations that occur throughout a female migraineur's life, so that appropriate, stratified therapies can be implemented. In doing so, whether it is migraine onset at menarche in an adolescent young woman, or migraine worsening in a perimenopausal female migraineur, quality of life can be ensured.

The trigeminal autonomic cephalalgias (TACs) are a group of primary headache syndromes all marked by unilateral headache and ipsilateral cranial autonomic features. The TACs include cluster headache, paroxysmal hemicrania, short-lasting unilateral neuralgiform headache attacks with conjunctival injection and tearing, and hemicrania continua. Pathophysiology includes the trigeminal pain system, autonomic system, hypothalamus, and more recently an identified role for the vagus nerve. Diagnosis is made after looking at headache frequency, duration, and accompanying symptoms. Each TAC has its own unique treatment, which is discussed in depth.

"Other Primary Headaches" in the ICHD-3 encompasses activity-related headaches, headaches due to direct physical stimuli, epicranial headaches and a miscellanea, including hypnic headache and new daily-persistent headache. They can be primary or secondary and their etiologies differ depending on headache type. For instance, activity-related headaches can be induced by Valsalva maneuvers ("cough headache") or prolonged exercise ("exercise and sexual headaches"). Almost half of cough headaches are secondary to posterior fossa abnormality, whereas only 20% of exertional/sexual headaches are secondary, with subarachnoid hemorrhage the most frequent etiology. This article reviews the clinical diagnosis and management of these heterogeneous headaches.

NEUROLOGIC CLINICS

RELATED SERIES

Neuroimaging Clinics
Psychiatric Clinics
Child and Adolescent Psychiatric Clinics

THE CLINICS ARE AVAILABLE ONLINE!
Access your subscription at:
www.theclinics.com

NEUROLOGIC CLINICS

FORTHCOMING ISSUES

February 2020
Neuroimaging
Laszlo L. Mechtler, Editor

May 2020
Treatment of Movement Disorders
Joseph Jankovic, Editor

August 2020
Case Studies in Neuromuscular Disorders
Aziz Shaibani, Editor

RECENT ISSUES

August 2019
Circadian Rhythm Disorders
Phyllis C. Zee, Editor

May 2019
Vasculitis and the Nervous System
David S. Younger, Editor

February 2019
Neurology of Pregnancy
Mary Angela O'Neal, Editor

RELATED SERIES

Neuroimaging Clinics
Psychiatric Clinics
Child and Adolescent Psychiatric Clinics

THE CLINICS ARE AVAILABLE ONLINE!
Access your subscription at:
www.theclinics.com

Preface
Migraine and other Primary Headaches

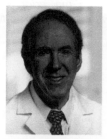

Randolph W. Evans, MD
Editor

This issue of *Neurologic Clinics* reviews migraine and other primary headaches. Secondary headaches were reviewed in *Neurologic Clinics* in 2014. *Neurologic Clinics* last covered primary headaches in 2009. Since then, there have been many advances, including most recently, monoclonal antibodies to CGRP, gepants, ditans, and neuromodulating devices.

Primary headaches are the cause of about 90% of all headaches. The burden is substantial. The most common primary headache seen in neurologic practice is migraine, with about 40 million people affected in the United States and up to 1 billion people affected worldwide per year. Somewhere between 3 and 7 million people have chronic migraine in the United States yearly. These numbers include many of you, as migraine affects over 50% of neurologists and 70% of headache specialists. Cluster headache has a prevalence of about 0.1% of the population, affecting about 250,000 people yearly in the United States. Other primary headaches reviewed in this issue are rare (with the exception of the common primary stabbing headache), including the following: hemicrania continua; primary cough, exercise, and association with sexual activity; primary thunderclap; cold-stimulus headache; external pressure headache; nummular headache; hypnic headache; and new daily persistent headache.

This issue covers many migraine topics, including the following: pathophysiology; transient neurologic dysfunction in migraine; vestibular migraine; diagnostic testing for migraine; acute and preventive treatment of migraine; migraine in the emergency department; inpatient migraine management; behavior medicine for migraine; pediatric migraine; and migraine in women. Two articles review trigeminal autonomic cephalalgias and other primary headaches. I hope this issue updates and expands your knowledge of our exciting and expanding field.

I thank our distinguished contributors for their outstanding articles. I also thank Stacy Eastman, *Neurologic Clinics* editor, Don Mumford, senior developmental editor, and

Neurol Clin 37 (2019) xiii–xiv
https://doi.org/10.1016/j.ncl.2019.07.011
0733-8619/19/© 2019 Published by Elsevier Inc.

the Elsevier production team for outstanding work. Finally, I am grateful for the support of my wife, Marilyn, and our children, Elliott, Rochelle (and husband Corry), and Jonathan.

Randolph W. Evans, MD
1200 Binz Street, #1370
Houston, TX 77004, USA

E-mail address:
revansmd@gmail.com

Migraine

Epidemiology, Burden, and Comorbidity

Rebecca C. Burch, MD[a],*, Dawn C. Buse, PhD[b],
Richard B. Lipton, MD[c]

KEYWORDS

- Migraine • Chronic migraine (CM) • Prevalence • Incidence
- Headache-related disability • Comorbidity • Progression • Risk factors

KEY POINTS

- Migraine is common, and occurs in about 12% of the US population overall, 18% of women, and 6% of men, each year. Global estimates are generally higher.
- Chronic migraine affects 1% to 2% of the global population; 2.5% of persons with episodic migraine progress to CM each year. Risk factors for progression may be modifiable or nonmodifiable.
- Migraine is associated with many medical comorbidities including cardiovascular disease, psychiatric disease, and sleep disorders.
- Migraine is the second most disabling condition worldwide and may affect occupational, academic, social, family, and personal domains of life.
- Chronic migraine is associated with higher headache-related disability/impact, medical and psychiatric comorbidities, health care resource use and direct and indirect costs, and lower socioeconomic status and health-related quality of life.

INTRODUCTION

Epidemiology, the study of diseases in populations, is essential to our understanding of every aspect of migraine. Migraine epidemiology informs clinical care of patients, shapes our understanding of migraine pathophysiology, and defines the burden of illness.[1,2] The epidemiologic, population-based perspective complements the view obtained in clinic-based studies, because many people with migraine do

Disclosure Statement: See last page of article.
[a] Department of Neurology, John R. Graham Headache Center, Brigham and Women's Hospital, Harvard Medical School, 1153 Centre Street, Suite 4H, Jamaica Plain, MA 02130, USA;
[b] Albert Einstein College of Medicine, 1250 Waters Place, 8th floor, Bronx, NY 10461, USA;
[c] Albert Einstein College of Medicine, Montefiore Headache Center, 1300 Morris Park Avenue, Van Etten 3C12, Bronx, NY 10461, USA
* Corresponding author.
E-mail address: rburch@bwh.harvard.edu
; @RebeccaCBurch (R.C.B.); @dawnbuse (D.C.B.)

not seek medical care and, of those that do, many are not diagnosed or optimally treated.

The population view facilitates an assessment of barriers to consultation, diagnosis, and treatment in various populations setting the stage for making improvements.[3,4] Understanding prevalence as a function of age and sex informs how likely migraine might be in a particular patient. Understanding how migraine manifests in different demographic groups can improve diagnosis of people with atypical presentations.[5]

Information about comorbidities provides the backdrop in which migraine typically appears. Clinically, epidemiology describes conditions that may confound the diagnosis, contribute to the overall burden of illness in patients with migraine, and affect therapeutic choices for acute and preventive treatment. Patterns of disease expression and comorbidity also provide a window into possible disease mechanisms.

In this article, we review the prevalence and incidence, societal, and individual burden, comorbidities, and natural history of episodic migraine (EM) and chronic migraine (CM). We also describe what is known about the transition from EM to CM (chronification or progression).

Migraine Prevalence and Incidence

The prevalence of EM has been assessed in many studies. We focus here on 3 large-scale, US population studies conducted over a 15-year period because they have relatively high participation rates, sampled demographically representative samples of the US population and used similar methods. These studies are the American Migraine Study I (AMS-I, 1989), the American Migraine Study II (AMS-II, 1999), and the American Migraine Prevalence and Prevention studies (AMPP, 2004).[6–8] In these studies, approximately 12% of respondents, including 18% of women, and 6% of men, reported migraine in the previous year. The most recent and largest of these 3 studies was the AMPP study.[8] For this longitudinal study, started in 2004, surveys were mailed to a sample of 120,000 US households selected to represent the population according to census data for age, sex, race, income, and region of the country. Stratified by gender, 17.4% of women and 5.7% of men had EM, and 0.91% met criteria for CM (1.29% of women; 0.48% of men).[5,8]

The prevalence of migraine or severe headache is also assessed by annual US government health studies.[9] Results from the National Health Interview Survey (NHIS) show that self-reported migraine and severe headache was reported by 15.3% of Americans overall, including 9.7% of men and 20.7% of women.[10] Review of annually collected data from this survey shows remarkable stability of prevalence over the last 19 years.[10] Migraine is significantly more common in women.[5] Results from the NHIS show that the 3-month prevalence ratio of migraine and severe headache ranged from 2 to 2.4 between 2005 and 2015.[11] The woman to man gender prevalence ratio varies with age. An analysis of AMPP study data showed that the adjusted woman to man prevalence ratios for migraine range from 1.5 to 1 for those 12 to 17 years old to 3.25 to 1 for those 18 to 29 years old.[5] Before puberty, migraine is more common in boys than girls. After puberty, the prevalence of migraine increases gradually in men and much more rapidly in women. The AMPP study estimates the prevalence of migraine in people aged 12 to 19 years to be 6.3% (boys 5.0%, girls 7.7%).[12] Throughout adolescence, the prevalence in boys (adjusted for socioeconomic factors) increases from 2.9% to 4.1%. The adjusted prevalence in girls peaks at age 17 years at 9.8%.

Migraine is not only more common in women than in men, it is also experienced as more severe. For example, in comparison with men with migraine, women with migraine report higher pain intensity, headache-related disability, and more associated symptoms. Women are also more likely to consult doctors, use urgent care and emergency treatment of headache, and use more prescription drugs.[10,13] Although rates of consultation for and diagnosis of migraine are higher in women than in men, men with diagnosed migraine are more likely to be treated.[5,13] In the US population-based National Hospital Ambulatory Medical Care Survey, women were about twice as likely as men to visit the emergency department for a complaint of headache or pain in the head.[10]

North American studies consistently find an inverse relationship between migraine prevalence and socioeconomic status, as measured by income or education, whereas European studies have conflicting findings. US population-based studies have found correlations between lower household income and higher migraine prevalence rates.[7,14,15] The NHIS studies also found that prevalence of migraine or severe headache was highest in those with an annual family income less than $35,000, and a linear correlation between increasing annual income bracket and decreasing headache and migraine prevalence.[10] Migraine and severe headache were also more prevalent in those with Medicare or Medicaid rather than private insurance. In contrast, studies from the Netherlands, Denmark, and Canada did not find this inverse relationship.[16-18] The social causation hypothesis could account for these findings. Under this hypothesis, factors associated with low income, such as stressful lifestyle or poor diet, could increase the rate of migraine onset. Another possibility is the social selection hypothesis, which states that illness itself interferes with social or occupational function and causes low income. Research showing that people from low-income households have a higher rate of migraine incidence supports the social causation hypothesis.[6]

After adjusting for socioeconomic status, migraine prevalence in the United States varies by race. The AMPP study found that prevalence is highest in white women and men (20.4%, 8.6%), intermediate in African Americans (16.2%, 7.2%), and lowest in Asian Americans (9.2%, 4.2%).[14] Results from the 2005 to 2012 surveys also show that prevalence of migraine or severe headache is highest in whites (21% women, 10% men) compared with blacks (19.6%, 9.3%) or Hispanics (20.6%, 8.4%).[19] The 2014 NHIS survey included an initiative to specially survey typically underrepresented populations. In that year, the 3-month prevalence of migraine or severe headache was highest in American Indians and Alaska Natives (19.2%), followed by whites (15.5%), blacks or African Americans (15%), Hispanic or Latinos (14.9%), Native Hawaiian or Pacific Islanders (13.2%), and Asians (10.1).[10]

An analysis from the 2016 Global Burden of Disease (GBD) study, including data from 132 countries, estimated that worldwide 1.04 billion people had migraine, corresponding to a prevalence of 14.4% overall, 18.9% in women, and 9.8% in men.[20] The "Lifting the Burden: The Global Campaign to Reduce the Burden Worldwide," developed in concert with the World Health Organization, is a major initiative to assess migraine prevalence around the world by compiling research globally. This project has found migraine prevalence highest in Europe and lowest in Africa and China (Table 1).[21,22] These differences by region of the world and race could be explained by methodological differences among studies, genetic, biological, environmental, social, or other factors.

Prevalence estimates reported in Lifting the Burden analyses have generally been higher than those from the AMS, AMPP, and NHIS studies. This may be related to methodological differences between the US and global studies. Both the AMPP and the NHIS required respondents to self-report their diagnoses and/or symptoms meeting diagnostic criteria and to endorse "severe headache" (or migraine, in the case of the NHIS) in the past year (AMPP) or 3 months (NHIS). This may have resulted

Table 1
Comparison of migraine 1-year prevalence worldwide

Region	Overall Prevalence (%)	Headache >15 d/mo (%)
Global	15	1.7–4
United States	11.7 overall 5.6 men 17.1 women	1
Americas	10.6	4
Russia and Eastern Europe	16–20	10
European Union	35	7
Sub-Saharan Africa	18–23	3–12
Southeast Asia	25–33	3–8
Western Pacific (China)	9	1–2

Adapted from Saylor D, Steiner TJ. The Global Burden of Headache. Semin Neurol 2018;38(2):182-190; and WHO Atlas of headache disorders and resources in the world 2011. May 2012. https://www.who.int/mental_health/management/atlas_headache_disorders/en/. Accessed January 11, 2019.

in some people with mild to moderate migraine being missed in the AMPP survey. The studies conducted as part of the Lifting the Burden initiative used door-to-door personal interviews to determine migraine diagnoses in members of a household. This may result in a more accurate diagnosis of migraine or could, alternatively, result in overdiagnosis because of false-positives. A UK study that used in-person interviews but also used a severe headache screening question found migraine prevalence similar to that in the United States. This suggests that screening for severe headache may underestimate migraine prevalence.[23]

Migraine incidence is less well studied than prevalence. A 12-year longitudinal study conducted in Copenhagen found migraine incidence to be 8.1 per 1000 person-years, with a woman to man ratio of 6.2 to 1.[24] Incidence declined with age, peaking in 25- to 34-year-old women at 23 per 1000 person-years and in men at about 10 per 1000 person-years. In the 55- to 64-year-old age group, incidence was less than 5 per 1000 person-years. AMPP study researchers used reported age of onset among prevalent cases to model age-incidence profiles using the reconstructed cohort method.[25] The cumulative lifetime incidence was 43% in women and 18% in men. Migraine incidence peaked in the 20- to 24-year-old age group in women (18.2 per 1000 person-years) and in the 15- to 19-year-old age group in men (6.2 per 1000 person-years). Values for cumulative incidence are far higher than the 1-year period prevalence of migraine in the same population, probably indicating a high rate of migraine remission.

Chronic Migraine: Prevalence and Incidence

Global estimates of CM prevalence generally range from 1.4% to 2.2%.[26] A systematic review of studies including transformed migraine (a term that was previously used to describe migraine that transitioned from episodic to chronic) and CM found that these conditions were more prevalent in Europe, followed by the Western Pacific and then the Americas.[26] In this analysis the prevalence of CM in adolescents was estimated at 0.76% (confidence interval [CI], 0.05–1.48), with a gradual increase with increasing age through the teenage years. Prevalence was higher in teenage girls than boys (1.39% vs. 0.15%). AMPP study analyses reported a CM prevalence of 0.91% overall (1.29% of girls; 0.48% of boys).[15] Relative to 12- to 17-year-olds, the age- and sex-specific prevalence for CM peaked in the decade of the 1940s at 1.89% for women and 0.79% (prevalence ratio = 3.35; 95% CI, 1.99–5.63) for men. CM was also much more common in women than men, with a sex prevalence ratio of 4.57 (95% CI, 3.13–6.67). The prevalence of CM was inversely related to household income. CM represented 7.7% of migraine cases overall (excluding probable migraine), and the proportion generally increased with age.

There are few data available on CM incidence in the population, as CM usually progresses from EM. Analyses of data from the AMPP study show that between 2.5% and 3% of people with EM in 1 year meet criteria for CM the following year.[27]

Burden of Migraine

Migraine is a highly burdensome condition for people, families, and society. An analysis of 2016 GBD data estimated that migraine caused 45.1 million years lived with disability (YLDs) in that year.[20] At the level of specific diseases, migraine was the second most disabling condition after low back pain.[20] Migraine can affect the function of the individual in multiple roles and settings including occupational, academic, social, familial, and personal.[28–30] The societal burden is magnified in that migraine prevalence is highest in the second, third, fourth, and fifth decades of life. In the GBD study, disability was highest in women between the ages of 15 and 49 years, with 20.3 million YLDs in this group because of migraine.[20] This is a time when work productivity is often at its peak and when people with migraine may be caring for children or elderly parents, further increasing the possible effect on quality of life and disability.

The burden of migraine occurs during (ictal) and between (interictal) attacks.[31] The ictal burden is related to experience of the migraine itself, including head pain, exacerbation by movement or activity, nausea, vomiting, and sensitivity to environmental stimuli. All of these symptoms limit function during attacks. The interictal burden of migraine manifests as difficulty in planning events owing to the possible occurrence of migraine, and as fear of the next attack (anticipatory anxiety). Migraine has a significant negative impact on health-related quality of life (HRQoL).[32] HRQoL is inversely related to headache-related disability and headache day frequency. HRQoL can improve with treatment of the migraine and psychological or behavioral treatment, and is an important target for intervention.

Assessment of disability is essential for optimized treatment planning.[33] The American Migraine Communication Study I showed that physicians underestimate the associated disability and impact of migraine and often do not assess the need for preventive therapy.[34] Assessment of headache-related disability allows health care providers to tailor treatment plans to disease severity and thus improve treatment outcomes.[35] A range of validated patient-reported outcomes (PROs) exist to aid in the management of migraine.[36] Disability and HRQoL can be measured by generic and disease-specific instruments. The Migraine Disability Assessment Scale (MIDAS) is a brief tool that is scored in units of lost days because of headache over 3 months in the domains of work and school, household work and chores, and family, social, and leisure activities.[35] Scores range from 0 to 270 and are graded by level of headache-related disability: grade I, little or no disability (0–5); grade II, mild disability (6–10); grade III, moderate disability (11–20); grade IV, severe disability (≥21). grade IV has been further subdivided into 2 categories to improve sensitivity in patients with CM: grade IV-A, severe disability (21–40), and grade IV-B, very severe disability (41–270).[30] The Headache Impact Test (HIT-6) is a shorter version of a longer web-based adaptive test and assesses activity limitations in several domains as well as pain severity, fatigue, frustration, and difficulty with concentration.[37] The Migraine Physical Function Impact Diary and Migraine Functional Impact Questionnaire are recent, novel patient-reported outcome measures for assessing the impact of migraine on physical function that followed 2009 US Food and Drug Administration guidance on development of PROs for inclusion in clinical trials to support labeling claims.[38–41] In addition, studies have also shown that simply asking "Tell me about your headaches and how they affect your life" is effective in establishing a dialog about headache that improves health care provider and patient satisfaction and appropriate treatment, and shortens visit length.[42] HRQoL can be measured with general or migraine-specific instruments.

The economic burden of migraine can be either direct (ie, medical costs) or indirect, including lost productive time.[43,44] Past studies have found that indirect costs made up the bulk of the economic burden of migraine, but more recent studies show the reverse.[45,46] People with migraine had individual direct and indirect costs estimated at nearly $9000 per year higher than demographically similar people without migraine.[46] In a survey of lost productive time because of common pain conditions in the US workforce over a 2-week period, Stewart[47] found that headache was the most commonly reported pain condition (followed by back pain and arthritis), leading to loss in productive time of 3.5 ± 0.1 hours per week. Using a large employer database, Hawkins and colleagues[44] determined that employees with recognized migraine each cost the employer approximately $2600 more annually than employees without migraine, because of absenteeism and short-term disability and workers' compensation claims.

Both clinic-based and population-based studies have demonstrated that, in comparison with those with EM, persons with CM have greater headache-related disability, headache impact, and decrements in HRQoL; lower socioeconomic status; higher rates of comorbid medical and psychiatric conditions; increased health care resource use; and higher direct and indirect costs.[15,37,48–52] In the 2005 AMPP survey, respondents with CM had statistically significant lower levels of household income, were less likely to be employed full time, and more likely to be occupationally disabled than those with EM.[53] In addition, persons with CM (relative to EM) had much higher rates of headache-related disability (assessed with the MIDAS). Among persons with CM, 24.8% had MIDAS scores that were in MIDAS grade IV-B ("very severe" headache-related disability) in comparison with just 3.2% of those in the EM group. Similar results from the AMPP study were seen for the HIT-6.[37] People with CM were significantly more likely to experience "severe" headache impact (72.9% vs. 42.3% of those with EM), as were people who were younger, experienced more migraine symptoms (other than pain) and at greater intensity, reported more severe head pain, and met criteria for depression.

Results from the Chronic Migraine Epidemiology and Outcomes (CaMEO) study also show greater disability in people with CM.[54] grade IV MIDAS scores were seen in 32.0% of men and 38% of women. Moderate or severe disability, shown by grade III or IV MIDAS scores, was seen in 71% of men and 82.6% of women with CM, compared with 26.7% of men and 37.9% of women with EM. The International Burden of Illness study confirms that this phenomenon is not restricted to the United States.[30] This study also found that those with CM reported greater health care resource use, including twice as many primary care visits, 3 times as many neurologist visits, and 1.5 times as many emergency department visits using the EM group for comparison.

Comorbidities of Migraine

Many medical conditions are more common in people with migraine compared with the general population (**Table 2**).[55] Neurologic comorbidities include epilepsy, stroke,

Table 2
Comorbidities of migraine

Vascular	Myocardial infarction Stroke Raynaud's phenomenon
Neurologic	Epilepsy Multiple sclerosis Restless legs syndrome Sleep disorders including insomnia
Psychiatric	Bipolar disorder Childhood adverse experiences Depression Generalized anxiety disorder Panic disorder Posttraumatic stress disorder
Nonmigraine pain conditions	Fibromyalgia Temporomandibular joint disorder
Other	Allergic rhinitis Asthma Systemic lupus erythematosus

restless legs syndrome (RLS), sleep disorders, ischemic stroke, and multiple sclerosis. Medical comorbidities include asthma, allergic rhinitis, vascular conditions (such as angina and claudication) and events (such as myocardial infarction), and nonheadache pain disorders, including temporomandibular joint disorder and fibromyalgia. Psychiatric comorbidities include depression, anxiety, panic disorder, posttraumatic stress disorder, and suicidality, among other conditions. Both clinic- and population-based studies have demonstrated higher rates of comorbid conditions in persons with CM (relative to EM).[53,54,56,57] Several theories have been proposed to explain underlying mechanisms that could promote comorbid conditions, including the notion that 1 disease may cause the other, latent brain state models, shared environment, and shared genetic origins.[1]

Cardiovascular disease
Cardiac disease is common in people with migraine, and many studies have shown that migraine is a risk factor for cardiovascular disease, and both cause mortality. An analysis of AMPP survey data found that 2.6 million people in the United States had EM and at least 1 cardiac event, condition (such as angina), or procedure (such as endarterectomy).[58] The AMPP survey also found that Framingham Risk Scores increased linearly with age in people with migraine. The proportion of migraineurs with a high Framingham Risk Score ranged from 0% for men and women aged 22% to 39%, to 15.2% of women and 53% of men in the ≥60 age group.[58] A 2015 meta-analysis included 15 observational studies and found an increased risk of myocardial infarction and angina (1.33, 95% CI, 1.08–1.64, and 1.29, 95% CI, 1.17–1.43, respectively) in people with migraine compared with those without migraine.[59] Data from prospective cohort studies, including the Nurses' Health Study, Women's Health Study, and Physicians' Health Study also support the association between cardiovascular disease and migraine and have shown 1.4- to 1.7-fold increases in the risk of major cardiovascular disease, myocardial infarction, angina/coronary revascularization procedures, and cardiovascular disease mortality in people with migraine versus those without.[60–62]

A 2017 meta-analysis of prospective cohort studies included 11 studies and 2,221,888 patients found a relative risk (RR) of 1.64 (95% CI, 1.22–2.20) for ischemic stroke.[63] The evidence base for hemorrhagic stroke is less robust, with an RR of 1.15 (95% CI, 0.85–1.56) in this analysis. Earlier meta-analyses found that the risk of stroke associated with migraine with aura was roughly doubled, but there was no increased risk associated with migraine without aura.[64] Interestingly, it seems that migraine is a more significant risk factor in people under the age of 45 who have an otherwise low cardiac risk factor burden. The risk of stroke in people with migraine is also higher in women, and in women who use estrogen-containing contraceptives.[65]

Migraine with aura is a risk factor for brain lesions.[66] These lesions include deep white matter lesions, subtentorial white matter lesions, and stroke-like posterior circulation areas. In the population-based CAMERA study of persons with migraine with aura, migraine without aura, and controls, posterior circulation stroke-like lesions were more likely in the migraine with aura group and more common in those with more attacks of migraine with aura.[66] The adjusted odds ratio (OR) for migraine with aura was 13.7 (95% CI, 1.7–112) and was even higher in patients with migraine with aura having more than 1 attack per month, with an OR of 15.8 (95% CI, 1.8–140). Longer duration of disease was also associated with an increased risk. Follow-up imaging at an average interval of 9 years found a statistically significant increase in the number of deep white matter lesions, particularly in the migraine without aura group of women.[67]

Psychiatric conditions

Migraine is comorbid with several psychiatric disorders including depression, anxiety disorders, bipolar disorder, posttraumatic stress disorder, personality disorders, and suicide attempts.[57] The prevalence of several psychiatric disorders was determined in a sample of over 36,000 subjects in a Canadian population-based cohort.[68] Major depression, bipolar disorder, panic disorder, and social phobia were all at least twice as prevalent in migraine subjects, and were independent of demographic and socioeconomic variables. Persons with migraine and one of the psychiatric comorbidities had lower HRQoL than those having either disorder alone.

Several population-based studies have found that depression is 2 to 2.5 times more common in migraineurs compared with the general population.[68–70] Approximately 40% of people with migraine also report depression.[70] The relationship between migraine and depression is bidirectional, with each condition increasing the risk of the other.[71] Anxiety disorders are also common, and the cumulative lifetime incidence of anxiety disorders in migraine is about 50%.[57] Migraine is associated with a 4- to 5-fold increase in the risk of general anxiety disorder and 3 to 10 times the risk of panic disorder.[56,72] Obsessive-compulsive disorder is also more common in people with migraine. Depression and anxiety commonly co-occur.

Rates of psychiatric comorbidity increase with increasing headache frequency and are highest among people with CM.[53,56] A large Norwegian population study assessed depression and anxiety disorders in more than 50,000 persons with migraine, other nonmigraine headache, and headache-free controls.[73] When participants were classified by tertiles of headache frequency, the adjusted OR of depression and anxiety increased linearly. Participants reporting 15 or more days of migraine per month had an adjusted OR of 6.4 (95% CI, 4.4–9.3) for depression and 6.9 (95% CI, 5.1–9.4) for anxiety. The CaMEO study found that the OR for depression was 3.05 (95% CI, 2.74–3.40) in people with CM compared with those with EM, and the OR for generalized anxiety disorder was 2.40 (2.16–2.67) in CM versus EM.[74]

Sleep disorders

There is a bidirectional relationship between sleep disorders and migraine. A study of 1283 patients in a tertiary headache center found that at least half reported at least occasional sleep disturbances.[75] Sleep disruption is one of the most commonly reported migraine triggers.[76] Sleep duration is shortened in people with migraine and is associated with headache severity.[77] The third HUNT study, a Norwegian population-based survey, assessed sleep with the Karolinska Sleep Questionnaire (KSQ) and the Epworth Sleepiness Scale (ESS).[78] Of the 297 participants, those with migraine were 3 times more likely to have an ESS score ≥ 10 compared with those without headache. A high KSQ score was 5 times more likely among those with migraine. Estimates of the increased risk of RLS in people with migraine range from OR of 1.2 to 4.2 depending on study design.[79] Symptoms of RLS may be more severe in people with migraine.[80] Studies are conflicting as to whether obstructive sleep apnea is more common in people with migraine, but it seems to be more common among people with CM compared with people with EM, and when present in people with EM it is a risk factor for migraine chronification.[79,81,82]

Comorbidities of Chronic Migraine

Both clinic-based and population-based studies have demonstrated a higher burden of medical and psychiatric comorbidity in persons with CM relative to EM.[52,53,74] In the 2005 AMPP survey respondents with CM were approximately twice as likely to have depression, anxiety, and chronic pain compared with those with EM. Respiratory disorders including asthma, bronchitis and chronic obstructive pulmonary disease, and cardiac risk factors, including hypertension, diabetes, high cholesterol, and obesity were also significantly more likely to be reported by those with CM. Findings from the International Burden of Illness study showed a similar pattern.[83] In this comparison of study respondents with migraine in the United States and Canada, approximately one-half (United States 49.0%, Canada 50.9%) of CM participants reported pain-related comorbidities, compared with only 26.7% and 25.2% of EM participants in the United States and Canada, respectively. Almost one-half (45.2%) of US CM participants reported a psychiatric disorder, compared with approximately one-third (29.0%) of EM participants.

Studies outside of North America have also found a high burden of comorbidity in people with CM. In the Taiwan National Health Insurance Research Database, patients with CM had a higher risk of medical comorbidities compared with patients with "other migraines": hyperlipidemia (RR = 1.32; P = .041) or asthma (RR = 1.77; P = .007); and psychiatric comorbidities: depression (RR = 1.88; $P\leq$.0001), bipolar disorder (RR = 1.81; P = .022), and anxiety disorders (RR = 1.48; $P\leq$.0001).[52] A Scottish database analysis of almost 1.5 million primary care patients evaluated the prevalence of 31 medical conditions in those with CM versus those without.[84] They found that 25 of the 31 conditions were more common in people with CM, and that 11.7% of people with CM had 5 or more comorbidities versus 4.9% of controls. Anxiety and depression were also 3 times more common in the CM population in this study.

Latent class analysis of data from the CaMEO study identified 8 natural groupings of migraine patients according to comorbidity profiles.[85] These subgroups differed in ways that were not used to identify the subgroups, including age, illness severity, and prognosis. This suggests that the comorbidity profiles of a person with migraine may signify a particular biological subtype. In addition, rates of progression from episodic to CM were found to differ by class, with hazard ratios for CM onset ranging from 5.34 (95% CI, 3.89, 7.33; $P\leq$.001) for the "Most Comorbidities" class to 1.53

(95% CI, 1.17, 2.01; $P<.05$) for the "Respiratory" class relative to the "Fewest Comorbidities" class.[86]

The Natural History of Migraine

Longitudinal population studies, as well as clinic-based observational studies, have informed our understanding of the natural history and the prognosis of migraine.[87,88] Researchers posit 4 partially overlapping clinical trajectories in persons with EM: complete remission, partial remission, persistence, and progression. Partial remission is associated with decreased migraine attack frequency and severity, and migraine accompanying symptoms such as nausea and photophobia may also decrease. People with CM may revert to EM or EM may decrease from high to low frequency. High-frequency, moderate-frequency, and low-frequency EM are now being studied as possibly distinct epidemiologic entities, so partial remission is often a clinically meaningful improvement.[89]

Progression, transformation, or chronification occur when migraine attack frequency increases crossing the $\geq$15 days per month CM boundary.[90] Migraine-associated symptom profiles and headache-related disability typically increase as well. Clinical progression is often associated with the experience of cutaneous allodynia and sensitization at the level of the trigeminal nucleus caudalis; signs of physiologic progression.[91] Longitudinal population studies estimate that around 2.5% to 3% of people with EM progress to CM each year.[27] This small subgroup of persons with EM who progress to CM may provide important clues into the mechanisms of progression.

Course of episodic migraine

An analysis of AMPP study data over the course of 2 years provides insight into the natural course of EM. Of the respondents who initially had EM, 82.8% still had EM in the following year, 2.5% had developed CM, and 14.0% had other outcomes (eg, remission, probable migraine, or tension-type headache.)[27]

Course of chronic migraine

Three-year longitudinal data from the AMPP survey were also used to track outcomes of patients with CM.[92] Almost 34% had CM in all 3 studied years (ie, persistent CM), whereas 26.1% had CM in the initial year but had other headache conditions (eg, low-frequency EM, no headache, probable migraine, episodic tension-type headache, or other episodic headache) in the subsequent 2 years (ie, remitted CM). Forty percent fluctuated from CM to EM and back to CM. Multivariate models found that predictors of remission included lower baseline headache days per month frequency (15–19 d/mo vs. 25–31 headache d/mo; OR = 0.29; 95% CI, 0.11–0.75) and the absence of cutaneous allodynia (OR = 0.45; 95% CI, 0.23–0.89).[92] Surprisingly, preventive medication use was associated with lower remission rates (OR = 0.41; 95% CI, 0.23–0.75), but this effect lost significance when headache day frequency was included. This finding may suggest that people with the most severe disease may be more likely to take preventive medication. Interventional studies in people with CM revealed improvement in headache frequency and severity after modification of risk factors, described below in more detail.

Fluctuations in migraine frequency over the course of a year were evaluated in the CaMEO study.[93] Respondents reported headache frequency every 3 months for 15 months. Of those who met criteria for CM at baseline, only 26.6% met criteria at every subsequent time point. Most (73.4%) met criteria for EM for at least one time point. The researchers also plotted the fluctuations in headache frequency in each individual and found substantive variation in headache days per month over the course of the study. This fluctuation shows that there is meaningful short-term variability in headache frequency. Modeling studies have also found that a significant proportion of fluctuation in the frequency of headache days may be attributed to random variation.[94] Random variation accounted for chronification rates of 0.6% to 1.3% and remission rates of 10.3% to 23.5%. This finding is important in interpreting many clinical phenomena, including response to preventive treatment and the effect of modifying risk factors on progression rates, because headache frequency has a natural fluctuation independent from any intervention. It also cautions against basing the classification of migraine as EM or CM based on only one time point. A diagnosis based on frequency over a longer time period may be more helpful.

Course of migraine in adolescents

A 3-year observational study of 209 adolescents (seventh through ninth grade) with ICHD-2-defined migraine in Thailand showed improvement in 12% of boys and 16% of girls, no improvement in 1% of boys and girls, and deterioration in 3% of boys and 7% of girls.[95] Avoidance of precipitating causes or unknown reasons/spontaneous remission accounted for most improvement. Stress-related daily school activities and inadequate rest were reported as common precipitating factors among students with nonimproving or worsening outcomes. Wang and colleagues[96] evaluated the outcome of adolescents aged 12 to 14 years with Chronic Daily Headache (CDH). At the 8-year follow-up, only 12% still had CDH. Sixty-eight percent of the cohort reported some or substantial improvement in headache frequency, whereas 20% reported no change and 12% reported worsening. Presence of CDH for more than 2 years, onset before 13 years of age, CDH presence at the 2001 follow-up, and migraine with and without aura all significantly predicted worsening of headache frequency at the 8-year follow-up.

Risk Factors for Chronic Migraine Onset

An estimated 2.5% to 3% of people with EM transition to CM each year.[27] A systematic review of studies that identify risk factors for the new onset of CM or related chronic headache diagnoses, such as transformed migraine and CDH, was recently published.[90] Of 1879 identified articles, 17 met inclusion and exclusion criteria. The strength of evidence was evaluated for each identified risk factor and rated as fair, moderate, or strong, using a modified version of AB Hill criteria for causation.[97] Risk factors were identified in the constructs sociodemographics, lifestyle factors and habits, headache features, comorbid and concomitant diseases and conditions, and pharmacologic treatment-related factors, and were categorized as nonmodifiable, potentially modifiable, and owing to putative factors. Putative factors include proinflammatory states and prothrombotic states. Development of central sensitization and increased activation of the trigeminal nociceptive pathways may be drivers of the new onset of CM or CDH. Among potentially modifiable risk factors, strong evidence was found for increased risk of progression with higher baseline headache frequency, comorbid depression, and medication overuse or high-frequency use. Moderate evidence was found for obesity, persistent-frequent migraine-associated nausea, cutaneous allodynia, snoring, and acute migraine treatment efficacy. Moderate evidence was also found for the nonmodifiable risk factors of comorbid asthma and noncephalic pain (**Table 3**). Risk factors for new onset CM and CDH in children and adolescents were similar to those identified in adults. The lack of strong evidence or any evidence does not imply that there is not a relationship between a particular risk factor and new onset CM or related

Table 3
Risk factors for progression from episodic to chronic migraine or CDH and the strength of evidence

| Risk Factors | | Strength of | |
Category	Variable	Evidence[a]	Modifiable Status
Sociodemographics, lifestyle factors and habits	Female gender	Fair	Nonmodifiable
	Low family SES	Fair	Nonmodifiable
	Daily caffeine intake	Fair	Potentially modifiable
	Obesity	Moderate	Potentially modifiable
	Major life events	Fair	Nonmodifiable
Headache features and symptoms	Headache day frequency	Strong	Potentially modifiable
	Persistent-frequent nausea associated with migraine	Moderate	Potentially modifiable
	Cutaneous allodynia	Moderate	Putative factor
Comorbid and concomitant diseases and conditions	Depression	Strong	Potentially modifiable
	Asthma	Moderate	Potentially modifiable
	Noncephalic pain	Moderate	Potentially modifiable
	Head and neck injury	Fair	Potentially modifiable
	Snoring	Moderate	Potentially modifiable
	Insomnia	Fair	Potentially modifiable
Pharmacologic treatment related	Acute medication use/overuse (type and frequency)	Strong	Potentially modifiable
	Acute migraine treatment efficacy	Moderate	Potentially modifiable

[a] Strength of evidence based on modified AB Hill criteria for causation.

disease; but may indicate little or no research, or that research did not have sufficient methodological rigor. In addition, it is likely that additional risk factors exist which have not yet been identified.

Effects of Modifying Risk Factors for Chronification among Persons with Chronic Migraine

A few studies have examined outcomes among persons with CM when they intervened with risk factors. Bond and colleagues[98] assessed 24 "severely-obese" patients with migraine before and 6 months after bariatric surgery. The mean number of headache days was reduced from an average of 11.1 preoperatively to 6.7 postoperatively ($P<.05$), after a mean percent excess weight loss of 49.4%. They also observed a reduction in headache pain severity and the number of patients reporting moderate to severe disability. Calhoun and Ford[99] tested the effects of a cognitive-behavioral intervention designed to improve sleep on CM status. In a randomized, placebo-controlled study, they tested whether behavioral sleep modification (BSM) would result in improvement in headache frequency and intensity and with remission from CM to EM in 43 women with transformed migraine (ie, CM). Compared with the control group, the BSM group reported statistically significant reductions in headache frequency and headache intensity, and was more likely to remit to EM. By the study end, 48.5% of those who participated in BSM had reverted to EM. In addition, intervention for other risk factors for CM should be tested to determine if progression to CM can be avoided, and if treatment of risk factors can lead to remission from CM to EM or no migraine.

SUMMARY

Migraine affects an estimated 40 million people in the United State and 1.02 billion people worldwide. Is the second most disabling condition worldwide. CM is less common than EM but is associated with higher disability, more comorbidity, and higher health care use. Approximately 2.5% to 3% of patients with EM progress to CM each year. Because only a subset of people with EM progress to CM in any given year, progression likely occurs as a function of genetic and environmental risk factors. Understanding the risk factors which differentiate people with migraine who progress to CM from those who do not, may provide insights into the mechanisms, prevention, and treatment of CM. Many risk factors for migraine progression have been identified, but the effect on progression of modifying these risk factors is not as clearly understood.

The studies included in this review have encompassed a range of methodologies, from door-to-door surveys in single towns to national mail-based surveys to mining of routinely collected data repositories. The increase of electronic databases is likely to be the future of migraine epidemiology, with electronic medical record systems and insurance claims data generating large-scale data sources. The first migraine-specific patient data registry, the American Registry for Migraine Research is now underway. Future areas for research include longitudinal studies evaluating the effect of modifying migraine risk factors; response to specific treatments in specific populations; and ways to reduce the disability associated with migraine.

DISCLOSURE STATEMENT

R.C. Burch has nothing to disclose. D.C. Buse, PhD, has received grant support and honoraria from Allergan, Avanir, Amgen, Biohaven, Lilly, Teva, and Promius. She is on the editorial board of Current Pain and Headache Reports. Dr R.B. Lipton is the Edwin S. Lowe Professor of Neurology at the Albert Einstein College of Medicine in New York. He receives research support from the NIH: 2PO1 AG003949 (Multiple Principal Investigator), 5U10 NS077308 (Principal Investigator), RO1 NS082432 (Investigator), 1RF1 AG057531 (Site Principal Investigator), RF1 AG054548 (Investigator), 1RO1 AG048642 (Investigator), R56 AG057548 (Investigator), K23 NS09610 (Mentor), K23AG049466 (Mentor), 1K01AG054700 (Mentor). He also receives support from the Migraine Research Foundation and the National Headache Foundation. He serves on the editorial board of Neurology, senior advisor to Headache, and associate editor to Cephalalgia. He has reviewed for the NIA and NINDS, holds stock options in eNeura Therapeutics and Biohaven Holdings; serves as consultant, advisory board member, or has received honoraria from: the American Academy of Neurology, Alder, Allergan, American Headache Society, Amgen, Autonomic Technologies, Avanir, Biohaven, Biovision, Boston Scientific, Dr Reddy's, Electrocore, Eli Lilly, eNeura Therapeutics, GlaxoSmithKline, Merck, Pernix, Pfizer, Supernus, Teva, Trigemina, Vector, and Vedanta. He receives royalties from Wolff's Headache, 7th and 8th Edition, Oxford Press University, 2009, Wiley and Informa.

REFERENCES

1. Lipton RB, Silberstein SD. Why study the comorbidity of migraine? Neurology 1994;44(10 Suppl 7):S4–5.

2. Lipton RB, Bigal ME. Ten lessons on the epidemiology of migraine. Headache 2007;47(Suppl 1):S2–9.

3. Minen M, Shome A, Halpern A, et al. A migraine management training program for primary care providers: an overview of a survey and pilot study findings, lessons learned, and considerations for further research. Headache 2016;56(4):725–40.

4. Patwardhan MB, Samsa GP, Lipton RB, et al. Changing physician knowledge, attitudes, and beliefs about migraine: evaluation of a new educational intervention. Headache 2006;46(5):732–41.

5. Buse DC, Loder EW, Gorman JA, et al. Sex differences in the prevalence, symptoms, and associated features of migraine, probable migraine and other severe headache: results of the American Migraine Prevalence and Prevention (AMPP) Study. Headache 2013;53(8):1278–99.

6. Stewart WF, Lipton RB, Celentano DD, et al. Prevalence of migraine headache in the United States. Relation to age, income, race, and other sociodemographic factors. JAMA 1992;267(1):64–9.

7. Lipton RB, Stewart WF, Diamond S, et al. Prevalence and burden of migraine in the United States: data from the American Migraine Study II. Headache 2001; 41(7):646–57.

8. Lipton RB, Bigal ME, Diamond M, et al. Migraine prevalence, disease burden, and the need for preventive therapy. Neurology 2007;68(5):343–9.

9. NHIS - National Health Interview Survey Homepage. Available at: https://www.cdc.gov/nchs/nhis/index.htm. Accessed January 11, 2019.

10. Burch R, Rizzoli P, Loder E. The prevalence and impact of migraine and severe headache in the United States: figures and trends from government health studies. Headache 2018;58(4):496–505.

11. Smitherman TA, Burch R, Sheikh H, et al. The prevalence, impact, and treatment of migraine and severe headaches in the United States: a review of statistics from national surveillance studies. Headache 2013;53(3):427–36.

12. Bigal ME, Lipton RB, Winner P, et al. Migraine in adolescents: association with socioeconomic status and family history. Neurology 2007;69(1):16–25.

13. Lipton RB, Serrano D, Holland S, et al. Barriers to the diagnosis and treatment of migraine: effects of sex, income, and headache features. Headache 2013;53(1): 81–92.

14. Stewart WF, Lipton RB, Liberman J. Variation in migraine prevalence by race. Neurology 1996;47(1):52–9.

15. Buse DC, Manack AN, Fanning KM, et al. Chronic migraine prevalence, disability, and sociodemographic factors: results from the American migraine prevalence and prevention study. Headache 2012;52(10):1456–70.

16. Launer LJ, Terwindt GM, Ferrari MD. The prevalence and characteristics of migraine in a population-based cohort: the GEM study. Neurology 1999;53(3): 537–42.

17. Rasmussen BK. Migraine and tension-type headache in a general population: psychosocial factors. Int J Epidemiol 1992;21(6):1138–43.

18. O'brien B, Goeree R, Streiner D. Prevalence of migraine headache in Canada: a population-based survey. Int J Epidemiol 1994;23(5):1020–6.

19. Loder S, Sheikh HU, Loder E. The prevalence, burden, and treatment of severe, frequent, and migraine headaches in US minority populations: statistics from National Survey studies. Headache 2015;55(2):214–28.

20. GBD 2016 Headache Collaborators. Global, regional, and national burden of migraine and tension-type headache, 1990-2016: a systematic analysis for the Global Burden of Disease Study 2016. Lancet Neurol 2018;17(11):954–76.

21. Saylor D, Steiner TJ. The global burden of headache. Semin Neurol 2018;38(2): 182–90.
22. WHO | Atlas of headache disorders and resources in the world 2011. 2012. Available at: https://www.who.int/mental_health/management/atlas_headache_disorders/en/. Accessed January 11, 2019.
23. Steiner TJ, Scher AI, Stewart WF, et al. The prevalence and disability burden of adult migraine in England and their relationships to age, gender and ethnicity. Cephalalgia 2003;23(7):519–27.
24. Lyngberg AC, Rasmussen BK, Jørgensen T, et al. Incidence of primary headache: a Danish epidemiologic follow-up study. Am J Epidemiol 2005;161(11): 1066–73.
25. Stewart WF, Wood C, Reed ML, et al, AMPP Advisory Group. Cumulative lifetime migraine incidence in women and men. Cephalalgia 2008;28(11): 1170–8.
26. Natoli JL, Manack A, Dean B, et al. Global prevalence of chronic migraine: a systematic review. Cephalalgia 2009;30(5):599–609.
27. Bigal ME, Serrano D, Buse D, et al. Acute migraine medications and evolution from episodic to chronic migraine: a longitudinal population-based study. Headache 2008;48(8):1157–68.
28. Leonardi M, Steiner TJ, Scher AT, et al. The global burden of migraine: measuring disability in headache disorders with WHO's Classification of Functioning, Disability and Health (ICF). J Headache Pain 2005;6(6):429–40.
29. Buse DC, Scher AI, Dodick DW, et al. Impact of migraine on the family: perspectives of people with migraine and their spouse/domestic partner in the CaMEO study. Mayo Clin Proc 2016. https://doi.org/10.1016/j.mayocp.2016.02.013.
30. Blumenfeld AM, Varon SF, Wilcox TK, et al. Disability, HRQoL and resource use among chronic and episodic migraineurs: results from the International Burden of Migraine Study (IBMS). Cephalalgia 2011;31(3):301–15.
31. Buse DC, Bigal MB, Rupnow M, et al. Development and validation of the Migraine Interictal Burden Scale (MIBS): a self-administered instrument for measuring the burden of migraine between attacks. Neurology 2007;68(Suppl 1):A89.
32. Abu Bakar N, Tanprawate S, Lambru G, et al. Quality of life in primary headache disorders: a review. Cephalalgia 2016;36(1):67–91.
33. Holmes WF, Anne MacGregor E, Sawyer JPC, et al. Information about migraine disability influences physicians' perceptions of illness severity and treatment needs. Headache 2001;41(4):343–50.
34. Lipton RB, Hahn SR, Cady RK, et al. In-office discussions of migraine: results from the American Migraine Communication Study. J Gen Intern Med 2008; 23(8):1145–51.
35. Stewart WF, Lipton RB, Kolodner K, et al. Reliability of the migraine disability assessment score in a population-based sample of headache sufferers. Cephalalgia 1999;19(2):107–14.
36. Buse DC, Sollars CM, Steiner TJ, et al. Why HURT? A review of clinical instruments for headache management. Curr Pain Headache Rep 2012;16(3):237–54.
37. Buse D, Manack A, Serrano D, et al. Headache impact of chronic and episodic migraine: results from the american migraine prevalence and prevention study. Headache 2011;52(1):3–17.
38. Kawata AK, Hsieh R, Bender R, et al. Psychometric evaluation of a novel instrument assessing the impact of migraine on physical functioning: the migraine physical function impact diary. Headache 2017;57(9):1385–98.

39. Hareendran A, Mannix S, Skalicky A, et al. Development and exploration of the content validity of a patient-reported outcome measure to evaluate the impact of migraine- the migraine physical function impact diary (MPFID). Health Qual Life Outcomes 2017;15(1):224.
40. Hareendran A, Skalicky A, Mannix S, et al. Development of a new tool for evaluating the benefit of preventive treatments for migraine on functional outcomes - the migraine functional impact questionnaire (MFIQ). Headache 2018;58(10): 1612–28.
41. Website. Food and Drug Administration. Guidance for industry patient-reported outcome measures: use in medical product development to support labeling claims. FDA; 2009. Available at: http://www.fda.gov/downloads/Drugs/.../Guidances/UCM193282.pdf. Accessed January 9, 2019.
42. Hahn SR, Lipton RB, Sheftell FD, et al. Healthcare provider-patient communication and migraine assessment: results of the American Migraine Communication Study, phase II. Curr Med Res Opin 2008;24(6):1711–8.
43. Baigi K, Stewart WF. Headache and migraine: a leading cause of absenteeism. Handb Clin Neurol 2015;131:447–63.
44. Hawkins K, Wang S, Rupnow M. Direct cost burden among insured US employees with migraine. Headache 2008;48(4):553–63.
45. Messali A, Sanderson JC, Blumenfeld AM, et al. Direct and indirect costs of chronic and episodic migraine in the United States: a web-based survey. Headache 2016;56(2):306–22.
46. Bonafede M, Sapra S, Shah N, et al. Direct and indirect healthcare resource utilization and costs among migraine patients in the United States. Headache 2018; 58(5):700–14.
47. Stewart WF. Lost productive time and cost due to common pain conditions in the US workforce. JAMA 2003;290(18):2443.
48. Meletiche DM, Lofland JH, Young WB. Quality-of-life differences between patients with episodic and transformed migraine. Headache 2001;41(6):573–8.
49. Bigal ME, Rapoport AM, Lipton RB, et al. Assessment of migraine disability using the migraine disability assessment (MIDAS) questionnaire: a comparison of chronic migraine with episodic migraine. Headache 2003;43(4):336–42.
50. Bigal ME, Serrano D, Reed M, et al. Chronic migraine in the population: burden, diagnosis, and satisfaction with treatment. Neurology 2008;71(8):559–66.
51. Stewart WF, Wood GC, Manack A, et al. Employment and work impact of chronic migraine and episodic migraine. J Occup Environ Med 2010;52(1):8–14.
52. Chen Y-C, Tang C-H, Ng K, et al. Comorbidity profiles of chronic migraine sufferers in a national database in Taiwan. J Headache Pain 2012;13(4):311–9.
53. Buse DC, Manack A, Serrano D, et al. Sociodemographic and comorbidity profiles of chronic migraine and episodic migraine sufferers. J Neurol Neurosurg Psychiatry 2010;81(4):428–32.
54. Lipton RB, Manack Adams A, Buse DC, et al. A comparison of the chronic migraine epidemiology and outcomes (CaMEO) study and American migraine prevalence and prevention (AMPP) study: demographics and headache-related disability. Headache 2016;56(8):1280–9.
55. Scher AI, Bigal ME, Lipton RB. Comorbidity of migraine. Curr Opin Neurol 2005; 18(3):305–10.
56. Buse DC, Silberstein SD, Manack AN, et al. Psychiatric comorbidities of episodic and chronic migraine. J Neurol 2012;260(8):1960–9.
57. Minen MT, Begasse De Dhaem O, Kroon Van Diest A, et al. Migraine and its psychiatric comorbidities. J Neurol Neurosurg Psychiatry 2016;87(7):741–9.

58. Lipton RB, Reed ML, Kurth T, et al. Framingham-based cardiovascular risk estimates among people with episodic migraine in the US population: results from the American Migraine Prevalence and Prevention (AMPP) Study. Headache 2017;57(10):1507–21.
59. Sacco S, Ornello R, Ripa P, et al. Migraine and risk of ischaemic heart disease: a systematic review and meta-analysis of observational studies. Eur J Neurol 2015; 22(6):1001–11.
60. Kurth T, Winter AC, Eliassen AH, et al. Migraine and risk of cardiovascular disease in women: prospective cohort study. BMJ 2016;353:i2610.
61. Kurth T, Schürks M, Logroscino G, et al. Migraine, vascular risk, and cardiovascular events in women: prospective cohort study. BMJ 2008;337:a636.
62. Kurth T, Gaziano JM, Cook NR, et al. Migraine and risk of cardiovascular disease in men. Arch Intern Med 2007;167(8):795–801.
63. Hu X, Zhou Y, Zhao H, et al. Migraine and the risk of stroke: an updated meta-analysis of prospective cohort studies. Neurol Sci 2017;38(1):33–40.
64. Schürks M, Rist PM, Bigal ME, et al. Migraine and cardiovascular disease: systematic review and meta-analysis. BMJ 2009;339:b3914.
65. Sheikh HU, Pavlovic J, Loder E, et al. Risk of stroke associated with use of estrogen containing contraceptives in women with migraine: a systematic review. Headache 2018;58(1):5–21.
66. Kruit MC, van Buchem MA, Hofman PAM, et al. Migraine as a risk factor for subclinical brain lesions. JAMA 2004;291(4):427–34.
67. Palm-Meinders IH, Koppen H, Terwindt GM, et al. Structural brain changes in migraine. JAMA 2012;308(18):1889–97.
68. Jette N, Patten S, Williams J, et al. Comorbidity of migraine and psychiatric disorders–a national population-based study. Headache 2008;48(4):501–16.
69. Breslau N, Lipton RB, Stewart WF, et al. Comorbidity of migraine and depression: investigating potential etiology and prognosis. Neurology 2003;60(8):1308–12.
70. Lipton RB, Hamelsky SW, Kolodner KB, et al. Migraine, quality of life, and depression: a population-based case-control study. Neurology 2000;55(5):629–35.
71. Breslau N, Davis GC, Schultz LR, et al. Joint 1994 Wolff Award Presentation. Migraine and major depression: a longitudinal study. Headache 1994;34(7):387–93.
72. Smitherman TA, Kolivas ED, Bailey JR. Panic disorder and migraine: comorbidity, mechanisms, and clinical implications. Headache 2013;53(1):23–45.
73. Zwart JA, Dyb G, Hagen K, et al. Depression and anxiety disorders associated with headache frequency. The Nord-Trøndelag Health Study. Eur J Neurol 2003;10(2):147–52.
74. Adams AM, Serrano D, Buse DC, et al. The impact of chronic migraine: The Chronic Migraine Epidemiology and Outcomes (CaMEO) Study methods and baseline results. Cephalalgia 2015;35(7):563–78.
75. Kelman L, Rains JC. Headache and sleep: examination of sleep patterns and complaints in a large clinical sample of migraineurs. Headache 2005;45(7):904–10.
76. Pellegrino ABW, Davis-Martin RE, Houle TT, et al. Perceived triggers of primary headache disorders: a meta-analysis. Cephalalgia 2018;38(6):1188–98.
77. Houle TT, Butschek RA, Turner DP, et al. Stress and sleep duration predict headache severity in chronic headache sufferers. Pain 2012;153(12):2432–40.
78. Hagen K, Åsberg AN, Stovner L, et al. Lifestyle factors and risk of migraine and tension-type headache. Follow-up data from the Nord-Trøndelag Health Surveys 1995-1997 and 2006-2008. Cephalalgia 2018;38(13):1919–26.

79. Vgontzas A, Pavlović JM. Sleep disorders and migraine: review of literature and potential pathophysiology mechanisms. Headache 2018;58(7):1030–9.

80. van Oosterhout WPJ, van Someren EJW, Louter MA, et al. Restless legs syndrome in migraine patients: prevalence and severity. Eur J Neurol 2016;23(6):1110–6.

81. Buse DC, Rains JC, Pavlovic JM, et al. Sleep disorders among people with migraine: results from the chronic migraine epidemiology and outcomes (CaMEO) study. Headache 2019;59(1):32–45.

82. Kristiansen HA, Kværner KJ, Akre H, et al. Migraine and sleep apnea in the general population. J Headache Pain 2011;12(1):55–61.

83. Stokes M, Becker WJ, Lipton RB, et al. Cost of health care among patients with chronic and episodic migraine in Canada and the USA: results from the International Burden of Migraine Study (IBMS). Headache 2011;51(7):1058–77.

84. McLean G, Mercer SW. Chronic migraine, comorbidity, and socioeconomic deprivation: cross-sectional analysis of a large nationally representative primary care database. J Comorb 2017;7(1):89–95.

85. Lipton RB, Fanning KM, Buse DC, et al. Identifying natural subgroups of migraine based on comorbidity and concomitant condition profiles: results of the chronic migraine epidemiology and outcomes (CaMEO) study. Headache 2018;58(7):933–47.

86. Lipton RB, Fanning KM, Buse DC, et al. Migraine progression in subgroups of migraine based on comorbidities: results of the CaMEO study. Neurology, in press.

87. Bigal ME, Lipton RB. Clinical course in migraine: conceptualizing migraine transformation. Neurology 2008;71(11):848–55.

88. Bigal ME, Lipton RB. The prognosis of migraine. Curr Opin Neurol 2008;21(3):301–8.

89. Silberstein SD, Lee L, Gandhi K, et al. Health care resource utilization and migraine disability along the migraine continuum among patients treated for migraine. Headache 2018;58(10):1579–92.

90. Buse DC, Greisman JD, Baigi K, et al. Migraine progression: a systematic review. Headache 2018. https://doi.org/10.1111/head.13459.

91. Boyer N, Dallel R, Artola A, et al. General trigeminospinal central sensitization and impaired descending pain inhibitory controls contribute to migraine progression. Pain 2014;155(7):1196–205.

92. Manack A, Buse DC, Serrano D, et al. Rates, predictors, and consequences of remission from chronic migraine to episodic migraine. Neurology 2011;76(8):711–8.

93. Serrano D, Lipton RB, Scher AI, et al. Fluctuations in episodic and chronic migraine status over the course of 1 year: implications for diagnosis, treatment and clinical trial design. J Headache Pain 2017;18(1):101.

94. Houle TT, Turner DP, Smitherman TA, et al. Influence of random measurement error on estimated rates of headache chronification and remission. Headache 2013;53(6):920–9.

95. Visudtibhan A, Thampratankul L, Khongkhatithum C, et al. Migraine in junior high-school students: a prospective 3-academic-year cohort study. Brain Dev 2010;32(10):855–62.

96. Wang S-J, Fuh J-L, Lu S-R. Chronic daily headache in adolescents: an 8-year follow-up study. Neurology 2009;73(6):416–22.

97. Hill AB. The environment and disease: association or causation? Proc R Soc Med 1965;58:295–300.
98. Bond DS, Vithiananthan S, Nash JM, et al. Improvement of migraine headaches in severely obese patients after bariatric surgery. Neurology 2011;76(13):1135–8.
99. Calhoun AH, Ford S. Behavioral sleep modification may revert transformed migraine to episodic migraine. Headache 2007;47(8):1178–83.

An Update
Pathophysiology of Migraine

Peter J. Goadsby, MD, PhD*, Philip R. Holland, PhD

KEYWORDS

- Migraine • Headache • Trigeminal • Trigeminovascular system
- Homeostatic networks • Pain • Aura • Cortical spreading depression

KEY POINTS

- Migraine is the most common disabling primary headache globally.
- Attacks typically present with unilateral throbbing headache and associated symptoms including, nausea, multisensory hypersensitivity, and marked fatigue.
- The diverse symptomatology highlights the complexity of migraine as a whole nervous system disorder involving somatosensory, autonomic, endocrine, and arousal networks.
- An attempt to describe the entirety of migraine has limitations, so the authors focus on recent advances in the understanding of its pathophysiology.
- They also address the underlying neuroanatomical basis for migraine-related headache, associated symptomatology, and discuss key clinical and preclinical findings that indicate that migraine likely results from dysfunctional homeostatic mechanisms.
- Whereby, abnormal central nervous system responses to extrinsic and intrinsic cues may lead to increased attack susceptibility.

INTRODUCTION

An understanding of the pathophysiology of migraine should be based on the anatomy and physiology of the pain-producing structures of the cranium integrated with knowledge of central nervous system modulation of these pathways (**Fig. 1**). Headache in general, and in particular migraine[1] and cluster headache,[2] is better understood now than it has been the case for the last 4 millennia.[3,4] Attacks commonly present as bouts of moderate to severe unilateral throbbing headache lasting 4 to 72 hours[5]; however, the head pain component of migraine represents only one single, albeit, highly disabling facet of the disorder.[1] Attacks commonly initiate with characteristic premonitory symptoms (marked fatigue, photophobia, difficulty concentrating, and

Disclosure Statement: This work was supported by the FP7 project EUROHEADPAIN (no. 602633), The Wellcome Trust (Synaptopathies; 104033) and the Medical Research Council (MR/P006264/1).

Headache Group, Basic and Clinical Neurosciences, Institute of Psychiatry, Psychology and Neuroscience, King's College London, UK
* Corresponding author. Wellcome Foundation Building, King's College Hospital, London SE5 9PJ, UK.
E-mail address: peter.goadsby@kcl.ac.uk

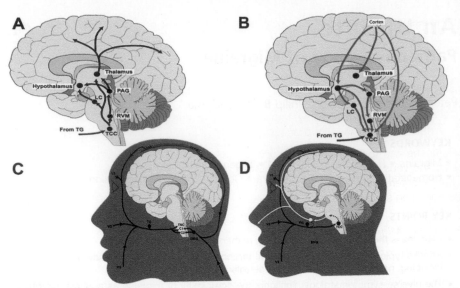

Fig. 1. Pathophysiology of migraine. Peripheral sensory inputs are conveyed via trigeminal afferents that arise in the trigeminal ganglion (TG) to the trigeminocervical complex (TCC) that represents the main interface for trigeminal pain processing between the peripheral and central nervous systems. Projection neurons then ascend in the trigeminothalamic tract, synapsing on thalamocortical relay neurons in multiple thalamic nuclei. En route to the thalamus, collateral projections also target several nuclei, including the rostral ventromedial medulla (RVM), locus coeruleus (LC), periaqueductal gray (PAG) and hypothalamus. Thalamocortical relay neurons then convey the sensory information to multiple cortical regions (A). This trigeminal pain processing network receives descending modulatory inputs at several levels. At the level of the TCC, direct projections from multiple cortical regions and indirect projections via the hypothalamus, PAG, RVM, and LC exert potent modulatory effects on neuronal firing (B). The TCC receives its peripheral sensory inputs from primary afferents innervating the intracranial and extracranial structures of all 3 dermatomes of the head (mandibular [V3], maxillary [V2], and ophthalmic [V1]) as well as convergent inputs from the posterior dura and cervical dermatomes (C). In addition to the ascending trigeminothalamic projections from the TCC, a trigeminal autonomic reflex exists between the trigeminal sensory afferents and the superior salivatory nucleus that regulates parasympathetic outflow to the face via the sphenopalatine ganglion (SPG). The dotted lines represent the potential interfaces between the trigeminal and parasympathetic arms of the trigeminal autonomic reflex (D) that remain to be fully characterized.

neck stiffness) that are highly predictive of an ensuing headache,[6,7] may include aura symptoms (20%–30% of cases),[8] and are associated with nausea and multimodal sensory alterations resulting in an aversion to touch (allodynia), light (photophobia), sound (phonophobia), and smell (osmophobia). In addition, there can also be considerable cranial autonomic involvement, including lacrimation, reddening of the eye, and facial flushing present during migraine attacks,[9–11] while such features are characteristic, and more prominent, of the trigeminal autonomic cephalalgias, a group of related primary headache disorders.[5]

MIGRAINE: EXPLAINING THE CLINICAL FEATURES

Migraine is in essence a familial episodic disorder whose key marker is headache with certain associated features. It is these features that give clues to its pathophysiology and has provided insights that have led to new treatments.

The essential elements of the puzzle include the following:

- Genetics of migraine
- The premonitory (prodromal) phase
- Migraine aura
- Anatomy, physiology, and pharmacology of the nociceptive trigeminovascular system
- Subcortical modulatory systems that influence trigeminal pain transmission and other sensory modality processing.

Migraine is a form of sensory processing disturbance with wide ramifications for central nervous system function, and although pain is used as the exemplar symptom, a brain-centered explanation provides a likely way to provide a generic explanation for the condition's manifestations.

Genetics of Migraine

One of the most important aspects of the pathophysiology of migraine is the inherited nature of the disorder.[12] It is clear from clinical practice that many patients have first degree relatives who also suffer from migraine.[3,13] Transmission of migraine from parents to children has been reported as early as the seventeenth century,[14] and numerous published studies have reported a positive family history.[15]

Genetic epidemiology

Studies of twin pairs are the classic method to investigate the relative importance of genetic and environmental factors. A Danish study included 1013 monozygotic and 1667 dizygotic twin pairs of the same gender, obtained from a population-based twin register.[16] The pairwise concordance rate was significantly higher among monozygotic than dizygotic twin pairs ($P<.05$). Several studies have attempted to analyze the possible mode of inheritance in migraine families and conflicting results have been obtained.[17–19] Both twin studies and population-based epidemiologic surveys strongly suggest that migraine without aura is a multifactorial disorder, caused by a combination of genetic and environmental factors. An unexplained but epidemiologically well-established predisposition relates to methylenetetrahydrofolate reductase gene mutation C677T that is certainly overrepresented in migraine with aura.[20] The presence of aura seems to be associated, in rarer inherited cases, such as CADASIL (cerebral autosomal dominant arteriopathy with subcortical infarcts and leukoencephalopathy [21]) or autosomal dominant retinal vasculopathy with cerebral leukodystrophy,[22] with structural protein dysfunction and perhaps with an embryonic syndrome that includes patent foramen ovale.[23] Such a view makes the small excess stroke risk for young migraineurs unsurprising[24] and suggests a common genetics as opposed to a pathophysiologic link for migraine pain.

Familial hemiplegic migraine

In approximately 50% of the reported families, familial hemiplegic migraine (FHM) has been assigned to chromosome 19p13.[25,26] Few clinical differences have been found between chromosome 19-linked and unlinked FHM families. Indeed, the clinical phenotype does not associate particularly with the known mutations.[27] The most striking exception is cerebellar ataxia, which occurs in approximately 50% of the chromosome 19-linked, but in none of the unlinked families.[25,26,28–30] Another less striking difference includes the fact that patients from chromosome 19-linked families are more likely to have attacks that can be triggered by minor head trauma or are that associated by coma.[31]

The biological basis for the linkage to chromosome 19 is mutations[32] involving the $Ca_v2.1$ (P/Q) type voltage-gated calcium channel[33] *CACNA1A* gene. Known as FHM-I, this mutation is responsible for about 50% of identified families. One consequence of this mutation may be enhanced glutamate release. Mutations in the *ATP1A2* gene[34,35] have been identified to be responsible for about 20% of FHM families. Interestingly, the phenotype of some FHM-II involves epilepsy.[36,37] The gene codes for a Na^+/K^+ adenosine triphosphatase and the mutation results in a smaller electrochemical gradient for Na^+. One effect of this change is to reduce or inactivate astrocytic glutamate transporters leading to a build-up of synaptic glutamate. It has also been suggested that alternating hemiplegia of childhood can be due to *ATP1A2* mutations.[38] The latter cases are most unconvincing for migraine. Dichgans and colleagues[39] reported a missense mutation (Q1489K) in *SCN1A* in 3 German families, thus characterizing the genetic defect of what is now known as FHM-III. This mutation affects a highly conserved amino acid in a part of the channel that contributes to its rapid closure after opening in response to membrane depolarization (fast inactivation). This represents a gain of function: instead of the channel rapidly closing, allowing the membrane to repolarize fully after an action potential, the mutated channel allows a persistent sodium influx.

Taken together, the known mutations suggest that migraine, or at least the neurologic manifestations currently called the aura, are ionopathies.[12,40] Linking the channel disturbance for the first time to the aura process has demonstrated that human mutations expressed in a knock-in mouse produce a reduced threshold for cortical spreading depression,[41] which has some interesting implications for understanding that process.[42]

Migraine Aura

Migraine aura is defined as a focal neurologic disturbance manifest as visual, sensory, or motor symptoms.[5] It is seen in about 30% of patients,[43] and it is clearly neurally driven.[44,45] The case for the aura being the human equivalent of the cortical spreading depression (CSD) of Leao[46,47] has been well made.[48] In humans visual aura has been described as affecting the visual field, suggesting the visual cortex, and it starts at the center of the visual field, propagating to the periphery at a speed of 3 mm/min,[49] and has been mapped in detail.[50] This is very similar to spreading depression described in rabbits.[47] Blood flow studies in patients have also shown that a focal hyperemia tends to precede the spreading oligemia,[51] and again this is similar to what would be expected with spreading depression. After this passage of oligemia, the cerebrovascular response to hypercapnia in patients is blunted while autoregulation remains intact.[52–54] Again this pattern is repeated with experimental spreading depression.[55–57] An interesting recent study suggested that female mice are more susceptible generally to CSD than male mice,[58] which would be consistent with the excess risk of migraine in females after menarche that is, still with them, on a population basis, into menopause and afterward. Human observations have rendered the arguments reasonably sound that human aura has as its equivalent in animals cortical spreading depression.[59] An area of controversy surrounds whether aura in fact triggers the rest of the attack and is indeed painful.[60] Based on the available experimental and clinical data, this investigator is not at all convinced that aura is painful,[61] but this does not diminish its interest or the importance of understanding it. Indeed, therapeutic developments may shed even further light on these relationships.

Therapeutic manipulation of aura: Tonabersat is a CSD inhibitor that entered clinical trials in migraine. It was not effective for migraine,[62] although was effective for aura.[63] Tonabersat (SB-220453) inhibits CSD, CSD-induced nitric oxide (NO) release, and cerebral vasodilation.[64,65] Tonabersat does not constrict isolated human blood vessels[66] but does inhibit trigeminally induced craniovascular effects.[67] Remarkably topiramate, a proven preventive agent in migraine,[68–70] also inhibits CSD in cat and rat,[71] and in the rat with prolonged dosing.[72] Tonabersat is inactive in the human NO-model of migraine,[73] as is propranolol,[74] although valproate showed some activity in that model.[75] Topiramate inhibits trigeminal neurons activated by nociceptive intracranial afferents[76] but not by a mechanism local to the trigeminocervical complex.[77] The model predicts that agents interacting with Na^+-based mechanisms might be effective,[78] as would glutamate-AMPA receptor mechanisms, but not GABAergic mechanisms, at least directly.[71] Glutamate N-methyl-D-aspartate–mediated effects have been reported to be important in CSD[55] and in an open-label study on migraine aura.[79] These may suggest some way forward for the management of at least the most disabled group who have persistent or prolonged aura.

The Premonitory (Prodromal) Phase of Migraine

Clinical manifestations of this phase that occurs in the hours or indeed days before the attack include: neck discomfort, tiredness, yawning, concentration impairment, mod change, food cravings, and alterations in urinary frequency. The symptoms point to subcortical structures.[7] Here the authors focus on the hypothalamus as a key potential structure involved, although migraine is clearly a network disorder. Because the premonitory phase leads into the pain phase, some aspects of pain modulation necessarily are swept into this section.

Hypothalamus

Hypothalamic activation was originally associated with the trigeminal autonomic cephalalgias, including cluster headache[80–83]; however, it is now well established that it is activated during the earliest premonitory phases of migraine,[84,85] during the headache phase,[86,87] and remains active even after the attenuation of the headache with sumatriptan.[87] The hypothalamus has reciprocal connections with the trigeminocervical complex,[88–90] as well as important projections terminating in the nucleus of the solitary tract, rostral ventromedial medulla, periaqueductal gray, and nucleus raphe magnus.[91] Given this widespread connectivity, a recent functional neuroimaging study identified potential important alterations in hypothalamic connectivity across the migraine phases.[85] During the interictal (attack-free) state the hypothalamus showed greater coupling to the spinal trigeminal nucleus; however, as the patient progressed into the attack this coupling switched to the periaqueductal gray, suggesting that the hypothalamus may act to differentially regulate descending modulation of trigeminovascular processing in a state-dependent manner.[92] In agreement with a pivotal role of the hypothalamus in the regulation of migraine-related head pain, a recent neuroimaging study has proposed a 2-stage model for hypothalamic involvement in episodic and chronic migraine, respectively.[93] In the premonitory phase and during episodic migraine, hypothalamic activation is observed in the more anterior regions; however, in those patients who have transitioned to chronic migraine (more than 15 headache days per month[5]), the hypothalamic activation is observed in the more posterior regions. The investigators hypothesize that different hypothalamic regions are involved in the initiation/triggering of attacks as compared with the maintenance of attacks during the chronic phase.

Nociceptive modulation The differential role of the hypothalamus is supported by the widespread activation of several hypothalamic nuclei in response to dural nociceptive stimulation, including the posterior, anterior, ventromedial, and paraventricular regions.[94,95] As such, dysregulation of hypothalamic nuclei with important roles in descending modulation of trigeminal nociceptive activation and homeostatic regulation may shift the threshold for attack initiation facilitating the transition from a more episodic state to a chronic state. Such divergent effects of altered hypothalamic function have been demonstrated preclinically in rodents. Within the posterior hypothalamic region, Bartsch and colleagues[97] demonstrated that dysregulation of orexinergic neural networks that project widely in the central nervous system, including the periaqueductal gray, locus coeruleus, and trigeminocervical complex, can have divergent effects on trigeminal nociceptive processing.[97] Local posterior hypothalamic microinjection of orexin A demonstrated an antinociceptive effect, and orexin B conversely induced a pronociceptive effect on trigeminocervical nociceptive processing. In agreement with this, Roberts and colleagues[90] further identified a similar bidirectional regulation of trigeminovascular processing from the paraventricular nucleus of the hypothalamus. The paraventricular nucleus has direct projections to the superior salivatory nucleus (regulating parasympathetic outflow to the face) and the superficial dorsal horn of the trigeminocervical complex. Gamma-aminobutyric acid ($GABA_A$) and 5-$HT_{1B/D}$ agonists along with pituitary adenylate cyclase-activating peptide antagonists microinjected into the paraventricular nucleus inhibited trigeminovascular activation, whereas $GABA_A$ antagonists and pituitary adenylate cyclase-activating peptide facilitated trigeminovascular activation. Of particular importance to migraine, the modulatory effects were state dependent, in that exposure of the rats to acute restraint stress decreased the $GABA_A$-mediated inhibitory effects, with no impact on the facilitation. As such, the hypothalamus may play a key role in state-dependent regulation (eg, in response to alterations in stress perception[98]) of migraine susceptibility.

Homeostatic changes The hypothalamus is established as the master regulator of homeostatic mechanisms, responding to several internal (eg, energy balance[99]) and external cues (eg, light/dark cycles[100]) to optimize state-dependent behavioral outputs. The common occurrence of hypothalamic-related perturbations such as altered appetite regulation,[101] sleep-wake states,[102] nociceptive processing,[90,97,103] and bodily fluid balance[104] further highlight its prominent role in migraine. This is supported by the recent emergence of a potential role for circadian dysregulation in migraine,[105–107] under the control of the hypothalamic master clock in the suprachiasmatic nuclei,[108] as well as differential trigeminovascular modulation via hypothalamic-mediated neuroendocrine signaling.[109]

The Nociceptive Trigeminovascular System

Primary afferent input

Although headache is one of the most salient features of migraine, the exact basis for the initiation and cessation of recurrent attacks remains elusive. Despite this enigma, the underlying head pain processing pathways are relatively well studied[110] and share several homologies with nontrigeminal-mediated pain processing. Trigeminal afferents arising in the trigeminal ganglion innervate almost all cranial tissues including the intracranial and extracranial structures of the head and face,[111–113] with additional cervical afferents from the upper cervical dorsal root ganglion innervating the occipital regions. Although cranial innervation exists from all 3 divisions of the trigeminal nerve, the ophthalmic division is considered the most relevant for migraine, given the common distribution of head pain around the periorbital dermatome. These trigeminal afferents express calcitonin gene-related peptide (CGRP), substance P, neurokinin A, and pituitary adenylate cyclase-activating polypeptide,[114–117] the proportion of transmitter varying with target.[118] The afferents largely consist of thinly myelinated and unmyelinated Aδ- and C-fibers synapsing centrally on second-order trigeminothalamic relay neurons in the dorsal horn of the trigeminal nucleus caudalis and its cervical extensions (trigeminocervical complex).[119–123]

Parabrachial projections Although most of the trigeminovascular afferents project to the trigeminocervical complex, recent studies have implicated potential additional projections that may help explain both the presence of autonomic features and the heightened perception of painful stimuli to the face. Direct projections from trigeminal ganglion afferents have been demonstrated to synapse in the ipsilateral parabrachial nucleus of mice.[124] This is in addition to the established indirect parabrachial innervation from the trigeminocervical complex.[125–128] This suggests that 2 alternate pathways arising from craniofacial nociceptors innervate the parabrachial nucleus and may in part explain the heightened perception of pain in the head and face, as compared with noncephalic pain. This trigeminoparabrachial-limbic pathway is considered to process affective-motivational aspects of pain. Optogenetic inhibition of lateral parabrachial neurons reduced capsaicin-evoked facial allodynia, whereas their activation evokes aversive behaviors.[124] The importance of this convergent trigeminoparabrachial-limbic pathway remains to be fully elucidated; however, as will be discussed later in the article, migraine has been linked to dysfunctional bodily homeostatic mechanisms, whereby abnormal behavioral sensory responses are evoked in response to normal stimuli (eg, touch and light). The parabrachial nucleus is a key hub in the maintenance of energy balance.[99] CGRP-expressing neurons from the parabrachial nucleus project to the central nucleus of the amygdala, where they act to reduce appetite[129] and modulate conditioned taste aversion.[130] It has recently been demonstrated that this may include the convergence of trigeminal somatosensory and taste signals, specifically those parabrachial gustatory neurons responding to threatening stimuli such as high salt concentration and bitter-tasting stimuli.[131]

Sphenopalatine ganglion In addition to this trigeminal parabrachial innervation, the presence of CGRP-immunoreactive fibers and CGRP receptors in the sphenopalatine ganglion that conveys parasympathetic outflow to the head and face[110] raises the possibility of trigeminovascular afferents expressing CGRP project directly from the trigeminal ganglion to the sphenopalatine ganglion.[132,133] Alternatively, a direct trigeminocervical complex to superior salivatory nucleus pathway, which provides the primary parasympathetic projections to the sphenopalatine ganglion, forming a trigeminal autonomic reflex[134] has been postulated; however, direct ascending trigeminocervical complex to sphenopalatine ganglion/superior salivatory nucleus projection remains to be demonstrated.

The modulation of the activity of this trigeminal autonomic reflex may underlie autonomic-mediated attack thresholds in patients. It receives direct reciprocal projections from hypothalamic, parabrachial, limbic, and cortical regions [Hosoya, 1983 #126;Li, 2010 #12861;Noseda, 2017 #128][135] that play prominent roles in the regulation of appetite, energy balance, sleep wake cycles, and stress responses, which could result in state-dependent susceptibility (eg, based on circadian output from the suprachiasmatic nucleus). Although preclinical studies in rats have demonstrated that activation of the trigeminal autonomic reflex via stimulation of the superior salivatory nucleus leads to increased neuronal responses in the trigeminocervical complex,[136,137] the data do not conclude if transmission occurs directly between the superior salivatory nucleus and the trigeminocervical complex or if this may happen at a peripheral synapse that connects the trigeminal and parasympathetic pathways.

Evidence from human studies, albeit in cluster headache, which activated the parasympathetic outflow to the face via direct stimulation of the sphenopalatine ganglion, suggests that activation of the peripheral branch of the trigeminal autonomic reflex alone is insufficient to induce head pain.[138] Highlighting, a potential key role for the central trigeminocervical complex to superior salivatory nucleus reflex, that may in combination lead to altered attack triggering thresholds.

TRIGEMINOCERVICAL ASCENDING PATHWAYS

Sensory information from the trigeminocervical complex projects to several key nuclei throughout the brain,[88,89,95,121,139–145] with dural nociceptive projections largely targeting the ventroposteromedial thalamic nuclei[120,146–148] and spinal dorsal horn neurons largely targeting the ventroposterolateral nuclei. Although the ventroposteromedial nuclei are considered the major target of trigeminothalamic projections, trigeminal inputs also synapse in the posterior and intralaminar thalamic nuclei. In addition, trigeminovascular sensory information is relayed to key medullary (rostral ventromedial medulla, nucleus raphe magnus, and parabrachial), brainstem (ventrolateral periaqueductal gray, nucleus of the solitary tract, and locus coeruleus), and diencephalic (lateral, anterior, and posterior hypothalamic nuclei) regions.

The thalamus likely represents a key first stage for multimodal sensory integration[149] in migraine, with important roles in nociceptive, touch, visual, olfactory, and auditory sensation. As such, the thalamus has emerged as a potential target for modulating the multimodal sensory dysfunction of migraine. This is supported by evidence demonstrating the convergence of retinal (light sensitive) and trigeminovascular (dural nociceptive) projections in the posterior thalamus of rats, whereby light stimuli were observed to facilitate trigeminovascular nociceptive activation in thalamocortical relay neurons,[150] with important implications for the aversive nature of light in migraine (photophobia). Recently, a direct role for the ventroposteromedial nuclei in multimodal sensory integration has emerged. Detailed multielectrode recordings from the rat primary sensory/visual and ventroposteromedial nucleus/dorsal lateral geniculate nucleus simultaneously identified that bimodal (sensory and light) stimulation leads to potentiation of sensory-evoked activity in the ventroposteromedial nucleus and increased coupling and signaling between the ventroposteromedial nucleus and primary sensory cortex.[151] This multimodal sensory integration was specific to the ventroposteromedial nucleus and did not occur in the dorsal lateral geniculate nucleus. Given that the ventroposteromedial nucleus is the primary interface for trigeminal-mediated signaling, it is possible that such multimodal sensory integration could further explain the aversive nature of light, sound, and smell in migraine.[152] Further, the thalamus has been linked to the presence of extracephalic allodynia during migraine attacks, with both tactile and thermal stimuli enhancing pulvinar thalamic activity in patients with migrane suffering from extracephalic allodynia.[120,148] In agreement, preclinical studies in rats have identified trigeminothalamic sensitization in response to meningeal inflammation in the ventroposteromedial nucleus and posterior and lateral posterior nuclei.[148]

MODULATION OF TRIGEMINOVASCULAR PROCESSING

The head pain processing trigeminovascular system is subject to powerful modulation at several levels, largely originating from corticofugal projections to multiple brainstem regions, including the periaqueductal gray, pontine, raphe, and medullary reticular nuclei.[119,153] Although direct corticotrigeminocervical complex projections originate largely in the primary somatosensory cortex, visual and insular cortices have been shown to modulate trigeminocervical complex neuronal activity.

The Brainstem

The brainstem and more specifically the periaqueductal gray rose to prominence in migraine when Weiller and colleagues[154] identified that the dorsal midbrain was activated during spontaneous attacks. It was then further demonstrated that this activation was independent of ongoing trigeminal pain, because it remained after triptan-induced pain normalization.[87] Several studies have now confirmed brainstem activation in the region of the periaqueductal gray[84,87,155–157] and recently a potential role for the periaqueductal gray in chronic migraine has been highlighted due to an increased iron deposition in the periaqueductal gray of patients with chronic migraine as compared with episodic migraineurs or healthy controls.[158,159] In agreement with a frequency-dependent alteration in periaqueductal gray function, patients with a higher frequency of migraine attacks demonstrate increased periaqueductal gray connectivity with higher-order cortical structures involved in pain perception and decreased connectivity with higher-order structures such as the prefrontal cortex involved in descending pain modulation.[160] This potential periaqueductal gray involvement is further associated with the presence of cranial allodynia during attacks; individuals reporting greater allodynia demonstrate significantly reduced volumes of midbrain regions including the periaqueductal gray compared with healthy controls.[161] The periaqueductal gray has reciprocal connections with higher-order (cortical, thalamic, and hypothalamic), brainstem (medullary dorsal horn and rostral ventromedial medulla), and the trigeminocervical complexes.[162–164] Experimental evidence demonstrates distinct activation of the ventrolateral periaqueductal gray in response to noxious durovascular stimuli, whereas altered periaqueductal gray signaling can modulate trigeminovascular processing.[165–167] Local ventrolateral periaqueductal gray microinjection of CGRP enhances trigeminovascular nociception,[168] whereas the clinically relevant blockade of CGRP and activation of 5-HT$_{1B/D}$ receptors is inhibitory.[168,169] Although the exact circuitry of the periaqueductal gray's antinociceptive role in migraine remains to be fully elucidated, it is likely via the periaqueductal gray-rostral ventromedial medulla circuitry. This is supported by a recent study that identified altered rostral ventromedial medulla to trigeminocervical complex functional connectivity in the period immediately before attack onset. Out with the headache, during the interictal phase migraineurs conversely demonstrated an increased functional connectivity,[170] highlighting that alterations in specific brainstem nuclei may represent a key stage in the initiation of migraine attacks. The rostral ventromedial medulla receives reciprocal projections from the periaqueductal gray[171] and is ideally positioned to modulate bidirectionally trigeminal nociceptive processing. "On" and "off" cells in the rostral ventromedial medulla provide descending modulation of trigeminal nociception; experimental inflammation of the dura mater potentiates the activity of "on" cells, whereas "off" cells are acutely inhibited.[172] Further, cephalic and extracephalic allodynia development in response to dural inflammatory-mediated central sensitization can be inhibited by direct blockade of the rostral ventromedial medulla. Thus, direct modulation of the rostral ventromedial medulla can inhibit trigeminal and spinal nociception. However, it should be noted that the rostral ventromedial medulla projects bilaterally to all levels of the spinal cord and as such it is difficult to reconcile a specific role in head pain processing, especially given the prominent unilateral nature of many primary headaches.[155]

As described earlier, migraine attacks are commonly preceded by an array of premonitory features including marked fatigue.[6] Although the specific mechanisms for these premonitory symptoms remain to be fully characterized, the locus coeruleus has emerged as a key neural hub. It is the principal site of norepinephrine synthesis in the brain[173] and receives projections from the paraventricular and lateral hypothalamic nuclei,[174] the latter of which represent the densest orexinergic projections from the hypothalamus,[96] which is considered to act by promoting activity in the ascending arousal network to promote wakefulness. In turn, the orexinergic neurons receive direct inputs from the lateral parabrachial nucleus,[175] suggesting a potential network for the integration of sensory/discriminative pain processing and vigilance. This is in keeping with a recent study that identified further state-dependent regulation of freezing behaviors in mice.[176] Activation of locus coeruleus noradrenergic to lateral amygdala projections that receive direct orexinergic inputs increases freezing behaviors, whereas inhibition of this pathway diminished this response.[176] Importantly, prior fasting of mice, which results in increased orexinergic tone, was able to potentiate the freezing behaviors, suggesting that dysfunction of this hypothalamic brainstem network may link homeostatic challenges (eg, energy balance) to altered nociceptive processing. With respect to trigeminovascular nociceptive processing electrical lesioning of the locus coeruleus demonstrates robust reductions in durovascular-evoked nociceptive processing in the trigeminocervical complex, which is mimicked by local activation of α2-adrenoceptors.[177] In contrast, α1-adrenoceptor activation was pronociceptive, in agreement with prior experiments that highlighted divergent effects of locus coeruleus modulation on pain.[178,179] In addition to the effects on nociception, chronic ablation of the locus coeruleus increased the susceptibility of rats to cortical spreading depression,[177] the electrophysiological correlate of migraine aura.[180] Given the specific arousal-related mechanisms of the locus coeruleus[181] and its regulation by the sleep-wake regulating orexinergic neurons,[176] the abovementioned studies suggest a potential link between the regulation of sleep and migraine,[102,182] which is supported by their clinical and pathophysiologic interactions.[102]

Potential Modulation of Trigeminovascular Processing by Cortical Spreading Depression

As noted previously, in approximately 25% to 30% of patients attacks can occur in conjunction with migraine aura,[5] most commonly presenting as transient visual disturbances, but motor or somatosensory symptoms may occur. Although the exact role for aura in migraine remains a fiercely debated topic in the field,[180] recent evidence has emerged demonstrating that cortical spreading depression, which is the accepted underlying mechanism of aura, can have direct actions on trigeminovascular nociceptive processing.[183] Cortical spreading depression is a slowly moving depolarizing wave that propagates across the cortex affecting neural, glial, and vascular functions with resultant suppression of activity.[184] With respect to the local microenvironment cortical spreading depression results in dysregulation of adenosine triphosphate, glutamate, potassium, nitric oxide, and CGRP dynamics.[185] It is known that in rats a single cortical spreading depression event can lead to both acute and prolonged increases in trigeminovascular activity[183] and that this increased activation can be prevented by targeted inhibition of CGRP mechanisms.[186] Interestingly, CGRP does not trigger aura in patients with migraine with aura or those with FHM,[187,188] this is in agreement with preclinical data demonstrating that CGRP receptor blockers inhibit CSD-evoked pain behaviors with no effect on the CSD propagation or hemodynamic response,[189] despite potential CGRP and CGRP receptor involvement in cortical spreading depression ex vivo.[190] In comparison most of the other nonspecific prophylactic therapies for migraine show a clear effect in reducing cortical spreading depression frequency.[191] Although the direct link between cortical spreading depression and trigeminovascular activation remains debated, one study[190] postulated a potential mechanism for recurrent cortical spreading depression–induced activation of meningeal nociceptors. Mice exposed to repeated cortical spreading depression demonstrated opening of neuronal Pannexin 1 megachannels, resulting in the release of proinflammatory molecules from neurons and astrocytes.[192] Importantly, suppression of this Pannexin 1–dependent cascade inhibited cortical spreading depression–induced increased trigeminovascular activation, suggesting the possibility that cortical spreading depression could act to promote trigeminal-mediated nociception in migraine with aura.

Modulation of Trigeminovascular Processing by the Human Migraine Trigger Nitroglycerin

Nitroglycerin has emerged as the most prominent exogenous triggers for delayed migraine-like attacks in patients.[193] Initially known for its ability to trigger migraine-related headache, it is now understood that nitroglycerin can induce a diverse array of migraine-related symptoms including premonitory symptoms and cutaneous allodynia.[194,195] Functional magnetic resonance imaging studies have identified increased activity in the posterolateral hypothalamus, midbrain tegmental area, periaqueductal gray, dorsal pons, and several cortical regions during nitroglycerin-triggered premonitory symptoms.[84] Despite the abundance of its use, the exact mechanism of action of nitroglycerin and other clinically used migraine triggers remains unknown.[193] Preclinically, the use of nitroglycerin to model migraine-related phenotypes and therapeutic potential has grown considerably, with both acute and chronic administration models developed.[196] Initial studies in rodents highlighted a progressive reduction in hind paw[197] and subsequently orofacial[198] withdrawal thresholds in response to nitroglycerin, while more recently a dose-dependent sensitivity has been highlighted for transgenic migraine relevant mouse models. For example, mice harboring the human loss of function mutation of casein kinase 1 delta that is responsible for familial advanced sleep phases and comorbid migraine with aura demonstrate an increased sensitivity to 5 mg/kg nitroglycerin, whereas their wild-type littermates do not respond at this dose.[105] Given the ongoing debate about the role of the peripheral versus central mechanisms of migraine and other pain disorders,[199] much of the focus on nitroglycerin has centered around potential changes in the trigeminal ganglion. Recently, a multiphasic effect of nitroglycerin was demonstrated in mice,[200] whereby initial increases in nitric oxide subsequently led to the generation of increased reactive oxygen and carbonyl species within the trigeminal ganglion. The prolonged hypersensitivity was transient receptor potential cation channel, subfamily A, member 1–dependent via the generation of nicotinamide adenine dinucleotide phosphate oxidase 1 and 2. This interesting study highlights a potential divergent role for nitroglycerin in the modulation of trigeminovascular processing, with acute nitric oxide resulting in early sensitization of trigeminal afferents that may explain the mild initial headache observed in patients,[193] while alternate downstream mechanisms were critical for driving the prolonged hypersensitivity akin to the delayed migraine-like attacks in patients. Physiologically, the nitroglycerin-evoked hypersensitivity has been associated with increased trigeminovascular activation.[195] Intravenous nitroglycerin evokes a delayed sensitization of spontaneous and durovascular nociceptive-evoked trigeminocervical complex neuronal responses in rats, with increased Aδ- and C-fiber responses. Crucially, second-order trigeminocervical complex ascending neurons, which initially only responded with Aδ latencies, demonstrated the unmasking of a C-fiber response following nitroglycerin. This trigeminovascular sensitization was triptan sensitive, being inhibited by naratriptan, which in agreement with clinical data shows that nitroglycerin-induced migraine-like attacks are triptan sensitive.[195] With respect to the potential site of action of nitroglycerin a recent imaging study utilizing ultra-high field sodium imaging identified early changes in sodium concentrations in the brainstem and extracerebral cerebrospinal fluid before the onset of mechanical hypersensitivity.[201] This is in agreement with the human neuroimaging data, with key brainstem regions active during the premonitory phase of nitroglycerin-triggered attacks.[84] Although not discussed in detail in this article there is growing evidence for the utility of several human migraine triggers in preclinical models, including CGRP[202,203] and cilostazol,[204] although nitroglycerin remains the most commonly utilized.

REFERENCES

1. Goadsby PJ, Holland PR, Martins-Oliveira M, et al. Pathophysiology of migraine-a disorder of sensory processing. Physiol Rev 2017;97:553–622.
2. Hoffmann J, May A. Diagnosis, pathophysiology, and management of cluster headache. Lancet Neurol 2018;17(1):75–83.
3. Lance JW, Goadsby PJ. Mechanism and management of headache. 7th edition. New York: Elsevier; 2005.
4. Olesen J, Tfelt-Hansen P, Ramadan N, et al. The headaches. Philadelphia: Lippincott, Williams & Wilkins; 2005.
5. Headache Classification Committee of the International Headache Society (IHS). The international classification of headache disorders, 3rd edition. Cephalalgia 2018;38:1–211.
6. Giffin NJ, Ruggiero L, Lipton RB, et al. Premonitory symptoms in migraine: an electronic diary study. Neurology 2003;60:935–40.
7. Karsan N, Goadsby PJ. Biological insights from the premonitory symptoms of migraine. Nat Rev Neurol 2018;14:699–710.
8. Viana M, Sances G, Linde M, et al. Clinical features of migraine aura: Results from a prospective diary-aided study. Cephalalgia 2017;37:979–89.
9. Gelfand AA, Reider AC, Goadsby PJ. Cranial autonomic symptoms in pediatric migraine are the rule, not the exception. Neurology 2013;81:431–6.
10. Lai T-H, Fuh J-L, Wang S-J. Cranial autonomic symptoms in migraine: characteristics and comparison with cluster headache. J Neurol Neurosurg Psychiatry 2009;80:1116–9.
11. Obermann M, Yoon M-S, Dommes P, et al. Prevalence of trigeminal autonomic symptoms in migraine: a population-based study. Cephalalgia 2007;27:504–9.
12. Tolner EA, Houben T, Terwindt GM, et al. From migraine genes to mechanisms. Pain 2015;156(Suppl 1):S64–74.
13. Silberstein SD, Lipton RB, Goadsby PJ. Headache in clinical practice. 2nd edition. London: Martin Dunitz; 2002.
14. Willis T. Opera omnia. Amstelaedami. Henricum Wetstenium; 1682.
15. Russell MB. Genetic epidemiology of migraine and cluster headache. Cephalalgia 1997;17:683–701.
16. Ulrich V, Gervil M, Kyvik KO, et al. Evidence of a genetic factor in migraine with aura: a population based Danish twin study. Ann Neurol 1999;45:242–6.
17. Mochi M, Sangiorgi S, Cortelli P, et al. Testing models for genetic determination in migraine. Cephalalgia 1993;13:389–94.
18. Lalouel JM, Morton NE. Complex segregation analysis with pointers. Hum Hered 1981;31:312–21.

19. Russell MB, Iselius L, Olesen J. Investigation of the inheritance of migraine by complex segregation analysis. Hum Genet 1995;96:726–30.
20. Scher AI, Terwindt GM, Verschuren WM, et al. Migraine and MTHFR C677T genotype in a population-based sample. Ann Neurol 2006;59:372–5.
21. Joutel A, Corpechot C, Ducros A, et al. Notch3 mutations in CADASIL, a hereditary adult-onset condition causing stroke and dementia. Nature 1996;383:707–10.
22. Richards A, van den Maagdenberg AM, Jen JC, et al. C-terminal truncations in human 3'-5' DNA exonuclease TREX1 cause autosomal dominant retinal vasculopathy with cerebral leukodystrophy. Nat Genet 2007;39:1068–70.
23. Diener HC, Kurth T, Dodick D. Patent foramen ovale and migraine. Curr Pain Headache Rep 2007;11:236–40.
24. Kurth T. Migraine and ischaemic vascular events. Cephalalgia 2007;27:965–75.
25. Joutel A, Ducros A, Vahedi K, et al. Genetic heterogeneity of familial hemiplegic migraine. Am J Hum Genet 1994;55:1166–72.
26. Ophoff RA, Eijk Rv, Sandkuijl LA, et al. Genetic heterogeneity of familial hemiplegic migraine. Genomics 1994;22:21–6.
27. Ducros A, Denier C, Joutel A, et al. The clinical spectrum of familial hemiplegic migraine associated with mutations in a neuronal calcium channel. N Engl J Med 2001;345:17–24.
28. Joutel A, Bousser MG, Biousse V, et al. A gene for familial hemiplegic migraine maps to chromosome 19. Nat Genet 1993;5:40–5.
29. Haan J, Terwindt GM, Bos PL, et al. Familial hemiplegic migraine in The Netherlands. Clin Neurol Neurosurg 1994;96:244–9.
30. Teh BT, Silburn P, Lindblad K, et al. Familial cerebellar periodic ataxia without myokymia maps to a 19-cM region on 19p13. Am J Hum Genet 1995;56:1443–9.
31. Terwindt GM, Ophoff RA, Haan J, et al, The Dutch Migraine Genetics Research Group. Familial hemiplegic migraine: a clinical comparison of families linked and unlinked to chromosome 19. Cephalalgia 1996;16:153–5.
32. Ophoff RA, Terwindt GM, Vergouwe MN, et al. Familial hemiplegic migraine and episodic ataxia type-2 are caused by mutations in the Ca^{2+} channel gene CACNL1A4. Cell 1996;87:543–52.
33. Ertel EA, Campbell KP, Harpold MM, et al. Nomenclature of voltage-gated calcium channels. Neuron 2000;25(3):533–5.
34. Marconi R, De Fusco M, Aridon P, et al. Familial hemiplegic migraine type 2 is linked to 0.9Mb region on chromosome 1q23. Ann Neurol 2003;53:376–81.
35. De Fusco M, Marconi R, Silvestri L, et al. Haploinsufficiency of ATP1A2 encoding the Na^+/K^+ pump a2 subunit associated with familial hemiplegic migraine type 2. Nat Genet 2003;33:192–6.
36. Vanmolkot KRJ, Kors EE, Hottenga JJ, et al. Novel mutations in the Na^+,K^+-ATPase pump gene ATP1A2 associated with Familial Hemiplegic Migraine and Benign Familial Infantile Convulsions. Ann Neurol 2003;54:360–6.
37. Jurkat-Rott K, Freilinger T, Dreier JP, et al. Variability of familial hemiplegic migraine with novel A1A2 Na+/K+-ATPase variants. Neurology 2004;62:1857–61.
38. Swoboda KJ, Kanavakis E, Xaidara A, et al. Alternating hemiplegia of childhood or familial hemiplegic migraine?: A novel ATP1A2 mutation. Ann Neurol 2004;55:884–7.
39. Dichgans M, Freilinger T, Eckstein G, et al. Mutation in the neuronal voltage-gated sodium channel SCN1A causes familial hemiplegic migraine. Lancet 2005;366:371–7.

40. Goadsby PJ, Kullmann DK. Another migraine gene - further opportunities to understand an important disorder. The Lancet 2005;366:345–6.
41. van den Maagdenberg AMJM, Pietrobon D, Pizzorusso T, et al. A Cacna1a knock-in migraine mouse model with increased susceptibility to cortical spreading depression. Neuron 2004;41:701–10.
42. Goadsby PJ. Migraine aura: a knock-in mouse with a knock-out message. Neuron 2004;41:679–80.
43. Rasmussen BK, Olesen J. Migraine with aura and migraine without aura: an epidemiological study. Cephalalgia 1992;12:221–8.
44. Olesen J, Friberg L, Skyhoj-Olsen T, et al. Timing and topography of cerebral blood flow, aura, and headache during migraine attacks. Ann Neurol 1990;28: 791–8.
45. Cutrer FM, Sorensen AG, Weisskoff RM, et al. Perfusion-weighted imaging defects during spontaneous migrainous aura. Ann Neurol 1998;43:25–31.
46. Leao AAP. Pial circulation and spreading activity in the cerebral cortex. J Neurophysiol 1944;7:391–6.
47. Leao AAP. Spreading depression of activity in cerebral cortex. J Neurophysiol 1944;7:359–90.
48. Lauritzen M. Pathophysiology of the migraine aura. The spreading depression theory. Brain 1994;117:199–210.
49. Lashley KS. Patterns of cerebral integration indicated by the scotomas of migraine. AMA Arch Neurol Psychiatry 1941;46:331–9.
50. Hansen JM, Baca SM, VanValkenburgh P, et al. Distinctive anatomical and physiological features of migraine aura revealed by 18 years of recording. Brain 2013;136:3589–95.
51. Olesen J, Larsen B, Lauritzen M. Focal hyperemia followed by spreading oligemia and impaired activation of rCBF in classic migraine. Ann Neurol 1981;9: 344–52.
52. Sakai F, Meyer JS. Abnormal cerebrovascular reactivity in patients with migraine and cluster headache. Headache 1979;19:257–66.
53. Lauritzen M, Skyhoj-Olsen T, Lassen NA, et al. Regulation of regional cerebral blood flow during and between migraine attacks. Ann Neurol 1983;14:569–72.
54. Harer C, Kummer Rv. Cerebrovascular CO2 reactivity in migraine: assessment by transcranial Doppler ultrasound. J Neurol 1991;238:23–6.
55. Kaube H, Goadsby PJ. Anti-migraine compounds fail to modulate the propagation of cortical spreading depression in the cat. Eur Neurol 1994;34:30–5.
56. Lambert GA, Michalicek J, Storer RJ, et al. Effect of cortical spreading depression on activity of trigeminovascular sensory neurons. Cephalalgia 1999;19: 631–8.
57. Kaube H, Knight YE, Storer RJ, et al. Vasodilator agents and supracollicular transection fail to inhibit cortical spreading depression in the cat. Cephalalgia 1999;19:592–7.
58. Brennan KC, Romero-Reyes M, Lopez Valdes HE, et al. Reduced threshold for cortical spreading depression in female mice. Ann Neurol 2007;61:603–6.
59. Hadjikhani N, Sanchez del Rio M, Wu O, et al. Mechanisms of migraine aura revealed by functional MRI in human visual cortex. Proc Natl Acad Sci U S A 2001; 98:4687–92.
60. Moskowitz MA, Bolay H, Dalkara T. Deciphering migraine mechanisms: clues from familial hemiplegic migraine genotypes. Ann Neurol 2004;55:276–80.
61. Goadsby PJ. Migraine, aura and cortical spreading depression: why are we still talking about it? Ann Neurol 2001;49:4–6.

62. Goadsby PJ, Ferrari MD, Csanyi A, et al. Randomized double blind, placebo-controlled proof-of-concept study of the cortical spreading depression inhibiting agent tonabersat in migraine prophylaxis. Cephalalgia 2009;29:742–50.

63. Hauge AW, Asghar MS, Schytz HW, et al. Effects of tonabersat on migraine with aura: a randomised, double-blind, placebo-controlled crossover study. Lancet Neurol 2009;8:718–23.

64. Read SJ, Smith MI, Hunter AJ, et al. SB-220453, a potential novel antimigraine compound, inhibits nitric oxide release following induction of cortical spreading depression in the anaesthetized cat. Cephalalgia 1999;20:92–9.

65. Smith MI, Read SJ, Chan WN, et al. Repetitive cortical spreading depression in a gyrencephalic feline brain: inhibition by the novel benzoylamino-benzopyran SB-220453. Cephalalgia 2000;20:546–53.

66. MaassenVanDenBrink A, van den Broek RW, de Vries R, et al. The potential anti-migraine compound SB-220453 does not contract human isolated blood vessels or myocardium; a comparison with sumatriptan. Cephalalgia 2000;20:538–45.

67. Parsons AA, Bingham S, Raval P, et al. Tonabersat (SB-220453) a novel benzo-pyran with anticonvulsant properties attenuates trigeminal nerve-induced neuro-vascular reflexes. Br J Pharmacol 2001;132:1549–57.

68. Diener HC, Tfelt-Hansen P, Dahlof C, et al. Topiramate in migraine prophylaxis-results from a placebo-controlled trial with propranolol as an active control. J Neurol 2004;251:943–50.

69. Brandes JL, Saper JR, Diamond M, et al. Topiramate for migraine prevention: a randomized controlled trial. JAMA 2004;291:965–73.

70. Silberstein SD, Neto W, Schmitt J, et al. Topiramate in migraine prevention: results of a large controlled trial. Arch Neurol 2004;61:490–5.

71. Akerman S, Goadsby PJ. Topiramate inhibits cortical spreading depression in rat and cat: impact in migraine aura. Neuroreport 2005;16:1383–7.

72. Ayata C, Jin H, Kudo C, et al. Suppression of cortical spreading depression in migraine prophylaxis. Ann Neurol 2006;59:652–61.

73. Tvedskov JF, Iversen HK, Olesen J. A double-blind study of SB-220453 (Toner-basat) in the glyceryltrinitrate (GTN) model of migraine. Cephalalgia 2004;24:875–82.

74. Tvedskov JF, Thomsen LL, Iversen HK, et al. The effect of propranolol on glyceryltrinitrate-induced headache and arterial response. Cephalalgia 2004;24:1076–87.

75. Tvedskov JF, Thomsen LL, Iversen HK, et al. The prophylactic effect of valproate on glyceryltrinitrate induced migraine. Cephalalgia 2004;24:576–85.

76. Storer RJ, Goadsby PJ. Topiramate inhibits trigeminovascular neurons in the cat. Cephalalgia 2004;24:1049–56.

77. Storer RJ, Goadsby PJ. Topiramate has a locus of action outside of the trigemi-nocervical complex. Cephalalgia 2005;25:934.

78. Akerman S, Holland PR, Goadsby PJ. Mechanically-induced cortical spreading depression associated regional cerebral blood flow changes are blocked by Na+ ion channel blockade. Brain Res 2008;1229:27–36.

79. Kaube H, Herzog J, Kaufer T, et al. Aura in some patients with familial hemiple-gic migraine can be stopped by intranasal ketamine. Neurology 2000;55:139–41.

80. May A, Bahra A, Buchel C, et al. Hypothalamic activation in cluster headache attacks. The Lancet 1998;352:275–8.

81. May A, Buchel C, Bahra A, et al. Intra-cranial vessels in trigeminal transmitted pain: a PET Study. Neuroimage 1999;9:453–60.
82. Matharu MS, Cohen AS, Frackowiak RSJ, et al. Posterior hypothalamic activation in paroxysmal hemicrania. Ann Neurol 2006;59:535–45.
83. Matharu MS, Cohen AS, McGonigle DJ, et al. Posterior hypothalamic and brainstem activation in hemicrania continua. Headache 2004;44:747–61.
84. Maniyar FH, Sprenger T, Monteith T, et al. Brain activations in the premonitory phase of nitroglycerin triggered migraine attacks. Brain 2014;137:232–42.
85. Schulte LH, May A. The migraine generator revisited: continuous scanning of the migraine cycle over 30 days and three spontaneous attacks. Brain 2016; 139:1987–93.
86. Sprenger T, Maniyar FH, Monteith TS, et al. Midbrain activation in the premonitory phase of migraine: a $H_2^{15}O$-positron emission tomography study. Headache 2012;52:863–4.
87. Denuelle M, Fabre N, Payoux P, et al. Hypothalamic activation in spontaneous migraine attacks. Headache 2007;47:1418–26.
88. Malick A, Burstein R. Cells of origin of the trigeminohypothalamic tract in the rat. J Comp Neurol 1998;400:125–44.
89. Malick A, Strassman AM, Burstein R. Trigeminohypothalamic and reticulohypothalamic tract neurons in the upper cervical spinal cord and caudal medulla of the rat. J Neurophysiol 2000;84:2078–112.
90. Robert C, Bourgeais L, Arreto CD, et al. Paraventricular hypothalamic regulation of trigeminovascular mechanisms involved in headaches. J Neurosci 2013; 33(20):8827–40.
91. Settle M. The hypothalamus. Neonatal Netw 2000;19:9–14.
92. Graebner AK, Iyer M, Carter ME. Understanding how discrete populations of hypothalamic neurons orchestrate complicated behavioral states. Front Syst Neurosci 2015;9:111.
93. Schulte LH, Allers A, May A. Hypothalamus as a mediator of chronic migraine: Evidence from high-resolution fMRI. Neurology 2017;88(21):2011–6.
94. Benjamin L, Levy MJ, Lasalandra MP, et al. Hypothalamic activation after stimulation of the superior sagittal sinus in the cat: a Fos study. Neurobiol Dis 2004; 16:500–5.
95. Malick A, Burstein R. A neurohistochemical blueprint for pain-induced loss of appetite. Proc Natl Acad Sci U S A 2001;98:9930–5.
96. Peyron C, Tighe DK, van den Pol AN, et al. Neurons containing hypocretin (orexin) project to multiple neuronal systems. J Neurosci 1998;18:9996–10015.
97. Bartsch T, Levy MJ, Knight YE, et al. Differential modulation of nociceptive dural input to [hypocretin] Orexin A and B receptor activation in the posterior hypothalamic area. Pain 2004;109:367–78.
98. Lipton RB, Buse DC, Hall CB, et al. Reduction in percieved stress as a migraine trigger: testing the "let-down headache" hypothesis. Neurology 2014;82: 1395–401.
99. Waterson MJ, Horvath TL. Neuronal regulation of energy homeostasis: beyond the hypothalamus and feeding. Cell Metab 2015;22(6):962–70.
100. Buijs RM, Vargas NG. Synchrony between suprachiasmatic nucleus-driven signals and the light/dark cycle is essential for liver homeostasis. Hepatology 2017; 65(6):2110–2.
101. Parker JA, Bloom SR. Hypothalamic neuropeptides and the regulation of appetite. Neuropharmacology 2012;63(1):18–30.

102. Holland PR. Headache and sleep: shared pathophysiological mechanisms. Cephalalgia 2014;34:725–44.
103. Holland PR, Goadsby PJ. Cluster headache, hypothalamus, and orexin. Curr Pain Headache Rep 2009;13:147–54.
104. Thorn NA. Antidiuretic hormone synthesis, release, and action under normal and pathological circumstances. Adv Metab Disord 1970;4:39–73.
105. Brennan KC, Bates EA, Shapiro RE, et al. Casein kinase id mutations in familial migraine and advanced sleep phase. Sci Transl Med 2013;5:183ra56.
106. Holland PR, Goadsby PJ. Orexin and primary headache disorders. In: Lawrence AJ, de Lecea L, editors. Behavioural neuroscience of orexin/hypocretin. Current topics in behavioral neurosciences. New York: Springer, in press.
107. van Oosterhout W, van Someren E, Schoonman GG, et al. Chronotypes and circadian timing in migraine. Cephalalgia 2018;38(4):617–25.
108. Hastings MH, Maywood ES, Brancaccio M. Generation of circadian rhythms in the suprachiasmatic nucleus. Nat Rev Neurosci 2018;19(8):453–69.
109. Martins-Oliveira M, Akerman S, Holland PR, et al. Neuroendocrine signaling modulates specific neural networks relevant to migraine. Neurobiol Dis 2017; 101:16–26.
110. Akerman S, Holland P, Goadsby PJ. Diencephalic and brainstem mechanisms in migraine. Nat Rev Neurosci 2011;12:570–84.
111. Penfield W, McNaughton F. Dural headache and innervation of the dura mater. AMA Arch Neurol Psychiatry 1940;44:43–75.
112. Ray BS, Wolff HG. Experimental studies on headache. Pain sensitive structures of the head and their significance in headache. Arch Surg 1940;41:813–56.
113. McNaughton FL, Feindel WH. Innervation of intracranial structures: a reappraisal. In: Rose FC, editor. Physiological aspects of clinical neurology. Oxford (United Kingdom): Blackwell Scientific Publications; 1977. p. 279–93.
114. Edvinsson L, MacKenzie ET, McCulloch J, et al. Nerve supply and receptor mechanisms in intra- and extracerebral blood vessels. In: Olesen J, Edvinsson L, editors. Basic mechanisms of headache. Amsterdam: Elsevier Science Publishers; 1988. p. 127–44.
115. Uddman R, Edvinsson L, Ekman R, et al. Innervation of the feline cerebral vasculature by nerve fibers containing calcitonin gene-related peptide: trigeminal origin and co-existence with substance P. Neurosci Lett 1985;62:131–6.
116. Uddman R, Goadsby PJ, Jansen I, et al. Localization of pituitary adenylate cylase activating peptide (PACAP) in cerebral vessels. Colocalization with VIP, effects in cerebral blood vessels in vitro and in situ and on cerebral blood flow. J Cereb Blood Flow Metab 1993;13(Suppl 1):S633.
117. Uddman R, Edvinsson L. Neuropeptides in the cerebral circulation. Cerebrovasc Brain Metab Rev 1989;1:230–52.
118. O'Connor TP, van der Kooy D. Enrichment of a vasoactive neuropeptide (calcitonin gene related peptide) in trigeminal sensory projection to the intracranial arteries. J Neurosci 1988;8:2468–76.
119. Millan MJ. Descending control of pain. Prog Neurobiol 2002;66:355–474.
120. Burstein R, Yamamura H, Malick A, et al. Chemical stimulation of the intracranial dura induces enhanced responses to facial stimulation in brain stem trigeminal neurons. J Neurophysiol 1998;79:964–82.
121. Liu Y, Broman J, Edvinsson L. Central projections of the sensory innervation of the rat middle meningeal artery. Brain Res 2008;1208:103–10.
122. Liu Y, Broman J, Edvinsson L. Central projections of sensory innervation of the rat superior sagittal sinus. Neuroscience 2004;129:431–7.

123. Holland PR, Akerman S, Goadsby PJ. Modulation of nociceptive dural input to the trigeminal nucleus caudalis via activation of the orexin 1 receptor in the rat. Eur J Neurosci 2006;24:2825–33.

124. Rodriguez E, Sakurai K, Xu J, et al. A craniofacial-specific monosynaptic circuit enables heightened affective pain. Nat Neurosci 2017;20(12):1734–43.

125. Cechetto DF, Standaert DG, Saper CB. Spinal and trigeminal dorsal horn projections to the parabrachial nucleus in the rat. J Comp Neurol 1985;240(2):153–60.

126. Dallel R, Ricard O, Raboisson P. Organization of parabrachial projections from the spinal trigeminal nucleus oralis: an anterograde tracing study in the rat. J Comp Neurol 2004;470(2):181–91.

127. Panneton WM, Gan Q. Direct reticular projections of trigeminal sensory fibers immunoreactive to CGRP: potential monosynaptic somatoautonomic projections. Front Neurosci 2014;8:136.

128. Zhang Li ZH, Qiao Y, Zhang T, et al. VGLUT1 or VGLUT2 mRNA-positive neurons in spinal trigeminal nucleus provide collateral projections to both the thalamus and the parabrachial nucleus in rats. Mol Brain 2018;11(1):22.

129. Carter ME, Soden ME, Zweifel LS, et al. Genetic identification of a neural circuit that suppresses appetite. Nature 2013;503(7474):111–+.

130. Carter ME, Han S, Palmiter RD. Parabrachial calcitonin gene-related peptide neurons mediate conditioned taste aversion. J Neurosci 2015;35(11):4582–6.

131. Li J, Lemon CH. Mouse parabrachial neurons signal a relationship between bitter taste and nociceptive stimuli. J Neurosci 2019;39(9):1631–48.

132. Ivanusic JJ, Kwok MM, Ahn AH, et al. 5-HT(1D) receptor immunoreactivity in the sphenopalatine ganglion: implications for the efficacy of triptans in the treatment of autonomic signs associated with cluster headache. Headache 2011;51: 392–402.

133. Csati A, Tajti J, Tuka B, et al. Calcitonin gene-related peptide and its receptor components in the human sphenopalatine ganglion – interaction with the sensory system. Brain Res 2012;1435:29–39.

134. May A, Goadsby PJ. The trigeminovascular system in humans: pathophysiological implications for primary headache syndromes of the neural influences on the cerebral circulation. J Cereb Blood Flow Metab 1999;19:115–27.

135. Takeuchi Y, Fukui Y, Ichiyama M, et al. Direct amygdaloid projections to the superior salivatory nucleus: a light and electron microscopic study in the cat. Brain Res Bull 1991;27(1):85–92.

136. Akerman S, Holland PR, Lasalandra MP, et al. Oxygen inhibits neuronal activation in the trigeminocervical complex after stimulation of trigeminal autonomic reflex, but not via direct dural activation of trigeminal afferents. Headache 2009;49:1131–43.

137. Akerman S, Holland PR, Summ O, et al. A translational in vivo model of trigeminal autonomic cephalalgias: therapeutic characterization. Brain 2012;135(Pt 12):3664–75.

138. Guo S, Petersen A, Schytz HW, et al. Cranial parasympathetic activation induces autonomic symptoms but no cluster headache attacks. Cephalalgia 2018;38:1418–28.

139. Burstein R, Cliffer KD, Giesler GJ Jr. Direct somatosensory projections from the spinal cord to the hypothalamus and telencephalon. J Neurosci 1987;7(12): 4159–64.

140. Burstein R, Cliffer KD, Giesler GJ. Cells of origin of the spinohypothalamic tract in the rat. J Comp Neurol 1990;291(3):329–44.

141. Liu Y, Broman J, Zhang M, et al. Brainstem and thalamic projections from a craniovascular sensory nervous centre in the rostral cervical spinal dorsal horn of rats. Cephalalgia 2009;29:935–48.
142. Matsushita M, Ikeda M, Okado N. The cells of origin of the trigeminothalamic, trigeminospinal and trigeminocerebellar projections in the cat. Neuroscience 1982;7(6):1439–54.
143. Shigenaga Y, Nakatani Z, Nishimori T, et al. The cells of origin of cat trigeminothalamic projections: especially in the caudal medulla. Brain Res 1983;277(2): 201–22.
144. Veinante P, Jacquin MF, Deschenes M. Thalamic projections from the whisker-sensitive regions of the spinal trigeminal complex in the rat. J Comp Neurol 2000;420(2):233–43.
145. Williams MN, Zahm DS, Jacquin MF. Differential foci and synaptic organization of the principal and spinal trigeminal projections to the thalamus in the rat. Eur J Neurosci 1994;6:429–53.
146. Zagami AS, Lambert GA. Stimulation of cranial vessels excites nociceptive neurones in several thalamic nuclei of the cat. Exp Brain Res 1990;81:552–66.
147. Zagami AS, Lambert GA. Craniovascular application of capsaicin activates nociceptive thalamic neurons in the cat. Neurosci Lett 1991;121:187–90.
148. Burstein R, Jakubowski M, Garcia-Nicas E, et al. Thalamic sensitization transforms localized pain into widespread allodynia. Ann Neurol 2010;68(1):81–91.
149. Tyll S, Budinger E, Noesselt T. Thalamic influences on multisensory integration. Commun Integr Biol 2011;4(4):378–81.
150. Noseda R, Kainz V, Jakubowski M, et al. A neural mechanism for exacerbation of headache by light. Nat Neurosci 2010;13:239–45.
151. Bieler M, Xu X, Marquardt A, et al. Multisensory integration in rodent tactile but not visual thalamus. Sci Rep 2018;8(1):15684.
152. Schwedt TJ. Multisensory integration in migraine. Curr Opin Neurol 2013;26(3): 248–53.
153. Porreca F, Ossipov MH, Gebhart GF. Chronic pain and medullary descending facilitation. Trends Neurosci 2002;25(6):319–25.
154. Weiller C, May A, Limmroth V, et al. Brain stem activation in spontaneous human migraine attacks. Nat Med 1995;1:658–60.
155. Afridi S, Giffin NJ, Kaube H, et al. A PET study in spontaneous migraine. Arch Neurol 2005;62:1270–5.
156. Afridi S, Matharu MS, Lee L, et al. A PET study exploring the laterality of brainstem activation in migraine using glyceryl trinitrate. Brain 2005;128:932–9.
157. Bahra A, Matharu MS, Buchel C, et al. Brainstem activation specific to migraine headache. Lancet 2001;357:1016–7.
158. Dominguez C, Lopez A, Ramos-Cabrer P, et al. Iron deposition in periaqueductal gray matter as a potential biomarker for chronic migraine. Neurology 2019; 92(10):e1076–85.
159. Welch KM, Nagesh V, Aurora S, et al. Periaqueductal grey matter dysfunction in migraine: cause or the burden of illness? Headache 2001;41:629–37.
160. Dahlberg LS, Linnman CN, Lee D, et al. Responsivity of periaqueductal gray connectivity is related to headache frequency in episodic migraine. Front Neurol 2018;9:61.
161. Chong CD, Gaw N, Fu Y, et al. Migraine classification using magnetic resonance imaging resting-state functional connectivity data. Cephalalgia 2017;37:828–44.
162. Hoskin KL, Bulmer DCE, Lasalandra M, et al. Fos expression in the midbrain periaqueductal grey after trigeminovascular stimulation. J Anat 2001;198:29–35.

163. Keay KA, Bandler R. Vascular head pain selectively activates ventrolateral peri-aqueductal gray in the cat. Neurosci Lett 1998;245:58–60.
164. Oliveras JL, Woda A, Guilbaud G, et al. Inhibition of the jaw opening reflex by electrical stimulation of the periacqueductal gray matter in the awake, unrestrained cat. Brain Res 1974;72:328–31.
165. Knight YE, Goadsby PJ. The periaqueductal gray matter modulates trigemino-vascular input: a role in migraine? Neuroscience 2001;106:793–800.
166. Knight YE, Bartsch T, Goadsby PJ. Trigeminal antinociception induced by bicu-culline in the periaqueductal grey (PAG) is not affected by PAG P/Q-type calcium channel blockade in rat. Neurosci Lett 2003;336:113–6.
167. Knight YE, Bartsch T, Kaube H, et al. P/Q-type calcium-channel blockade in the periaqueductal gray facilitates trigeminal nociception: a functional genetic link for migraine? J Neurosci 2002;22(5):RC213.
168. Pozo-Rosich P, Storer RJ, Charbit AR, et al. Periaqueductal gray calcitonin gene-related peptide modulates trigeminovascular neurons. Cephalalgia 2015;35:1298–307.
169. Bartsch T, Knight YE, Goadsby PJ. Activation of 5-HT$_{1B/1D}$ receptors in the peri-aqueductal grey inhibits meningeal nociception. Ann Neurol 2004;56:371–81.
170. Marciszewski KK, Meylakh N, Di Pietro F, et al. Changes in brainstem pain mod-ulation circuitry function over the migraine cycle. J Neurosci 2018;38(49): 10479–88.
171. Basbaum AI, Fields HL. Endogenous pain control mechanisms: review and hy-pothesis. Ann Neurol 1978;4:451–62.
172. Edelmayer RM, Vanderah TW, Majuta L, et al. Medullary pain facilitating neurons mediate allodynia in headache-related pain. Ann Neurol 2009;65:184–93.
173. Schwarz LA, Luo L. Organization of the locus coeruleus-norepinephrine system. Curr Biol 2015;25(21):R1051–6.
174. Reyes BA, Valentino RJ, Xu G, et al. Hypothalamic projections to locus coeru-leus neurons in rat brain. Eur J Neurosci 2005;22(1):93–106.
175. Arima Y, Yokota S, Fujitani M. Lateral parabrachial neurons innervate orexin neu-rons projecting to brainstem arousal areas in the rat. Sci Rep 2019;9(1):2830.
176. Soya S, Takahashi TM, McHugh TJ, et al. Orexin modulates behavioral fear expression through the locus coeruleus. Nat Commun 2017;8(1):1606.
177. Vila-Pueyo M, Strother LC, Kefel M, et al. Divergent influences of the locus co-eruleus on migraine pathophysiology. Pain 2019;160:385–94.
178. Hickey L, Li Y, Fyson SJ, et al. Optoactivation of locus ceruleus neurons evokes bidirectional changes in thermal nociception in rats. J Neurosci 2014;34(12): 4148–60.
179. Drummond PD. A possible role of the locus coeruleus in complex regional pain syndrome. Front Integr Neurosci 2012;6:104.
180. Charles A. The migraine aura. Continuum (Minneap Minn) 2018;24(4, Headache):1009–22.
181. Chan AC, Carter PJ. Therapeutic antibodies for autoimmunity and inflammation. Nat Rev Immunol 2010;10(5):301–16.
182. Brennan KC, Charles A. Sleep and headache. Semin Neurol 2009;29(4):406–18.
183. Zhang X, Levy D, Kainz V, et al. Activation of central trigeminovascular neurons by cortical spreading depression. Ann Neurol 2011;69(5):855–65.
184. Kramer DR, Fujii T, Ohiorhenuan I, et al. Cortical spreading depolarization: path-ophysiology, implications, and future directions. J Clin Neurosci 2016;24:22–7.
185. Enger R, Tang W, Vindedal GF, et al. Dynamics of ionic shifts in cortical spreading depression. Cereb Cortex 2015;25(11):4469–76.

186. Melo-Carrillo A, Noseda R, Nir R, et al. Selective inhibition of trigeminovascular neurons by fremanezumab: a humanized monoclonal Anti-CGRP antibody. J Neurosci 2017;37(30):7149–63.
187. Hansen JM, Hauge AW, Olesen J, et al. Calcitonin gene-related peptide triggers migraine-like attacks in patients with migraine with aura. Cephalalgia 2010;30: 1179–86.
188. Hansen JM, Thomsen LL, Olesen J, et al. Calcitonin gene-related peptide does not cause migraine attacks in patients with familial hemiplegic migraine. Headache 2011;51(4):544–53.
189. Filiz A, Tepe N, Eftekhari S, et al. CGRP receptor antagonist MK-8825 attenuates cortical spreading depression induced pain behavior. Cephalalgia 2019;39: 354–65.
190. Tozzi A, de Iure A, Di Filippo M, et al. Critical role of calcitonin gene-related peptide receptors in cortical spreading depression. Proc Natl Acad Sci U S A 2012; 109(46):18985–90.
191. Costa C, Tozzi A, Rainero I, et al. Cortical spreading depression as a target for anti-migraine agents. J Headache Pain 2013;14:62.
192. Karatas H, Erdener SE, Gursoy-Ozdemir Y, et al. Spreading depression triggers headache by activating neuronal Panx1 channels. Science 2013;339:1092–5.
193. Ashina M, Hansen JM, BO AD, et al. Human models of migraine - short-term pain for long-term gain. Nat Rev Neurol 2017;13(12):713–24.
194. Afridi S, Kaube H, Goadsby PJ. Glyceryl trinitrate triggers premonitory symptoms in migraineurs. Pain 2004;110:675–80.
195. Akerman S, Karsan N, Bose P, et al. Nitroglycerin triggers triptan-responsive cranial allodynia and trigeminal neuronal hypersensitivity. Brain 2019;142: 103–19.
196. Demartini C, Greco R, Zanaboni AM, et al. Nitroglycerin as a comparative experimental model of migraine pain: from animal to human and back. Prog Neurobiol 2019;177:15–32.
197. Bates E, Nikai T, Brennan K, et al. Sumatriptan alleviates nitroglycerin-induced mechanical and thermal allodynia in mice. Cephalalgia 2010;30:170–8.
198. Farkas S, Bolcskei K, Markovics A, et al. Utility of different outcome measures for the nitroglycerin model of migraine in mice. J Pharmacol Toxicol Methods 2016; 77:33–44.
199. Eller-Smith OC, Nicol AL, Christianson JA. Potential mechanisms underlying centralized pain and emerging therapeutic interventions. Front Cell Neurosci 2018;12:35.
200. Marone IM, De Logu F, Nassini R, et al. TRPA1/NOX in the soma of trigeminal ganglion neurons mediates migraine-related pain of glyceryl trinitrate in mice. Brain 2018;141(8):2312–28.
201. Abad N, Rosenberg JT, Hike DC, et al. Dynamic sodium imaging at ultra-high field reveals progression in a preclinical migraine model. Pain 2018;159(10): 2058–65.
202. Mason BN, Kaiser EA, Kuburas A, et al. Induction of migraine-like photophobic behavior in mice by both peripheral and central CGRP mechanisms. J Neurosci 2017;37(1):204–16.
203. Wattiez AS, Wang M, Russo AF. CGRP in animal models of migraine. Handb Exp Pharmacol 2019;1–23.
204. Christensen CE, Younis S, Deen M, et al. Migraine induction with calcitonin gene-related peptide in patients from erenumab trials. J Headache Pain 2018; 19(1):105.

Transient Neurologic Dysfunction in Migraine

Rod Foroozan, MD^{a,}*, F. Michael Cutrer, MD^b

KEYWORDS

- Migraine • Aura • Persistent aura • Retinal migraine • Brainstem migraine
- Pathophysiology • Visual snow

KEY POINTS

- Ocular manifestations from migraine may occur with several different manifestations.
- Evidence has accumulated to consider visual snow syndrome as a separate entity than persistent migraine aura without infarction.
- The occurrence of focal neurologic symptoms that localize to the brainstem is now considered a separate migraine aura subtype.

INTRODUCTION

The sudden appearance of neurologic symptoms just before or at the beginning of an attack is an alarming feature of migraine in over a quarter of patients. Collectively, transient neurologic symptoms attributed to migraine are known as the migraine aura. Over the course of a patient's migraine history, auras can often lead to Emergency Department visits and neuroimaging investigation. They also figure prominently in historical medical descriptions of migraine, even though they often do not accompany every attack and do not occur at all in up to 70% of migraine sufferers. Although migraine is arguably the most common cause of concurrent neurologic symptoms and headache, it is not the only setting in which this occurs; care should be taken in the evaluation of "migrainous" neurologic symptoms to ensure that they are indeed consistent with migraine aura. This task is complicated to some degree by the recent addition of brainstem and retinal aura to the International Headache Society (IHS) criteria,[1] because their presumed extracortical origin differs from cortical localization of the classical visual, sensory, language, and motor symptoms. In 2009, we published an earlier version of "Transient Neurologic Dysfunction in Migraine." The following is an updated version with inclusion of new material that has become available since that time.

^a Baylor College of Medicine, 6565 Fannin NC-205, Houston, TX 77030, USA; ^b Mayo Clinic, 200 First Street, Southwest, Rochester, MN 55905, USA
* Corresponding author.
E-mail address: Foroozan@bcm.tmc.edu

Neurol Clin 37 (2019) 673–694
https://doi.org/10.1016/j.ncl.2019.06.002
0733-8619/19/© 2019 Elsevier Inc. All rights reserved.

neurologic.theclinics.com

GENERAL CLINICAL FEATURES OF MIGRAINE WITH AURA

Under the current IHS criteria, International Classification of Headache Disorders-3 (ICHD-3), published in early 2018, migraine with aura is divided into 4 major types: migraine with typical aura (visual, sensory and language disturbance), migraine with brainstem aura, hemiplegic migraine (HM), and retinal migraine. To meet diagnostic criteria for migraine with aura the patient must have attacks in which they experience headaches meeting criteria for migraine and

A. At least 2 attacks fulfilling criteria B and C
B. One or more of the following fully reversible aura symptoms:
    1. Visual
    2. Sensory
    3. Speech and/or language
    4. Motor
    5. Brainstem
    6. Retinal
C. At least 3 of the following 6 characteristics:
    1. At least 1 aura symptom spreads gradually over 5 minutes
    2. Two or more aura symptoms occur in succession
    3. Each individual aura symptom lasts 5 to 60 minutes
    4. At least 1 aura symptom is unilateral
    5. At least 1 aura symptom is positive
    6. The aura is accompanied, or followed within 60 minutes, by headache
D. Not better accounted for by another ICHD-3 diagnosis.

In the case of visual and sensory symptoms of the typical aura, there are certain characteristics that may be used to distinguish them from ischemia-related symptoms. Both sensory and visual auras have a slow migratory or spreading quality in which symptoms slowly spread across the affected body part or the visual field followed by a gradual return to normal function in the areas first affected after 20 to 60 minutes. This spreading quality is not characteristic of an ischemic event[2] in which neurologic deficits tend to appear somewhat suddenly and tend to be equally distributed within the relevant vascular territory. In stroke, the affected area can certainly expand as blood flow drops in additional vessels. However, ischemic change is a more stepwise and less smoothly spreading process. Although a migratory pattern is also seen in partial seizure disorders, its progression is generally much more rapid. Neither ischemia nor seizure is associated with the return of function in the areas first affected even as symptoms are simultaneously appearing in newly affected areas.

In addition, migraine aura often has a biphasic quality inherent in its neurologic symptoms with positive phenomena (eg, shimmering lights, zig-zagging visual disturbances, or tingling paresthesia) appearing first, only to be followed within a few minutes by negative symptoms (eg, scotoma, loss of visual image or numbness, or loss of sensation). Ischemic events do not tend to exhibit a bimodal progression of symptoms and—while there may be a biphasic progression in the course of a seizure—progression is likely to occur at a much faster rate. In the language aura, making the same biphasic analogy is more difficult. Whereas patients experiencing the language aura report both paraphasic errors and word retrieval errors (abnormal function), migraineurs seldom become mute (loss of function) during language aura. Assessing basic language function is complex given the importance of context. Obtaining accurate descriptions of language dysfunction during aura is also problematic because of the difficulties in laying down precise memories while language is disturbed.

In migraine aura, different neurologic symptoms tend to occur sequentially. Almost all patients experiencing more than 1 type of aura during a single attack first recount the appearance of 1 aura type (most often visual), which is then followed by another aura type. Some patients experience all 3 typical auras in sequence during a single attack. In almost 20 years of asking patients to describe their aura, none have reported the appearance of all aura types at the same time.[2] In contrast to migraine aura, the simultaneous manifestation of multiple types of neurologic symptoms is, however, quite common in cerebral ischemia.

In HM, motor symptoms do not have positive and negative phases. No twitching or migratory spasm is noted before weakness by patients with HM. However, the most prominent difference is the much greater average duration of motor weakness with HM. Patients with HM often have unilateral weakness for hours to days, which is much longer than the 60 minutes or less reported in the other aura types.[3] As our knowledge of the pathophysiological mechanisms of each aura type improves, so too will our understanding of whether or not the motor aura arises from a process analogous to those underlying the more common aura types. However, it should be noted that, in attacks of HM, more typical aura symptoms almost always occur.[1]

In brainstem aura (previously referred to as basilar or basilar-type), transient symptoms of vertigo, diplopia, tinnitus, hypacusis, dysarthria, ataxia, and decreased level of consciousness do not have the bimodal or spreading quality observed in the typical aura symptoms and make the distinction from ischemia more difficult. Visual disturbances in retinal migraine, including scintillation and scotomata, resemble typical visual aura, but they are monocular. When retinal migraine occurs in the absence of a typical migrainous headache, distinction from an ischemic retinal event can be problematic.

EPIDEMIOLOGY OF MIGRAINE AURA

In the mid-1990s, a Danish population-based nosographic analysis of migraine aura found that 163 of 4000 randomly sampled patients were identified with migraine.[4] In this sample, visual aura was by far the most common symptom, occurring in 99% of subjects; this was followed by sensory and then language auras. Only visual aura occurred in 64% of patients, whereas other aura types typically coincided with another aura type (usually visual).[5] Among 3091 patients with migraine with aura drawn from 7334 migraine patients entered into the Mayo Clinic Headache Registry, 2616 (84.6%) reported having at least 2 episodes of visual aura, 1319 (42.7%) language aura, 1118 (36.2%) sensory aura, and 418 (13.5%) motor aura. Also noted in this clinic-based cohort was a higher occurrence of nonvisual aura symptoms in the absence of visual disturbance. In a study of study of 362 patients with migraine with typical aura and/or brainstem aura (basilar-type), 38 patients reported brainstem aura symptoms for an estimated 10% among patients with migraine with typical aura.[6]

TRANSIENT NEUROLOGICAL DISTURBANCE IN MIGRAINE
Visual System and Retinal Disturbance in Migraine

Ocular manifestations associated with migraine
Migraine remains one of the most common disorders that cause transient visual loss. Afferent visual dysfunction remains the most common sensory symptom in migraine with aura, and we covered the commonly encountered visual symptoms in our previous review for this journal in 2009.[7] In addition to highlighting the updates in the criteria for migraine with visual manifestations, we included other clinical scenarios that have been linked to migraine and may be more common than initially considered: visual snow syndrome (VSS), benign unilateral episodic mydriasis, and isolated eye pain.

The direct link of these conditions to migraine is frequently difficult to confirm but remains an important consideration, particularly when other causes of these clinical entities are excluded.

Migraine with aura: updated criteria

Migraine with aura is a recurrent condition characterized by reversible neurologic symptoms, which typically develop over 5 to 20 minutes and resolve within 60 minutes. Migraine headache typically follows the aura, although less commonly pain may not be present. Visual symptoms are the most common sensory manifestation in migraine aura. Migraine with aura has been characterized by criteria put forward by the IHS, in the ICHD, which was revised in 2013 (with a beta version), and in the third edition (ICHD-3) in 2018.[8] The first section of the ICHD-3 deals with migraine and outlines the updated criteria for migraine with aura.

Migraine with visual aura was previously often labeled as "ocular" or "ophthalmic" migraine. In our previous review we highlighted different types of visual symptoms and included some illustrative examples, which we have reprinted here (**Figs. 1 and 2**).[7] Visual aura is the most common type of aura, occurring in over 90% of patients. It often appears as a zigzag figure near fixation that may gradually evolve in the right or left hemifield and develop scintillating edges. There is often a relative or absolute scotoma in the area of visual involvement, so that positive and negative visual symptoms may occur individually or together (**Fig. 3**). When visual field loss is present it is common for patients to interpret loss of vision of the hemifield in each eye to monocular visual loss in the eye with the temporal field (because it is larger than the nasal field) loss.

Other phenomena characteristically associated with visual aura include sparkles and flashes (photopsia) of light. Shimmering (such as "heat waves" on pavement) or rotation of images may be noted. When other types of aura are present, they are typically accompanied by visual aura. There is often marked variability in the clinical presentation of migraine, both among patients, and between episodes in individual patients.[9]

Migraine aura may occur in the absence of headache (previously termed acephalgic migraine or migrainous accompaniments). This has been labeled in the IHS as typical aura without headache. The aura fulfills all of the criteria for migraine with aura. This absence of headache pain often confuses patients and causes them to dismiss migraine as the potential cause. Visual dysfunction is the most common feature of migraine aura without headache, occurring 75% of the time.[10]

Retinal migraine

In our previous review we discussed retinal migraine at length.[7] Patients with retinal migraine have been thought to lose visual function because of vasospasm involving the ocular circulation. The condition should be monocular and causes a variety of symptoms including a shadow, graying out of vision, or photopsia. The duration of visual symptoms is typically less than 30 minutes.[10]

Some of the ambiguity in the diagnosis of transient visual loss from migraine comes from the difficulty patients have distinguishing monocular visual loss from visual loss within the same hemifield in both eyes.[11] In addition, monocular temporal visual symptoms from disorders of the visual cortex (temporal crescent syndrome) may cause confusion with disorders of involving the anterior visual pathways. As alternative theories of the pathogenesis of migraine have evolved, so has the notion that retinal migraine is a common cause of transient visual loss.

The IHS revised the criteria for the diagnosis of retinal migraine.[1] The criteria include:

Description: repeated attacks of monocular visual disturbance, including scintillations, scotomata, or blindness, associated with migraine headache.

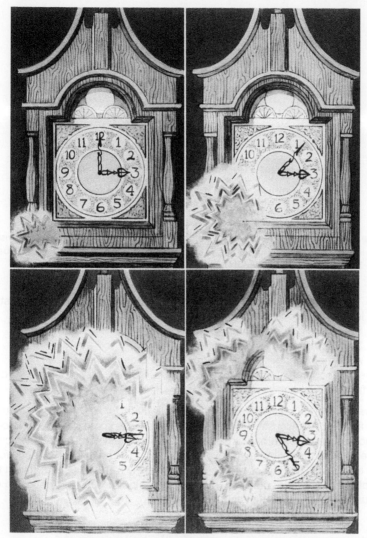

Fig. 1. Classical migrainous scintillating scotoma development and expansion of fortification figures. Initial small paracentral scotoma (top left). Enlarging scotoma for 7 minutes later (top right). Scotoma obscuring much of the central vision for 15 minutes later (bottom left). Break-up of scotoma at 20 minutes (bottom right). (*From* Hupp SL, Kline LB, Corbett JJ. Visual disturbances of migraine. Surv Ophthalmol 1989;33(4):221-36; with permission.)

Diagnostic criteria for retinal migraine (ICHD-3):

A. Attacks fulfilling criteria for migraine with aura and criterion B below.
B. Aura characterized by both of the following:
    1. Fully reversible, monocular, positive, and/or negative visual phenomena (eg, scintillations, scotomata, or blindness) confirmed during an attack by either or both of the following:
        a. Clinical visual field examination

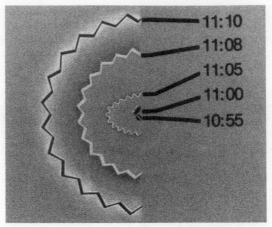

Fig. 2. Expansion of the visual aura of migraine from a "germ" in the paracentral visual field occurring over 15 minutes. (*From* Hupp SL, Kline LB, Corbett JJ. Visual disturbances of migraine. Surv Ophthalmol 1989;33(4):221-36; with permission.)

      b. The patient's drawing of a monocular field defect (made after clear instruction)
   2. At least 2 of the following:
      a. Spreading gradually over ≥5 minutes
      b. Symptoms last 5 to 60 minutes
      c. Accompanied, or followed within 60 minutes, by headache
C. Not better accounted for by another ICHD-3 diagnosis, and other causes of amaurosis fugax have been excluded.

    The revised IHS criteria eliminated the requirement for a normal eye examination between attacks. As discussed for migraine visual aura, some patients who complain of monocular visual disturbance have a homonymous hemianopia, which is not recognized unless they alternately cover each eye.[11] The revised IHS criteria for retinal migraine emphasize that the condition is an extremely rare cause of transient monocular visual loss. Therefore, patients should undergo a thorough evaluation to exclude other causes of monocular transient visual loss.

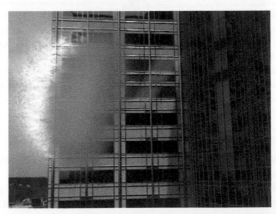

Fig. 3. A representation of the positive (scintillation) and negative (relative scotoma) symptoms that can occur during attacks of typical migraine visual aura.

The distinction between retinal migraine and ocular vasospasm may not be possible.[12] Patients with vasospasm involving the ocular circulation have been noted to respond favorably to calcium channel blockers.[13] Rarely, reports have included photographic and angiographic evidence of involvement of the ophthalmic vessels, including changes within the retinal vasculature.[14,15]

Retinal structure
Structural changes within the retina have been recognized using imaging modalities of the posterior segment. Ninety patients with migraine were found to have thinning of the ganglion cell layer, retinal nerve fiber layer, and choroid on spectral domain-optical coherence tomography.[16] Similar findings have been noted by other groups.[17,18] In 15 patients with migraine with aura, optical coherence tomographic angiography demonstrated an enlarged foveal avascular zone area.[19] The investigators postulated that this finding may increase the risk of ocular and systemic vascular complications in this group of patients.

Persistent migraine visual aura without infarction
Persistent migraine visual aura most commonly consists of positive visual phenomena. These most commonly are formed (shapes or figures) or unformed (lights or sparkles) visual hallucinations.[20] The hallucinations are less commonly more complex (metamorphopsia or palinopsia). The IHS revised criteria for persistent migraine visual aura includes that the findings must occur without infarction.[1]

Description: aura symptoms persisting for 1 week or more without evidence of infarction on neuroimaging.

Diagnostic criteria:

A. Aura fulfilling criterion B.
B. Occurring in a patient with migraine with aura and typical of previous auras, except that 1 or more aura symptom persists for $\geq$1 week.
C. Neuroimaging shows no evidence of infarction.
D. Not better accounted for by another ICHD-3 diagnosis.

The IHS noted that persistent aura symptoms are not common but have been documented. They are often bilateral and may last for months or years. Other ocular and neurologic conditions (seizures, toxic-metabolic conditions, retinopathy, and psychiatric disease) may cause these types of visual symptoms so that the diagnosis of persistent migraine visual aura without infarction is typically one of exclusion. The IHS did not provide clear guidelines as to which tests should be performed to exclude other conditions that may cause persistent visual symptoms. A thorough eye examination to exclude an ocular cause for the symptoms seems to be reasonable.

Visual snow syndrome
Whereas persistent migraine aura without infarction is thought to be a rare entity (noted as such by the IHS), descriptive patterns that have been believed to be associated with, but independent of, migraine are more common in practice. One is VSS, also referred to as primary persistent visual disturbance.[20] Patients may describe this as television static noted when there is impaired signal on an analog television,[21] or pixellation of vision.

Some patients notice symptoms only under certain lighting conditions or in certain circumstances; others notice them all of the time. The abnormal visual image occurs in both eyes and covers the entire visual field. Not all patients with these symptoms have a clear history of migraine, and in some the diagnosis of persistent migraine visual aura without infarction has been inferred because no other causes were evident. These visual symptoms have been thought to originate from a distinct clinical disorder, and some have suggested that they be regarded as separate from those of persistent migraine visual aura without infarction.[22,23] Patients may also have nonvisual symptoms such as tinnitus.

One group has developed criteria for the diagnosis of VSS, in part based on a review of 22 patients and an Internet survey of 275 self-assessed patients with the syndrome.[24] Migraine was noted in 59% of the patients. The authors proposed criteria for VSS and these have been incorporated into the appendix of the IHCD-3 under complications of migraine,[1] although the IHS recognized that it may be separate from the migraine spectrum.[1,24,25]

Description: dynamic, continuous, tiny dots in the entire visual field lasting longer than 3 months.

Diagnostic criteria:

A. Presence of at least 2 additional visual symptoms of the 4 following categories:
   1. Palinopsia
   2. Enhanced entopic phenomena
   3. Photophobia
   4. Nyctalopia
B. Symptoms are not consistent with typical migraine visual aura as defined by the IHS.
C. Symptoms are not better explained by another disorder.

Additional notes from the IHS criteria are as follows[1]:

1. Patients compare visual snow with television static ("television snow"). The dots are usually black or gray on a white background and gray or white on a black background. Patients also report transparent dots, white flashing dots and colored dots.
2. Palinopsia may be visual after-images and/or trailing of moving objects. Visual after-images are different from retinal after-images, which occur only after staring at a high-contrast image and are in the complementary color.
3. These phenomena, arising from the structure of the visual system itself, include excessive floaters in both eyes, excessive blue field entoptic phenomena (uncountable little gray/white/black dots or rings shooting over the visual field of both eyes when looking at homogeneous bright surfaces such as a blue sky), self-lighting of the eye (colored waves or clouds perceived when closing the eyes in the dark), and spontaneous photopsia (bright flashes of light).
4. As described under migraine with typical aura.
5. Normal ophthalmology tests (corrected visual acuity, dilated pupil funduscopy, visual field examination, and electroretinography) and no intake of psychotropic drugs.

In efforts to distinguish VSS from migraine, a different research group reviewed 105 articles on visual snow, persistent visual disturbances, migraine, palinopsia, nyctalopia, tinnitus, entoptic phenomena, photopsia, photophobia, and sensory processing.[26] They proposed that entoptic phenomena and VSS may be related to failure of inhibition of cortical or subcortical filtering, which normally prevents visual stimuli from coming to consciousness. Although they noted overlap between VSS and persistent migraine aura without infarction, the authors suggested that VSS is characterized by: constant flickering in the entire visual field, palinopsia, nyctalopia (impaired visual function in dim light), and monocular entoptic phenomena, whereas migraine aura occurs with the gradual development of symptoms, occurs with fortification spectra, is characterized by teichopsia (sensation of bright shimmering colors), and is typically homonymous.

The cause of this syndrome has remained unclear, although abnormal cortical processing has been the most likely candidate thus far. Areas with increased brain metabolism in a group of 17 patients with VSS, of whom 14 had migraine, in comparison with healthy controls, were identified using [^{18}F]-2-fluoro-2-deoxy-D-glucose positron emission tomography and statistical parametric mapping.[27] After adjusting for typical migraine aura, comparison patients with VSS—most of whom had comorbid migraine—with age-matched and sex-matched controls showed brain hypermetabolism in the right lingual gyrus and in the cerebellum. This suggests that the visual symptoms occur on the basis of a neurologic issue likely mediated through the effects of the visual association cortex. Cortical hyperexcitability was suggested in 16 patients with visual snow when compared with 18 controls.[28] Four visual tasks performed included: center-surround contrast matching, luminance increment detection in noise, and global form and global motion coherence thresholds. The patients with VSS demonstrated reduced center-surround contrast suppression and increased luminance increment thresholds in noise when compared with controls, consistent with increased excitability in primary visual cortex.[28]

Persistent aura may resolve spontaneously in some patients and continue in others. Patients with VSS often remain stable throughout life and without evidence of progressive visual loss or structural abnormalities in the anterior visual pathways. Therefore, reassurance that VSS may be a condition based on abnormal visual perception, rather than a progressive neurologic disorder characterized by loss of vision, is helpful.[26] Medical treatment of VSS has focused on agents used to treat seizures and migraine, without clear success for any particular agent.[29–31] Other therapeutic approaches have included tinted lenses with a specific colored filter (often blue-yellow), which have been reported to improve symptoms in some patients.[32] Interest in the condition led to a multidisciplinary conference, which included patients with VSS and their family members, on May 5, 2018.[33]

Episodic pupillary mydriasis

The clinical presentation of a dilated pupil typically sparks alarm and results in a thorough evaluation for a neurogenic cause. However, in the absence of ptosis and ophthalmoplegia (and including normal ocular alignment), transient isolated unilateral pupillary dilation (also referred to as a springing pupil) had been described as a benign phenomenon[34] in patients with migraine, typically in middle age,[35] although it has also been reported in children.[36] In 7 patients, the episodes of mydriasis usually occurred with a typical migraine headache. A subsequent report of 24 patients (7 seen by the author and 17 reviewed by clinical survey) noted migraine in 58% of patients.[37] The mydriasis occurred unilaterally in all patients in whom laterality was reported, although in 2 patients it could occur in either eye (and this sequential pupil involvement has been noted in other reports).[38] The median frequency of the episodes was 2.5 per month and the median duration was 12 hours (range 10 minutes to 7 days). Fourteen patients noted headache or orbital pain with the episodes of mydriasis. Other series have noted similar findings.[38–40] One report described benign unilateral episodic mydriasis that occurred 3 years before the onset of migraine with visual aura.[41] The authors suggested that the transient mydriasis could be considered as an unusual form of migrainous aura.

As a caveat, 1 series of 2 patients noted carotid occlusion and carotid dissection ipsilateral to the episodes of apparently benign episodic unilateral mydriasis, although the investigators acknowledged that it was unknown if the episodes were causal or coincidental to the disease of the internal carotid artery.[42]

Proposed mechanisms for benign episodic unilateral mydriasis have included impaired parasympathetic activity (likely mediated through a transient deficit in the ciliary ganglion) and increased sympathetic activity. The ciliary ganglion has been implied as a potential site of the deficit in a report of 9 patients with episodic mydriasis.[43] Seven women and 2 men, with a mean age of 34 years, were included. The patients presented during 1 hemicranial migraine attack ipsilateral to the mydriasis, which persisted for a mean of 3 months, while migraine headaches remained with their typical intermittent course. Cholinergic supersensitivity was noted with 0.125% topical pilocarpine in all patients. The authors suggested that cholinergic supersensitivity, similar to that of the isolated tonic (Adie) pupil, indicated dysfunction of the ipsilateral ciliary ganglion parasympathetic fibers. In other reports, the results from topical pharmacologic testing have failed to produce conclusive results and often the episodes do not last long enough to study the effects of topical agents.

Eye pain

The source of eye pain, which is frequently accompanied by inflammation of the anterior segment resulting in a red eye, can often be determined with slit lamp biomicroscopy. An eye examination will help exclude conditions such as angle-closure glaucoma (including that associated with Topiramate).[44,45] However, slit lamp examination will be unrevealing in some patients.[46,47] In a review of 2603 patients from 2 institutions, an inflammatory ocular condition (including conjunctivitis, keratitis, and uveitis) accounted for 69% of patients with eye pain.[48] Migraine was noted to be the cause in 3% of patients from the ophthalmology clinic but in 51% of patients from the neurology clinic.

Dry eye syndrome is one of the most common causes of eye pain, and an increased prevalence of dry eye syndrome has been noted in patients with migraine.[49,50] Dry eye symptoms and findings were greater in 46 patients with migraine when compared with 50 healthy controls. Abnormalities of the tear film have been noted in 30 patients with migraine when compared with 30 control subjects.[51] Improvement in symptoms of dry eye in patients with chronic migraine has been noted after botulinum toxin A injection into the procerus, corrugators, frontalis, temporalis, occipitalis, cervical, paraspinals, and trapezius muscles.[52] The injections also improved photophobia, and the effects on dry eye were independent of baseline tear film volume. The benefits of botulinum toxin injection were postulated to be due to modulation of shared trigeminal neural pathways.

Subtle abnormalities of the ocular biometric parameters, including in the cornea, have been noted in patients with migraine. Using confocal microscopy, corneal nerve fiber density was found to be significantly lower in 19 migraine patients compared with controls in 1 study,[53] and 36 patients with migraine and photophobia in another report by different investigators.[54] In 58 patients with migraine, corneal sensation was evaluated with a Cochet-Bonnet esthesiometer in 5 different regions of the cornea. Patients with migraine were found to have increased corneal sensation, suggesting that corneal sensation is altered in patients with migraine.[55]

Pain in the superonasal orbit may be caused by inflammation of the superior oblique tendon or the cartilaginous trochlea through which it passes. In some patients with pain over the trochlea[56] but without an obvious inflammatory cause, the terms "trochlear migraine" and "primary trochlear headache" have been used.[57,58] Injections of anesthetic and corticosteroids may result in long-lasting pain relief and may improve superior oblique function in those in whom it is impaired.[59]

Summary of visual disturbance

Visual symptoms from migraine are classically transient. The aura may include positive and negative symptoms that occur within the homonymous visual field and characteristically last in the range of 30 minutes. Transient monocular visual symptoms associated with migraine (with criteria updated by the ICHD-3) are likely rare disorders that may be indistinguishable from vasospasm of the ophthalmic circulation. Structural imaging has demonstrated changes in retinal architecture in patients with migraine. Enough evidence has accumulated to consider VSS as a separate entity than persistent migraine aura without infarction, and VSS seems to be based on abnormal cortical processing. Patients with benign episodic unilateral mydriasis and isolated eye pain often have a history of migraine, suggesting a potential association if not a causal relationship.

Sensory System Dysfunction in Migraine

The migraine sensory aura is quite alarming to patients and may result in medical consultation. Sensory aura most often starts as unilateral tingling or "paresthesia" in a hand or distal arm, which then slowly migrates proximally, only to jump from the arm to the ipsilateral face before reaching the shoulder. The crawling, tingling sensation moves from the cheek and side of the nose, across the perioral region and lips, then spreads inside the mouth, to involve the ipsilateral buccal mucosa and half of the tongue.[2] Paresthesia or a "feeling of needles and pins" is usually the first sensory symptom, leaving numbness in its wake,[60] although auras that consist primarily of numbness also occur. In a study of 51 patients with sensory aura, Russell and Olesen[4] reported that the hand (96% of cases) and face (67%) were the body parts most commonly affected, whereas the leg (24%) and torso (18%) were much less likely to be involved. The sensory symptoms, recorded in this particular series of individuals, progressed for less than 30 minutes (82%). The unilateral symptoms of sensory aura are frequently quite distressing for patients, especially at their first appearance, because of their similarity to those of stroke or transient ischemic attack. Although the presence of migraine aura does, in fact, seem to be an independent risk factor of ischemic stroke in women who have a low level of other cardiovascular risk factors,[61] the overall increase in absolute risk attributable to migraine with aura when compared with other factors is modest. There are clinical features that help to distinguish sensory aura from stroke. The spread of paresthesia across the face and into the mouth to affect half the tongue is a classical feature of migraine sensory aura and is rarely seen in cases of cerebrovascular ischemia.[62]

Language System Dysfunction in Migraine

Many patients find language disturbance during migraine aura difficult to describe, so it may be overlooked in the medical history unless specifically asked about. Whereas speech disturbance may result from numbness and tingling in the mouth and/or tongue, as the sensory aura gradually migrates intraorally, this is distinct from language aura. In language aura, patients have impaired language comprehension, marked word finding difficulties, and a decreased ability to read or write. This implies more than just a pure sensory or proprioceptive disturbance. It is considered a lateralizing symptom affecting 1 side of the brain,[1] which is consistent with other types of typical aura (visual, sensory, and language). Interestingly, language aura seems to occur with a higher frequency in patients with HM than in those with typical aura only (approximately 20% in typical aura vs. 47% in HM).[63] In another series of patients with language aura, 76% had paraphasic errors, 72% had other production problems, and 38% had impaired comprehension.[4] Fortunately, the distressing symptoms of language disturbance tend to persist for less than 30 minutes in most patients.[4] A recent questionnaire based on case series reported other instances of symptomatic cortical dysfunction including proper name anomia, ideational apraxia, and proposagnosia.[64]

Motor System Dysfunction in Migraine

Although uncommon, motor aura is a frightening symptom because of the possibility that the hemiparesis represents an ischemic brain event. Migraine with motor aura was the first migraine syndrome to be linked to genetic mutation and has been extensively studied. The motor aura typically lasts longer (typically up to 72 hours) than the other aura symptoms, but should be fully reversible.[3] In some rare instances, however, the motor weakness of familial hemiplegic migraine (FHM) may persist for weeks or even result in permanent neurologic deficit.[65,66] The extent of the unilateral weakness is variable and can present from mild clumsiness to complete hemiplegia.[4] The weakness of HM tends to start in 1 limb and progress over time.[4] Patients with HM almost always experience typical aura (visual, sensory, or language) symptoms in addition to unilateral weakness. Sensory disturbance is the most common.[4] When multiple aura symptoms are seen, they occur in a sequential fashion.

Variants in 3 different genes have been linked to families with HM: CACNA1A gene (neuronal calcium channel) for FHM 1, ATP1A2 (glial sodium/potassium pump subunit) for FHM 2, and SCN1A (neuronal voltage-gated sodium channel subunit) for FHM 3.[67–69] Among these affected families, there is variability in both the phenotype and penetrance. In some cases, gene mutations implicated in FHM have been identified in asymptomatic family members.[70,71] Nonfamilial sporadic cases have also been identified. FHM mutations have been associated with hyperexcitability in experimental models, suggesting an altered threshold for initiation of cortical spreading depression (CSD).[72,73]

Brainstem Dysfunction in Migraine

In the most recent ICHD-3 criteria, transient neurologic symptoms that localize to the brainstem were included as a separate type of aura. Many of these symptoms had been a part of what was previously called basilar artery migraine,[74] Bickerstaff's migraine,[75] or basilar-type migraine,[6] although additional symptoms previously associated with basilar artery (including bilateral paresthesia and visual scintillations affecting the bilateral visual fields) were not included in the new criteria. To diagnose brainstem aura under the new criteria, 2 of the following symptoms must be present: dysarthria, vertigo (but not all dizziness), tinnitus, hypacusis (not ear fullness), diplopia (not including blurred vision), ataxia, or decreased level of consciousness.[1] If any motor weakness is present then HM should be diagnosed.[1] In many patients with brainstem aura, other typical aura symptoms may also occur[6] and should also be diagnosed as having migraine with typical aura.

In a Danish population-based study of 38 patients with brainstem aura, the brainstem symptoms ranged widely in duration from less than 5 minutes to greater than 24 hours.[6] In order of reported frequency, the brainstem symptoms included: vertigo (61%), dysarthria (53%), diplopia (45%), tinnitus (45%), bilateral visual symptoms (40%), bilateral paresthesia (24%), impaired level of consciousness (24%), and hypacusis (21%).

PATHOPHYSIOLOGY OF MIGRAINE AURA

Because the focal neurologic symptoms of aura could be localized to a specific brain area, aura has figured prominently in migraine pathophysiological research. Until the 1980s, the vasogenic theory of migraine was used to explain the aura. It was postulated that the aura occurred as the consequence of an initial vasoconstrictive phase in the migraine attack.[76] However, as early as the 1940s, proponents of the neurogenic theory of migraine hypothesized that the aura was the clinical manifestation of a spreading abnormality which moved over the visual cortex at a rate of 3 to 5 mm per minute. This spreading abnormality was believed to be atypical for ischemia. Around the same time, Leao, a neurophysiologist, described an electrophysiological phenomenon, characterized by cortical hyper-excitation followed by suppression, which originated and migrated over areas of contiguous cortex in experimental animals at a slow rate of 3 to 4 mm per minute, after chemical or mechanical stimulations.[77] This phenomenon, which Leao called CSD, has been proposed as the cause of migraine aura, based on its slow rate of cortical spread, which is similar to that extrapolated for migraine aura across visual cortex. The fact that both CSD and aura move across neurovascular boundaries strengthens this hypothesis. The neurogenic theory proposes that the decreases in blood flow observed during migraine aura are the direct consequence of reduced metabolic demand in abnormally functioning neurons, rather than vasoconstriction. Evidence from functional imaging techniques, applied during the aura phase in humans, has generally supported the neurogenic theory.

Functional Neuroimaging and the Migraine Aura

Beginning in the early 1980s, various functional imaging techniques[78–80] used during aura symptoms have supported a CSD or CSD-like phenomenon as the underlying mechanism of the migraine aura. These early studies have been consistent with more recent arterial spin labeling-based perfusion studies.[76] One of the most recent of these studies applied blood oxygen level-dependent (BOLD) imaging to aura. BOLD imaging is based on known increases in MRI signal intensity that occur in response to decreases in local deoxyhemoglobin concentration.[81] In this study, BOLD imaging was performed before, during, and after exercise-induced visual auras.[82] BOLD imaging was also carried out during aura symptoms in 2 spontaneous auras as well. During visual aura, there was a loss of cortical activation to visual stimuli in the occipital lobe contralateral to the visual field in which the scotoma was reported by the patient. As the visual symptoms resolved, cortical activation within the affected occipital lobe returned to normal. In the study of the induced aura, BOLD imaging was initiated after exercise but before the onset of symptoms, was carried out continuously during the visual symptoms, and was continued well into the headache phase after complete resolution of the visual symptoms. With the onset of the aura symptoms, loss of cortical activation to visual stimulation was observed first in V3a, an area of the visual association cortex rather than in the primary visual cortex. Over the next 30 to 40 minutes, the portion of the visual cortex that was unresponsive to visual stimulation expanded to involve the neighboring occipital cortex at a rate of 3.5 mm per minute, eventually encompassing large areas of the ipsilateral primary visual and association cortices. The BOLD functional MRI findings observed during human migraine aura are similar to those that have been seen in CSD induced in animal experiments,[83] indicating that a human process analogous to CSD might be the source of migraine visual aura. The findings from 2 cases of spontaneous migraine visual aura studied with BOLD imaging were the same as those observed during later time points in the exercise-induced aura. Findings from functional MRI carried out in patients experiencing prolonged or persistent aura have been inconsistent.[22,84–86]

Many subsequent imaging studies of migraine pathophysiology have focused on changes in cortical thickness in patients who have migraine with aura compared with patients without aura. Studies about a decade ago reported increased cortical thickness of visual and somatosensory areas in migraine patients compared with healthy controls.[87,88] However, later relatively small studies have shown conflicting results.[89–91] In a recent large study with subjects recruited from the Danish Twin Registry, 166 female patients with migraine with aura were compared with 30 nonaffected co-twins and 137 healthy controls. MRI studies of brain were performed and assessed for cortical thickness in the Brodmann areas of the visual cortex (V1, V2, V3A, and MT) and the somatosensory cortex. They found that, compared with controls, patients with migraine with aura had thicker cortices in areas V2 and V3A, while differences in V1, MT, and somatosensory cortex the remaining areas examined were not statistically significant.[92]

Altered cortical function in migraine with aura

There is accumulating evidence that altered cortical function accounts for differences in patients who experience migraine aura have altered cortical function. Such differences may account for their susceptibility to recurrent episodes of aura. In the 1980s and 1990s, ^{31}P magnetic resonance spectroscopic (MRS) studies suggested altered phosphocreatinine/inorganic phosphate ratios (index of brain phosphorylation potential),[93,94] indicating altered neuronal energy metabolism. Other MRS studies have shown low magnesium levels in the occipital cortex of migraine aura sufferers,[95] suggesting lowered thresholds for induction of a CSD or CSD-like phenomenon via disinhibition of N-methyl-D-aspartate receptor activity.[96] Interestingly, a more recent MRS study of migraine aura revealed that patients who experienced purely visual aura had baseline increased lactate levels, which showed no changed despite prolonged visual stimulation between migraine attacks. Conversely, patients who reported experiencing episodes of visual aura symptoms plus an additional aura type (sensory, language, or motor), had levels of brain lactate which were not increased compared with those in healthy controls, but increased rather sharply with prolonged visual stimulation.[97] The cause(s) of these unexpected findings are not clear.

Electrophysiological studies that have used various evoked potential modalities, have consistently demonstrated a decrease in habituation in the cortex of migraineurs with aura after repeated stimulation compared with normal controls.[98] The most recent of these studies used nociceptive blink reflex responses and showed a deficit in patients with migraine aura, albeit this deficit was less pronounced than that seen in migraine without aura.[99] This altered habituation response has led to the hypothesis that a deficiency in habituation related to abnormal functioning in the subcortico-cortical aminergic pathways is critical in the vulnerability to aura.[100] Other electrophysiological evidence from transcranial magnetic stimulation-based studies also suggests altered cortical excitability in migraineurs who experience aura.[101] Although all of the details of altered cortical processing in patients who experience the aura are not yet available, the body of evidence indicating that such differences exist is growing. There is currently a portable transcranial magnetic stimulation device that has been approved for acute and preventative treatment of migraine, lending credence to this line of research.[102]

Genetic factors

At this point in time, it seems clear that the propensity to experience recurrent episodes of migraine aura are to a large extent genetically determined. Several genetic loci have been linked to typical migraine with aura (**Table 1**). Although the FHM studies are not included in the table, one should remember that patients with FHM may also experience typical auras.

Table 1
Loci with reported association with migraine aura

Chromosome/ Locus	Gene/Protein	Migraine Type	References
1 p36	MTHF-R	MA	Kara et al,[108] 2003; Roecklein et al,[109] 2013
4 q24	?	MA	Wessman et al,[110] 2002
6 p12-p21	?	MA and MO	Carlsson et al,[111] 2002
6 q25.1	Estrogen receptor 1	MA and MO	Colson et al,[112] 2004
9q21-q22	?	MA	Tikka-Kleemola et al,[113] 2010
10q25.3	KCNK18	MA	LaFrenière et al,[114] 2010
11 q22-23	Progesterone receptor	MA and MO	Colson et al,[103] 2005
11 q23	Dopamine D2 (DRD2) Ncol	MA	Peroutka et al,[115] 1998
11 q23	DRD2 Ncol	MA	Peroutka et al, [116] 1997
11 q24	?	MA	Cader et al,[117] 2003
15 q11-q13	?GABA-A	MA	Russo et al,[118] 2005
17 q11.1-q12	Human serotonin transporter (SLC6A4)	MA and MO	Ogilvie et al,[119] 1998

The genetic determinants of migraine aura probably consist of many loci, which, based on the presence of certain polymorphisms, confer greater or lesser susceptibility to aura. Each of these potential "susceptibility genes" individually have a low-to-moderate effect.[103] It is then the vector sum of these effects that determine overall level of susceptibility to aura and many of the clinical features of migraine syndrome in general. It is also possible that, when susceptibility-conferring polymorphisms occur in the same individual, they might act synergistically to produce the migraine phenotype. Such complex genetic interactions will probably be difficult to detect by traditional single-locus linkage analysis.

To address this issue, there have been 3 large genome-wide association studies (GWAS) of migraine.[104–106] The first of these focused on migraine with aura and yielded a single locus associated with migraine with aura at 8q22.1, which was near the MTDH gene.[104]

Based on the sample populations for these studies, large meta-analyses have been published as additional samples were added. The most recent of these was published in August of 2018 and was based on 59,674 migraine cases and 316,078 nonmigraine control subjects from 22 GWAS studies.[107] Because of the large sample number rendered from pooling the subjects from many studies, the meta-analysis identified 38 distinct loci, 28 of which had not been previously reported. However, when subgroup analyses were carried out using stricter requirements for phenotyping to identify subjects as having migraine with aura versus migraine without aura, the sample sizes decreased considerably compared with the main analysis (6332 cases vs. 144,883 controls for migraine with aura and 8348 cases vs. 139,622 controls for migraine without aura). For the migraine without aura subset, 7 of the previously identified genomic loci reached statistical significance. Unfortunately, no loci were associated with migraine with aura in the migraine with aura subset analysis.[107] This indicates that, in migraine with aura, much of the genetic susceptibility may be driven by uncommon or rare variants that are less likely to be identified in GWAS until large numbers of samples from carefully phenotyped subjects with migraine with aura are available.

SUMMARY

Neurologic symptoms that accompany headache in over a quarter of migraine patients are classically transient and were thought to occur as the result of cortical phenomena. The addition of brainstem aura and retinal aura to the ICHD-3 criteria brings more heterogeneity to the presumed localization of aura symptoms. Visual symptoms of typical migraine aura are by far the most common type. The visual aura may include positive and negative symptoms, which occur within the homonymous visual field and characteristically last in the range of 30 minutes. Persistent migraine visual aura is uncommon and may be a distinct entity from primary persistent visual disturbance (visual snow). Transient monocular visual symptoms associated with migraine, now referred to as "retinal migraine," are considered a subtype of migraine. Migraine has rarely been associated with fixed visual loss (most commonly from stroke, ischemic optic neuropathy, or retinal vascular occlusion), but evidence for a cause-and-effect mechanism remains somewhat limited. Other aura symptoms include language disturbance and unilateral sensory symptoms. Because of the early identification of monogenic variation linked to the motor aura, it is now considered an integral part of a distinct migraine subtype known as HM. Although patients with HM also generally experience more typical visual, sensory, and language auras, the motor symptoms are of longer duration, and it is unclear whether they arise from an analogous phenomenon. The occurrence of focal neurologic symptoms that localize to the brainstem is now also considered a separate migraine aura subtype. Data from functional neuroimaging have suggested that the more typical aura symptoms may arise from a CSD-like process. The tendency for aura seems to be influenced by complex genetic factors that thus have been less readily associated with common variants by large GWAS studies than the headache phenotype.

REFERENCES

1. Headache Classification Committee of the International Headache Society (IHS). The International Classification of Headache Disorders, 3rd edition. Cephalalgia 2018;38(1):1–211.
2. Cutrer FM, Huerter K. Migraine aura. Neurologist 2007;13(3):118–25.
3. DeLange JM, Cutrer FM. Our evolving understanding of migraine with aura. Curr Pain Headache Rep 2014;18:453.
4. Russell MB, Olesen J. A nosographic analysis of the migraine aura in a general population. Brain 1996;119:335–61.
5. Russell MB, Iversen HK, Olesen J. Improved description of the migraine aura by a diagnostic aura diary. Cephalalgia 1994;14:107–17.
6. Kirchmann M, Thomsen LL, Olesen J. Basilar-type migraine: clinical, epidemiologic, and genetic features. Neurology 2006;66:880–6.
7. Foroozan R, Cutrer FM. Transient neurologic dysfunction in migraine. Neurol Clin 2009;27:361–78.
8. Tassorelli C, Diener HC, Dodick DW, et al. Guidelines of the International Headache Society for controlled trials of preventative treatment of chronic migraine in adults. Cephalalgia 2018;38:815–32. Changed to ICHD-3.
9. Hansen JM, Goadsby PJ, Charles AC. Variability of clinical features in attacks of migraine with aura. Cephalalgia 2016;36:216–24.
10. Hupp SL, Kline LB, Corbett JJ. Visual disturbances of migraine. Surv Ophthalmol 1989;33:221–36.
11. Leopore FE. Retinal migraine. J Neuroophthalmol 2007;27:242–3 [author reply: 4–5].

12. Hill DL, Daroff RB, Ducros A, et al. Most cases labeled as "retinal migraine" are not migraine. J Neuroophthalmol 2007;27:3–8.

13. Winterkorn JM, Kupersmith MJ, Wirtschafter JD, et al. Brief report: treatment of vasospastic amaurosis fugax with calcium-channel blockers. N Engl J Med 1993;329:396–8.

14. Doyle E, Vote BJ, Casswell AG. Retinal migraine: caught in the act. Br J Ophthalmol 2004;88:301–2.

15. El Youssef N, Maalouf N, Mourad A, et al. Teaching neuroimages: retinal migraine in action. Neurology 2018;90:e992.

16. Abdellatif MK, Fouad MM. Effect of duration and severity of migraine on retinal nerve fiber layer, ganglion cell layer, and choroidal thickness. Eur J Ophthalmol 2018;28:714–21. Accessed January 5, 2019.

17. Reggio E, Chisari CG, Ferrigno G, et al. Migraine causes retinal and choroidal structural changes: evaluation with ocular coherence tomography. J Neurol 2017;264:494–502.

18. Feng YF, Guo H, Huang JH, et al. Retinal nerve fiber layer thickness changes in migraine: a meta-analysis of case-control studies. Curr Eye Res 2016;41: 814–22.

19. Chang MY, Phasukkijwatana N, Garrity S, et al. Foveal and peripapillary vascular decrement in migraine with aura demonstrated by optical coherence tomography angiography. Invest Ophthalmol Vis Sci 2017;58:5477–84.

20. Liu GT, Schatz NJ, Galetta SL, et al. Persistent positive visual phenomena in migraine. Neurology 1995;45:664–8.

21. Available at: https://en.wikipedia.org/wiki/Visual_snow.

22. Jager HR, Giffin NJ, Goadsby PJ. Diffusion- and perfusion-weighted MR imaging in persistent migrainous visual disturbances. Cephalalgia 2005;25:323–32.

23. Schankin CJ, Goadsby PJ. Visual snow–persistent positive visual phenomenon distinct from migraine aura. Curr Pain Headache Rep 2015;19:23.

24. Schankin CJ, Maniyar FH, Digre KB, et al. 'Visual snow' - a disorder distinct from persistent migraine aura. Brain 2014;137:1419–28.

25. Puledda F, Schankin C, Digre K, et al. Visual snow syndrome: what we know so far. Curr Opin Neurol 2018;31:52–8.

26. White OB, Clough M, McKendrick AM, et al. Visual snow: visual misperception. J Neuroophthalmol 2018;38:514–21.

27. Schankin CJ, Maniyar FH, Sprenger T, et al. The relation between migraine, typical migraine aura and "visual snow". Headache 2014;54:957–66.

28. McKendrick AM, Chan YM, Tien M, et al. Behavioral measures of cortical hyperexcitability assessed in people who experience visual snow. Neurology 2017;88: 1243–9.

29. Rothrock JF. Successful treatment of persistent migraine aura with divalproex sodium. Neurology 1997;48:261–2.

30. Chen WT, Fuh JL, Lu SR, et al. Persistent migrainous visual phenomena might be responsive to lamotrigine. Headache 2001;41:823–5.

31. Bou Ghannam A, Pelak VS. Visual snow: a potential cortical hyperexcitability syndrome. Curr Treat Options Neurol 2017;19:9.

32. Lauschke JL, Plant GT, Fraser CL. Visual snow: a thalamocortical dysrhythmia of the visual pathway? J Clin Neurosci 2016;28:123–7.

33. Pelak VS. The Visual Snow Conference: May 5, 2018, University of California San Francisco. J Neuroophthalmol 2018;38:e17–8.

34. Hallett M, Cogan DG. Episodic unilateral mydriasis in otherwise normal patients. Arch Ophthalmol 1970;84:130–6.

35. Woods D, O'Connor PS, Fleming R. Episodic unilateral mydriasis and migraine. Am J Ophthalmol 1984;98:229–34.
36. Yeo DCM, Wijetilleka S, Sharma B, et al. Benign episodic unilateral mydriasis in children: presentation and features in 2 young siblings. Can J Ophthalmol 2018; 53:e255–6.
37. Jacobson DM. Benign episodic unilateral mydriasis. Clinical characteristics. Ophthalmology 1995;102:1623–7.
38. Martin-Santana I, Gonzalez-Hernandez A, Tandon-Cardenes L, et al. Benign episodic mydriasis. Experience in a specialist neuro-ophthalmology clinic of a tertiary hospital. Neurologia 2015;30:290–4.
39. Manai R, Timsit S, Rancurel G. Unilateral benign episodic mydriasis. Rev Neurol (Paris) 1995;151:344–6 [in French].
40. Sarkies NJ, Sanders MD, Gautier-Smith PC. Episodic unilateral mydriasis and migraine. Am J Ophthalmol 1985;99:217–8.
41. Maggioni F, Mainardi F, Malvindi ML, et al. The borderland of migraine with aura: episodic unilateral mydriasis. J Headache Pain 2011;12:105–7.
42. Chamberlain PD, Sadaka A, Berry S, et al. Intermittent mydriasis associated with carotid vascular occlusion. Eye (Lond) 2018;32:457–9.
43. Barriga FJ, Lopez de Silanes C, Gili P, et al. Ciliary ganglioplegic migraine: migraine-related prolonged mydriasis. Cephalalgia 2011;31:291–5.
44. Friedman DI, Gordon LK, Quiros PA. Headache attributable to disorders of the eye. Curr Pain Headache Rep 2010;14:62–72.
45. Fraunfelder FW, Fraunfelder FT, Keates EU. Topiramate-associated acute, bilateral, secondary angle-closure glaucoma. Ophthalmology 2004;111:109–11.
46. Fiore DC, Pasternak AV, Radwan RM. Pain in the quiet (not red) eye. Am Fam Physician 2010;82:69–73.
47. Digre KB. More than meets the eye: the eye and migraine - what you need to know. J Neuroophthalmol 2018;38:237–43.
48. Bowen RC, Koeppel JN, Christensen CD, et al. The most common causes of eye pain at 2 tertiary ophthalmology and neurology clinics. J Neuroophthalmol 2018; 38:320–7.
49. Koktekir BE, Celik G, Karalezli A, et al. Dry eyes and migraines: is there really a correlation? Cornea 2012;31:1414–6.
50. Sarac O, Kosekahya P, Yildiz Tasci Y, et al. The prevalence of dry eye and Sjogren syndrome in patients with migraine. Ocul Immunol Inflamm 2017;25:370–5.
51. Shetty R, Deshpande K, Jayadev C, et al. The impact of dysfunctional tear films and optical aberrations on chronic migraine. Eye Vis (Lond) 2017;4:4.
52. Diel RJ, Hwang J, Kroeger ZA, et al. Photophobia and sensations of dryness in patients with migraine occur independent of baseline tear volume and improve following botulinum toxin A injections. Br J Ophthalmol 2018. https://doi.org/10.1136/bjophthalmol-2018-312649.
53. Kinard KI, Smith AG, Singleton JR, et al. Chronic migraine is associated with reduced corneal nerve fiber density and symptoms of dry eye. Headache 2015;55:543–9.
54. Shetty R, Deshmukh R, Shroff R, et al. Subbasal nerve plexus changes in chronic migraine. Cornea 2018;37:72–5.
55. Aykut V, Elbay A, Esen F, et al. Patterns of altered corneal sensation in patients with chronic migraine. Eye Contact Lens 2018;44(Suppl 2):S400–3.
56. Fernandez-de-Las-Penas C, Cuadrado ML, Gerwin RD, et al. Myofascial disorders in the trochlear region in unilateral migraine: a possible initiating or perpetuating factor. Clin J Pain 2006;22:548–53.

57. Yanguela J, Sanchez-del-Rio M, Bueno A, et al. Primary trochlear headache: a new cephalgia generated and modulated on the trochlear region. Neurology 2004;62:1134–40.
58. Pareja JA, Sanchez del Rio M. Primary trochlear headache and other trochlear painful disorders. Curr Pain Headache Rep 2006;10:316–20.
59. Smith JH, Garrity JA, Boes CJ. Clinical features and long-term prognosis of trochlear headaches. Eur J Neurol 2014;21:577–85.
60. Lord GDA. Clinical characteristics of the migrainous aura. In: Amery WK, Wauquier A, editors. The prelude to the migraine attack. London: Baillière Tindall; 1986. p. 87–98.
61. Kurth T, Schurks M, Logroscino G, et al. Migraine, vascular risk, and cardiovascular events in women: prospective cohort study. BMJ 2008;337:a636.
62. Fisher CM. Late-life migraine accompaniments: further experience. Stroke 1986; 17:1033–42.
63. Bradshaw P, Parsons M. Hemiplegic migraine, a clinical study. Q J Med 1965; 34:65–85.
64. Vincent MB, Hadjikhani N. Migraine aura and related phenomena: beyond scotomata and scintillations. Cephalalgia 2007;27(12):1368–77.
65. Schwedt TJ, Zhou J, Dodick DW. Sporadic hemiplegic migraine with permanent neurological defecits. Headache 2014;54:163–6.
66. Oberndorfer S, Wober C, Nasel C, et al. Familial hemiplegic migraine: follow-up findings of diffusion-weighted magnetic resonance imaging (MRI), perfusion-MRI and [99mTc] HMPAO-SPECT in a patient with prolonged hemiplegic aura. Cephalalgia 2004;24:533–9.
67. Ophoff RA, Terwindt GM, Vergouwe MN, et al. Familial hemiplegic migraine and episodic ataxia type-2 are caused by mutations in the Ca^{2+} channel gene CACNL1A4. Cell 1996;87:543–52.
68. Ducros A, Joutel A, Vahedi K, et al. Mapping of a second locus for familial hemiplegic migraine to 1q21-q23 and evidence of further heterogeneity. Ann Neurol 1997;42:885–90.
69. Dichigans M, Freilinger T, Eckstein G, et al. Mutation in the neuronal voltage-gated sodium channel SCN1A in familial hemiplegic migraine. Lancet 2005; 366:371–7.
70. deVries B, Freilinger T, Vanmolkot KR, et al. Systematic analysis of three FHM genes in 39 sporadic patients with hemiplegic migraine. Neurology 2007;69: 2170–6.
71. Riant F, Ducros A, Ploton C, et al. De novo mutations in APT1A2 and CACNA1A are frequent in early-onset sporadic hemiplegic migraine. Neurology 2010;75: 967–72.
72. Moskowitz MA, Bolay H, Dalkara T. Deciphering migraine mechanisms: clues from familial hemiplegic migraine genotypes. Ann Neurol 2004;55:276–80.
73. deVries B, Frants RR, Ferrari MD, et al. Molecular genetics of migraine. Hum Genet 2009;126:115–32.
74. Sturzenegger MH, Meienberg O. Basilar artery migraine: a follow-up study of 82 cases. Headache 1985;25:408–15.
75. Bickerstaff ER. Basilar artery migraine. Lancet 1961;i:15–7.
76. Wolf ME, Okazaki S, Eisele P, et al. Arterial spin labeling cerebral perfusion magnetic resonance imaging in migraine aura: an observational study. J Stroke Cerebrovasc Dis 2018;27(5):1262–6.
77. Leao AAP. Spreading depression of activity in the cerebral cortex. J Neurophysiol 1944;7:359–90.

78. Olesen J, Larsen B, Lauritzen M. Focal hyperemia followed by spreading oligemia and impaired activation of rCBF in classic migraine. Ann Neurol 1981;9:
344–52.

79. Lauritzen M, Skyhoj Olsen T, Lassen NA, et al. Changes of regional cerebral
blood flow during the course of classical migraine attacks. Ann Neurol 1983;
13:633–41.

80. Woods RP, Iacoboni M, Mazziotta JC. Bilateral spreading cerebral hypoperfusion during spontaneous migraine headache. N Engl J Med 1994;331:1689–92.

81. Sorensen AG, Rosen BR. Functional MRI of the brain. In: Atlas S, editor.
Magnetic resonance imaging of the brain and spine. 2nd edition. Philadelphia:
Lippincott-Raven Publishers; 1996.

82. Hadjikhani N, Sanchez Del Rio M, Wu O, et al. Mechanisms of migraine aura
revealed by functional MRI in human visual cortex. Proc Natl Acad Sci U S A
2001;98(8):4687–92.

83. James MF, Smith MI, Bockhorst KH, et al. Cortical spreading depression in gyrencephalic feline brain studied by magnetic resonance imaging. J Physiol 1999;
519 Pt 2:415–25.

84. Smith M, Cros D, Sheen V. Hyperfusion with vasogenic leakage by fMRI in
migraine with prolonged aura. Neurology 2002;58(8):1308–10.

85. Gekeler F, Holtmannspotter M, Straube A, et al. Diffusion-weighted magnetic
resonance imaging during the aura of pseudomigraine with temporary neurologic symptoms and lymphocytic pleocytosis. Headache 2002;42(4):294–6.

86. Relja G, Granato A, Ukmar M, et al. Persistent aura without infarction: description of the first case studied with both brain SPECT and perfusion MRI. Cephalalgia 2005;25(1):56–9.

87. Granziera C, DaSilva AFM, Snyder J, et al. Anatomical alterations of the visual
motion processing network in migraine with and without aura. PLoS Med
2006;3:e402.

88. DaSilva AFM, Granziera C, Snyder J, et al. Thickening in the somatosensory cortex of patients with migraine. Neurology 2007;69:1990–5.

89. Datta R, Detre JA, Aguirre GK, et al. Absence of changes in cortical thickness in
patients with migraine. Cephalalgia 2011;31:1452–8.

90. Messina R, Rocca MA, Colombo B, et al. Cortical abnormalities in patients with
migraine: a surface based analysis. Radiology 2013;268:170–80.

91. Hougaard A, Amin FM, Amgrim N, et al. Sensory migraine aura is not associated
with structural gray matter abnormalities. Neuroimage Clin 2016;11:322–7.

92. Gaist D, Hougaard A, Garde E, et al. Migraine with visual aura associated with
thicker visual cortex. Brain 2018;141:776–85.

93. Welch KMA, Levine SR, D'Andrea G, et al. Brain pH during migraine studied by
in-vivo 31-phosphorus NMR spectroscopy. Cephalalgia 1988;8:273–7.

94. Welch KMA, Levine SR, D'Andrea G, et al. Preliminary observations on brain
energy metabolites in migraine studied by in vivo 31-phosphorus NMR spectroscopy. Neurology 1989;39:538–41.

95. Welch KMA, Barkley GL, Ramadan NM, et al. NMR spectroscopic and magneto-
encephalographic studies in migraine with aura: support for the spreading
depression hypothesis. Pathol Biol (Paris) 1992;40(4):349–54.

96. van Harreveld A, Fifekova E. Mechanisms involved in spreading depression.
J Neurobiol 1973;4:375–87.

97. Sandor PS, Dydak U, Schoenen J, et al. MR-spectroscopic imaging during
visual stimulation in subgroups of migraine with aura. Cephalalgia 2005;25(7):
507–18.

98. Strigaro G, Cerino A, Falletta L, et al. Impaired visual inhibition in migraine with aura. Clin Neurophysiol 2015;126(10):1988–93.

99. Perrotta A, Anastasio MG, De Icco R, et al. Frequency-dependent habituation deficit of the nociceptive blink reflex in aura with migraine headache. Can migraine aura modulate trigeminal excitability? Headache 2017;57(6):887–98.

100. Schoenen J, Ambrosini A, Sándor PS, et al. Evoked potentials and transcranial magnetic stimulation in migraine: published data and viewpoint on their pathophysiologic significance. Clin Neurophysiol 2003;114(6):955–72.

101. Aurora SK, Welch KM, Al-Sayed F. The threshold for phosphenes is lower in migraine. Cephalalgia 2003;23(4):258–63.

102. McComas AJ, Upton ARM. Transcranial magnetic stimulation in migraine: a new therapy and new insights into pathogenesis. Crit Rev Biomed Eng 2016;44(5): 319–26.

103. Colson N, Lea R, Quinlan S, et al. Investigation of hormone receptor genes in migraine. Neurogenetics 2005;6:17–23.

104. Anttila V, Stefansson H, Kallela M, et al. Genome-wide association study of migraine implicates a common susceptibility variant on 8q22.1. Nat Genet 2010;42:869–73.

105. Chasman DI, Schurks M, Anttila V, et al. Genome-wide association study reveals three susceptibility loci for common migraine in the general population. Nat Genet 2011;43:695–8.

106. Freilinger T, Anttila V, de Vries B, et al. Genome-wide association analysis identifies susceptibility loci for migraine without aura. Nat Genet 2012;44:777–82.

107. Gormley P, Anttila V, Winsvold BS, et al. Meta-analysis of 375,000 individuals identifies 38 susceptibility loci for migraine. Nat Genet 2016;48(8):856–66.

108. Kara I, Sazci A, Ergul E, et al. Association of the C677T and A1298C polymorphisms in the 5,10 methylenetetrahydrofolate reductase gene in patients with migraine risk. Brain Res Mol Brain Res 2003;111:84–90.

109. Roecklein KA, Scher AI, Smith A, et al. Haplotype analysis of the folate-related genes MTHFR, MTRR, and MTR and migraine with aura. Cephalalgia 2013; 33(7):469–82.

110. Wessman M, Kallela M, Kaunisto MA, et al. A susceptibility locus for migraine with aura, on chromosome 4q24. J Hum Genet 2002;70:652–62.

111. Carlsson A, Forsgren L, Nylander PO, et al. Identification of a susceptibility locus for migraine with and without aura on 6p12.2-p21.1. Neurology 2002;59: 1804–7.

112. Colson NJ, Lea RA, Quinlan S, et al. The estrogen receptor 1 G594A polymorphism is associated with migraine susceptibility in two independent case/control groups. Neurogenetics 2004;5:129–33.

113. Tikka-Kleemola P, Artto V, Vepsäläinen S, et al. A visual migraine aura locus maps to 9q21-q22. Neurology 2010;74:1171–7.

114. Lafrenière RG, Cader MZ, Poulin JF, et al. A dominant-negative mutation in the TRESK potassium channel is linked to familial migraine with aura. Nat Med 2010; 16:1157–60.

115. Peroutka SJ, Price SC, Wilhoit TL, et al. Comorbid migraine with aura, anxiety, and depression is associated with dopamine D2 receptor (DRD2) NcoI alleles. Mol Med 1998;4(1):14–21.

116. Peroutka SJ, Wilhoit T, Jones K. Clinical susceptibility to migraine with aura is modified by dopamine D2 receptor (DRD2) NcoI alleles. Neurology 1997; 49(1):201–6.

117. Cader ZM, Noble-Topham S, Dyment DA, et al. Significant linkage to migraine with aura on chromosome 11q24. Hum Mol Genet 2003;12:2511–7.
118. Russo L, Mariotti P, Sangiorgi E, et al. A new susceptibility locus for migraine with aura in the 15q11-q13 genomic region containing three GABA-A receptor genes. Am J Hum Genet 2005;76:327–33.
119. Ogilvie AD, Russell MB, Dhall P, et al. Altered allelic distributions of the serotonin transporter gene in migraine without aura and migraine with aura. Cephalalgia 1998;18(1):23–6.

Vestibular Migraine

Thomas Lempert, MD[a],*, Michael von Brevern, MD, PhD[b]

KEYWORDS

- Migraine • Vestibular • Vestibular migraine • Vertigo • Dizziness

KEY POINTS

- Vestibular migraine is recognized as one of the most common causes of recurrent vertigo.
- Vestibular migraine manifests with spontaneous or positional vertigo, with head motion intolerance, visually induced dizziness, and dizziness with nausea.
- A history of migraine and migraine symptoms during the attacks provides the key to diagnosis.
- Vestibular testing shows mostly mild abnormalities and serves to exclude other causes of vertigo.
- Treatment is currently based on scarce evidence and includes explanation and reassurance, lifestyle changes, and prophylactic antimigraine drugs.

INTRODUCTION

That migraine may present with attacks of vertigo has been recognized since the early days of neurology.[1] The clinical features of vestibular migraine (VM) have been well elucidated in several large case series.[2–7] The interest in VM surged in the last 2 decades with 90% of PubMed-listed articles appearing after the turn of the century. In 2012, the International Headache Society and the Bárány Society representing the international neurootological community published a first consensus on diagnostic criteria for VM.[8]

EPIDEMIOLOGY

The lifetime prevalence of VM has been estimated at 1% in a population-based study.[9] Another population-based study reported a much higher figure, namely a 1-year prevalence of 2.7%.[10] In patients with recurrent vertigo of unknown origin, the prevalence of migraine ranges from 60% to 80%.[11] In contrast, VM occurs in 10% to 20% of patients presenting to headache clinics.[12,13]

Disclosure: The authors have no conflict of interest relating to this article.
[a] Department of Neurology, Schlosspark-Klinik, Heubnerweg 2, Berlin 14059, Germany;
[b] Neurologisches Zentrum, Clayallee 177, Berlin 14195, Germany
* Corresponding author.
E-mail address: thomas.lempert@schlosspark-klinik.de

Neurol Clin 37 (2019) 695–706
https://doi.org/10.1016/j.ncl.2019.06.003
0733-8619/19/© 2019 Elsevier Inc. All rights reserved.

neurologic.theclinics.com

CLINICAL FEATURES

The diagnosis of VM is based on recurrent vestibular symptoms, migraine history, temporal association of vertigo with migraine symptoms, and exclusion of other causes[8,14] (**Box 1**).

VM presents with various types of vertigo, including spontaneous vertigo, positional vertigo, visually induced vertigo, head motion–induced vertigo, and head motion–induced dizziness with nausea. Some patients experience a sequence of spontaneous vertigo transforming into positional or head motion–induced vertigo after several hours or days. Positional vertigo can be transient or persistent as long as the critical head position is maintained.[7,15] Altogether, 40% to 70% of patients experience positional vertigo in the course of the disease, but not necessarily with every attack.[2,16] Head motion–induced vertigo presents with imbalance, illusory motion, and nausea aggravated or provoked by head movements.[4] A persistent susceptibility to motion sickness is common in patients with VM.[17] Visually induced vertigo (ie, vertigo provoked by moving visual scenes, such as traffic or movies) can be another prominent feature of VM and may persist to some degree in between attacks.[4]

Nausea and imbalance are frequent but nonspecific accompaniments of acute VM. Attacks of VM may be severe enough to force patients to stay in bed for a day or two, where they lie still, avoiding the slightest head movement.

Many patients experience attacks both with and without headache.[3,5] Frequently, patients have an attenuated headache with their vertigo compared with the usual migraine. In some patients, vertigo and headache never occur together.[3,6] Along with the vertigo, patients may experience photophobia, phonophobia, osmophobia, and visual or other auras.[7] These phenomena are of diagnostic importance because they may represent the only apparent connection of vertigo and migraine. Patients need to be asked specifically about these migraine symptoms because they often do not volunteer them.

Auditory symptoms, including hearing loss, tinnitus, and aural pressure, related to acute attacks have been reported in 20% to 40% patients with VM.[7,18,19] Hearing loss is usually mild and transient, without or with only minor progression in the course

---

Box 1
Diagnostic criteria for vestibular migraine

Vestibular migraine
1. At least 5 episodes with vestibular symptoms of moderate or severe intensity, lasting 5 minutes to 72 hours
2. Current or previous history of migraine with or without aura according to the International Classification of Headache Disorders (ICHD-3)
3. One or more migraine features with at least 50% of the vestibular episodes:
   • Headache with at least 2 of the following characteristics: 1-sided location, pulsating quality, moderate or severe pain intensity, aggravation by routine physical activity
   • Photophobia and phonophobia
   • Visual aura
4. Not better accounted for by another vestibular or ICHD diagnosis

Probable vestibular migraine (not included in ICHD-3)
1. At least 5 episodes with vestibular symptoms of moderate or severe intensity, lasting 5 minutes to 72 hours
2. Only 1 of the criteria B and C for vestibular migraine is fulfilled (migraine history or migraine features during the episode)
3. Not better accounted for by another vestibular or ICHD diagnosis

of the disease. About 20% develop mild bilateral downsloping sensorineural hearing loss over the years.[20]

Duration of episodes is highly variable: about 30% of patients have episodes lasting minutes, 30% have attacks for hours, and another 25% have attacks over several days. The remaining 15% have attacks lasting seconds only, which tend to occur repeatedly during head motion, visual stimulation, or after changes of head position. In these patients, episode duration is defined as the total period during which short attacks recur. At the other end of the spectrum, there are patients who may take 4 weeks to fully recover from an episode. However, the core episode rarely exceeds 72 hours.[3–7] Asking for migraine-specific precipitants of vertigo attacks may provide valuable diagnostic information; for example, provocation by menstruation, deficient sleep, excessive stress, specific foods, and sensory stimuli (eg, bright or scintillating lights, intense smells, or noise).

CLINICAL FINDINGS

In most patients, the general neurologic and otologic examination is normal in the symptom-free interval. Neuroophthalmologic evaluation may reveal mild central deficits such as persistent positional nystagmus and saccadic pursuit, particularly in patients with a long history of VM.[20,21]

During the acute phase of VM, most patients have a central spontaneous nystagmus, central positional nystagmus, or a combination of the two.[16,22] Positional nystagmus is usually persistent and often horizontal, beating either toward the lower ear (geotropic nystagmus) or toward the upper ear (apogeotropic nystagmus).[22,23] Occasional patients have a peripheral type of spontaneous nystagmus and a unilateral deficit of the horizontal vestibulo-ocular reflex.[16] Imbalance is a regular finding during acute attacks, whereas transient mild to moderate hearing loss is less common.[16]

VESTIBULAR TESTING

There is no specific testing abnormality in VM, neither in the acute episode nor in the interval. However, laboratory testing can be useful to exclude other diseases and to reassure patients. For correct interpretation of testing results, it should be taken into account that minor signs of peripheral and central vestibular dysfunction are common in patients with VM in the symptom-free interval.[20,21]

The most consistent laboratory finding in VM is a unilaterally reduced caloric response. In most studies about 10% to 20% of patients with VM showed a unilateral canal paresis.[5,24] Caloric asymmetry is usually mild but in 2 studies about a quarter of patients with a canal paresis had an asymmetry of more than 50%.[20,25] Bilateral caloric hyporesponsiveness has been reported in up to 11% of patients with VM.[2] Of note, patients with VM are 4 times more likely to have an emetic response to caloric stimulation than patients with a vestibular disorder coexisting with migraine.[26]

A pathologic head impulse test as assessed by bedside-testing is a rare finding in VM.[18,20,27] Video head impulse testing shows a mildly reduced unilateral gain in 9% to 11% of patients with VM.[24,25,27] The video head impulse test is less sensitive for detection of a vestibular deficit in VM than caloric irrigation.[24,25]

Assessment of cervical vestibular-evoked myogenic potential (cVEMP) and ocular vestibular-evoked myogenic potential (oVEMP) in patients with VM has yielded conflicting results. Most studies have described either unilaterally or bilaterally reduced amplitudes compared with healthy controls in about two-thirds of patients with VM, indicating saccular and utricular dysfunction.[28–30] Other studies involving cVEMP and oVEMP found no differences between patients with VM and controls.[31,32]

Abnormal oVEMP seems to be more prevalent than abnormal cVEMP in VM.[33,34] The latencies of the response were normal in most studies.[28,29,35] Some studies reported differences of various parameters in cVEMP and oVEMP between patients with VM and Ménière's disease,[29–32] but these results are conflicting and await conformation.

Abnormal vestibular testing results are also found in patients with migraine without a history of vestibular symptoms. Unilateral caloric hyporesponsiveness occurs with similar frequency in patients with migraine with and without vertigo.[36,37] Likewise, a study comparing cVEMPs between groups of migraineurs with and without vertigo found no difference in amplitudes.[38]

PATHOPHYSIOLOGY

The cause of VM is still a matter of speculation. Genetic, neurochemical, and inflammatory mechanisms have been proposed, and all of them are derived from the presumed pathophysiology of migraine.[39] Migraine is currently conceptualized as a neurogenic disorder in genetically susceptible individuals, probably resulting from dysfunctions of brainstem and diencephalic nuclei that activate sensory nerve endings around the extracranial and intracranial arteries of the head.[40]

A strong genetic component in VM can be assumed, similar to common forms of migraine that have a polygenic basis, with at least 47 loci affecting the susceptibility.[41] A family history of migraine was reported by 70% and a family history of vertigo by 66% of the patients in a large prospective series.[7] The locus of familial VM has been linked to chromosomes 22q12 and 5q35, but no specific genetic defect has been identified.[42,43]

The variability of symptoms and clinical findings during and in between attacks suggests that migraine may interact both with the peripheral and the central vestibular systems. Spreading depression of the cerebral cortex, the presumed mechanism of the migraine aura, may play a role in patients with short attacks.[3] Spreading depression may produce vestibular symptoms when the multisensory cortical areas processing vestibular information become involved, which are mainly located in the temporoparietal junction. However, several features of VM, such as complex nystagmus pattern and interictal peripheral vestibular dysfunction, cannot be explained by cortical spreading depression.

Most of the neurotransmitters that are involved in the pathogenesis of migraine, such as calcitonin gene–related peptide, serotonin, noradrenaline, and dopamine, are also known to modulate the activity of central and peripheral vestibular neurons and could contribute to the pathogenesis of VM. It has been speculated that unilateral release of these substances causes a static vestibular imbalance leading to vertigo, whereas bilateral release induces a state of altered vestibular excitability causing a motion sickness type of dizziness.[3,4,44]

The key mechanism of headache in migraine is sterile inflammation of intracranial vessels. In mice, electrical stimulation of the trigeminal nerve and intravenous administration of serotonin causes plasma extravasation in the inner ear.[45,46] This mechanism may explain vestibular and cochlear symptoms caused by dysfunction of the inner ear in migraine. The observation that painful trigeminal stimulation can evoke nystagmus in patients with migraine, but not in patients without a history of migraine, points to a low threshold activation of the connections between the trigeminal and vestibular systems in migraine.[47]

Another candidate mechanism for VM is a dysfunction of ion channels expressed in the inner ear or in central vestibular structures. This hypothesis seems to be promising because rare paroxysmal disorders presenting with migraine and vertigo, such as familial hemiplegic migraine and episodic ataxia type 2, have been found to result from dysfunction of a voltage-gated calcium channel encoded by the CACNA1A gene. However, no such genetic defect has yet been identified in VM.[48,49]

Endolymphatic hydrops of the cochlea was identified by gadolinium-enhanced MRI in 6 out of 7 patients and in 3 out of 30 patients with VM.[50,51] It remains unclear whether these patients were misdiagnosed and have a variant of Ménière's disease or whether VM can be associated with hydrops.

Recently, cerebral imaging studies have been performed in patients with VM. Examination of 2 patients with VM during an attack with fluorodeoxyglucose PET has yielded increased metabolism of temporoparietoinsular areas and of both thalami, indicating activation of vestibulothalamocortical pathways.[52] Voxel-based morphometry has yielded conflicting results, with gray matter volume reduction of temporal and occipital lobes in 1 study and volume increase of these structures in another study.[53,54] Functional imaging with functional MRI during caloric irrigation has shown increased thalamic activation in patients with VM compared with patients with migraine and healthy individuals.[55] Although these findings may indicate the involvement of supratentorial vestibular structures in VM, the origin of vestibular dysfunction remains to be elucidated.

DIFFERENTIAL DIAGNOSIS

VM must be differentiated from other vestibular and nonvestibular disorders presenting with dizziness and vertigo. Distinction is mostly based on accompanying symptoms, temporal evolution, and precipitating factors (**Table 1**).

Ménière's Disease

The most challenging differential diagnosis of VM is Ménière's disease, particularly in the early course when permanent hearing loss may not yet be detectable. By definition, Ménière's disease presents with vertigo attacks lasting between 20 minutes and 12 hours, but attacks of shorter duration may also occur.[56] Cochlear symptoms, including hearing loss, tinnitus, and aural fullness, are required for the diagnosis. In the early stage of the disease these symptoms are often transient and become permanent later. Both hearing loss and tinnitus preferentially affect the low-frequency range. Hearing loss, tinnitus, and aural fullness may also occur in VM but hearing loss remains mild in the course of the disease.[7,20] Furthermore, when hearing loss develops in VM, it is typically bilateral, whereas involvement of both ears from the onset is very rare in patients with Ménière's disease.[57] The differentiation between the two disorders is complicated by the observation that migraine is more common in patients with Ménière's disease than in healthy controls.[58] Furthermore, migraine symptoms such as headache and photophobia are also frequent accompaniments in attacks of Ménière's disease.[58–60] There are patients fulfilling diagnostic criteria of both Ménière's disease and VM.[18,58,61]

Benign Paroxysmal Positional Vertigo

VM may present with positional vertigo, mimicking benign paroxysmal positional vertigo (BPPV). For differentiation, observation of nystagmus during the acute phase may be required. In VM, positional nystagmus is of a central type and differs from nystagmus patterns described in BPPV: usually it has no latency and beats persistently in a direction not aligned with a single semicircular canal. Symptomatic episodes tend to be shorter with VM (minutes to days rather than weeks) and more frequent (several times per year with VM rather than once every few years with BPPV).[15]

Table 1
Differential diagnosis of vestibular migraine

Disorder	Key Features
BPPV	Vertigo lasting seconds to 1 min provoked by changes in head position. Positive positional test with typical positional nystagmus (beating most often in a torsional-vertical plane)
Ménière's disease	Spontaneous vertigo lasting 20 min to 12 h with concurrent hearing loss, tinnitus, and aural fullness. Progressive hearing loss over years starting in 1 ear
Vertebrobasilar TIA	Acute attacks lasting mostly minutes, with brainstem symptoms including vertigo, ataxia, dysarthria, diplopia, or visual field defects (but isolated vertigo may also occur). Often associated with craniocervical pain. Usually elderly patients with vascular risk factors
Vascular compression of the eighth nerve	Brief attacks of vertigo (seconds) several times per day with or without cochlear symptoms, typically responsive to carbamazepine
Autoimmune inner ear disease	Frequent attacks of variable duration, often bilateral with rapidly progressing hearing loss
Insufficient compensation of unilateral vestibular loss	Brief and mild spells of vertigo during rapid head movements, oscillopsia with head turns to affected ear. Positive head impulse test to affected side
Schwannoma of the eighth nerve	Rarely presents with (mild) attacks of vertigo. Key symptoms are slowly progressive unilateral hearing loss and tinnitus. Abnormal BAER
Anxiety disorder	Provocation or exacerbation in specific situations (leaving the house, public transport, supermarket), avoidance behavior, often prominent fear of falling

Abbreviations: BAER, brainstem auditory evoked response; BPPV, benign paroxysmal positional vertigo; TIA, transient ischemic attack.

Transient Ischemic Attacks

Vertebrobasilar transient ischemic attacks (TIAs) must be considered in patients with spontaneous transient vertigo, even if accompanying brainstem symptoms are absent. Vertebrobasilar TIAs are often associated with occipital headache and may thus mimic VM.[62] Suggestive features include onset after the age of 60 years, a total history of attacks lasting less than a few months, vascular risk factors, sudden onset of symptoms, and evidence for vascular disorder in the vertebral or proximal basilar artery.

Psychiatric Dizziness Syndromes

Anxiety and depression may cause dizziness and likewise complicate a vestibular disorder. About 50% of patients with VM have comorbid psychiatric disorders.[63,64] Besides vestibular episodes, about one-third of patients with VM have persistent postural-perceptual dizziness.[18] Anxiety-related dizziness is characterized by situational worsening, autonomic activation, catastrophic thinking, and avoidance behavior and is not accompanied by severe nausea, vomiting, external vertigo (seeing the world move), or falls.

TREATMENT

Current treatment recommendations are based on observational studies, anecdotal experience, and expert opinion. However, well-conducted randomized clinical trials are lacking.[65] For acute and prolonged attacks, antiemetic drugs such as dimenhydrinate or benzodiazepines may be helpful to alleviate vertigo and nausea. There is only anecdotal evidence that triptans may be effective in acute VM. One small controlled study on zolmitriptan for acute VM was inconclusive.[66] Intravenous methylprednisolone (1000 mg/d for 1–3 days) terminated prolonged attacks or exacerbations with daily recurrences in a small clinical series of 4 patients.[67]

Prophylactic treatment is indicated when attacks of VM are frequent and severe (Table 2). A review identified 8 observational studies that showed marginal benefit with migraine prophylactic medications, which is difficult to distinguish from spontaneous improvement in the absence of control groups.[68] There is limited evidence for prophylactic treatment from an unblinded randomized trial using 10 mg of flunarizine (not marketed in the United States), which showed a significant decrease in frequency and severity of attacks compared with a control group receiving no preventive drug.[69] Beyond common migraine prophylactic agents, acetazolamide and lamotrigine may be effective.[70,71] There is no evidence that any prophylactic drug is more effective than others.[72] A drug is chosen primarily by comorbid conditions and expected side effects. In general, the medication is started at a low dose and then increased slowly. Patients should monitor frequency and severity of their attacks in a diary. It is essential to evaluate treatment response after 2 to 3 months. A 50% reduction in attack frequency is a realistic goal. A prophylactic drug that does not show efficacy in an individual patient should be stopped and replaced by another agent. There is no consensus on the duration of prophylactic drug treatment. If VM is well controlled for at least 6 months, medication can be slowly tapered and, if possible, discontinued.

Nonpharmaceutical treatment should not be neglected and may be even more effective than drugs in individual patients. A thorough explanation of the migraine origin of the attacks is important to relieve health fears and provide a foundation for self-management. Lifestyle modification (eg, avoidance of identified triggers, regular sleep schedules, adequate sleep, and regular meals) has a firm place in

Table 2
Prophylactic treatment of vestibular migraine (in the absence of firm evidence)

Drug	Daily Dose (mg)	Common Side Effects
Propranolol[77]	40–240	Fatigue, hypotension, impotence, depression, bronchial constriction
Metoprolol[78]	50–200	Fatigue, hypotension, impotence, depression, bronchial constriction
Topiramate[79]	50–100	Paresthesia, somnolence, weight loss, cognitive dysfunction
Valproic acid[78]	600–900	Weight gain, sedation, fetal malformation
Flunarizine[69]	5–10	Weight gain, sedation, depression
Amitriptylin[80]	50–100	Sedation, orthostatic hypotension, dry mouth, weight gain, constipation, urinary retention, conduction block
Pizotifen[81]	1.5–6	Weight gain, sedation
Acetazolamide[70]	250–750	Paresthesia, nausea, sedation, hypokalemia

migraine prophylaxis. There is evidence that migraine headaches can be reduced by aerobic exercise, and the efficacy is probably equal to prophylactic medication.[73] Likewise, regular exercise seems to reduce intensity and frequency of VM.[74] Selected patients, particularly those with chronic dizziness and imbalance, may profit from vestibular rehabilitation.[75] For patients with occasional and less severe attacks, explanation and reassurance may be sufficient to cope with the symptoms.

PROGNOSIS

A follow-up study 9 years after initial diagnosis found that almost 90% of patients were still symptomatic with recurrent vertigo but frequency of attacks was reduced in 56%.[20] Mild persistent unsteadiness developed in 18% of patients. Both cochlear symptoms during attacks (49%) and mild bilateral sensorineural hearing loss with a downsloping pattern on audiometry (18%) were more common on follow-up than at initial presentation. Rarely, bilateral vestibulopathy may develop in the course of VM.[76]

REFERENCES

1. Liveing E. On megrim: sick headache and some allied health disorders: a contribution to the pathology of nerve storms. London: Churchill; 1873. p. 129–48.
2. Kayan A, Hood JD. Neuro-otological manifestations of migraine. Brain 1984;107: 1123–42.
3. Cutrer FM, Baloh RW. Migraine-associated dizziness. Headache 1992;32:300–4.
4. Cass SP, Furman JM, Ankerstjerne JK, et al. Migraine-related vestibulopathy. Ann Otol Rhinol Laryngol 1997;106:182–9.
5. Dieterich M, Brandt T. Episodic vertigo related to migraine (90 cases): vestibular migraine. J Neurol 1999;246:883–92.
6. Neuhauser H, Leopold M, von Brevern M, et al. The interrelations of migraine, vertigo, and migrainous vertigo. Neurology 2001;56:436–41.
7. Teggi R, Colombo R, Albera R, et al. Clinical features, familial history and migraine precursors in patients with definite vestibular migraine: The VM phenotypes projects. Headache 2018;58:534–44.
8. Lempert T, Olesen J, Furman J, et al. Vestibular migraine: diagnostic criteria. J Vestib Res 2012;22:167–72.
9. Neuhauser HK, Radtke A, von Brevern M, et al. Migrainous vertigo: prevalence and impact on quality of life. Neurology 2006;67:1028–33.
10. Formeister EJ, Rizk HG, Kohn MA, et al. The epidemiology of vestibular migraine: a population-based survey study. Otol Neurotol 2018;39:1037–44.
11. Cha YH, Lee H, Santell LS, et al. Association of benign recurrent vertigo and migraine in 208 patients. Cephalalgia 2009;29:550–5.
12. Cho SJ, Kim BK, Kim BS, et al. Vestibular migraine in multicenter neurology clinics according to the appendix criteria in the third beta edition of the international classification of headache disorders. Cephalalgia 2016;36:454–62.
13. Yollu U, Uluduz DU, Yilmaz M, et al. Vestibular migraine screening in a migraine-diagnosed patient population, and assessment of vestibulocochlear function. Clin Otolaryngol 2017;42:225–33.
14. Headache Classification Committee of the International Headache Society (IHS). The international classification of headache disorders, 3rd edition. Available at: https://www.ichd-3.org/. Accessed January 8, 2019.
15. von Brevern M, Radtke A, Clarke AH, et al. Migrainous vertigo presenting as episodic positional vertigo. Neurology 2004;62:469–72.

16. von Brevern M, Zeise D, Neuhauser H, et al. Acute migrainous vertigo: clinical and oculographic findings. Brain 2005;128:365–74.
17. Murdin L, Chamberlain F, Cheema S, et al. Motion sickness in migraine and vestibular disorders. J Neurol Neurosurg Psychiatry 2015;86:585–7.
18. Neff BA, Staab JP, Eggers SD, et al. Auditory and vestibular symptoms and chronic subjective dizziness in patients with Ménière's disease, vestibular migraine, and Ménière's disease with concomitant vestibular migraine. Otol Neurotol 2012;33:1235–44.
19. Tabet P, Saliba I. Meniere's disease and vestibular migraine: updates and review of the literature. J Clin Med Res 2017;9:733–44.
20. Radtke A, von Brevern M, Neuhauser H, et al. Vestibular migraine: long-term follow-up of clinical symptoms and vestibulo-cochlear findings. Neurology 2012;79:1607–14.
21. Neugebauer H, Adrion C, Glaser M, et al. Long-term changes of central ocular motor signs in patients with vestibular migraine. Eur Neurol 2013;69:102–7.
22. Polensek SH, Tusa RJ. Nystagmus during attacks of vestibular migraine: an aid in diagnosis. Audiol Neurootol 2010;15:241–6.
23. Lechner C, Taylor RL, Todd C, et al. Causes and characteristics of horizontal positional nystagmus. J Neurol 2014;261:1009–17.
24. Kang WS, Lee SH, Yang CJ, et al. Vestibular function tests for vestibular migraine: clinical implication of video head impulse and caloric tests. Front Neurol 2016; 7:166.
25. Blödow A, Heinze M, Bloching MB, et al. Caloric stimulation and video-head impulse testing in Ménière's disease and vestibular migraine. Acta Otolaryngol 2014;134:1239–44.
26. Vitkovic J, Paine M, Rance G. Neuro-otological findings in patients with migraine- and nonmigraine-related dizziness. Audiol Neurootol 2008;13:113–22.
27. Mahringer A, Rambold HA. Caloric test and video-head-impulse: a study of vertigo/dizziness patients in a community hospital. Eur Arch Otorhinolaryngol 2014; 271:463–72.
28. Baier B, Dieterich M. Vestibular-evoked myogenic potentials in "vestibular migraine" and Ménière's disease. A sign of electrophysiological link? Ann N Y Acad Sci 2009;1164:324–7.
29. Zuniga MG, Janky KL, Schubert MC, et al. Can vestibular-evoked myogenic potentials help differentiate Ménière disease from vestibular migraine? Otolaryngol Head Neck Surg 2012;146:788–96.
30. Salviz M, Yuce T, Acar H, et al. Diagnostic value of vestibular-evoked myogenic potentials in Ménière's disease and vestibular migraine. J Vestib Res 2015;25: 261–6.
31. Taylor RL, Zagami AS, Gibson WP, et al. Vestibular evoked myogenic potentials to sound and vibration: characteristics in vestibular migraine that enable separation from Ménière's disease. Cephalalgia 2012;32:213–25.
32. Inoue A, Egami N, Fujimoto C, et al. Vestibular evoked myogenic potentials in vestibular migraine: do they help differentiating from Ménière's disease? Ann Otol Rhinol Laryngol 2016;125:931–7.
33. Zaleski A, Bogle J, Starling A, et al. Vestibular evoked myogenic potentials in patients with vestibular migraine. Otol Neurotol 2015;36:295–302.
34. Makowiec KF, Piker EG, Jacobson GP, et al. Ocular and cervical vestibular evoked myogenic potentials in patients with vestibular migraine. Otol Neurotol 2018;39:e561–7.

35. Boldingh MI, Ljostad U, Mygland A, et al. Vestibular sensitivity in vestibular migraine: VEMPs and motion sickness susceptibility. Cephalalgia 2011;31: 1211–9.

36. Casani AP, Sellari-Franceschini S, Napolitano A, et al. Otoneurologic dysfunction in migraine patients with or without vertigo. Otol Neurotol 2009;30:961–7.

37. Boldingh MI, Ljostad U, Mygland A, et al. Comparison of interictal vestibular function in vestibular migraine vs migraine without vertigo. Headache 2013;53: 1123–33.

38. Roceanu A, Allena M, de Pasqua V, et al. Abnormalities of the vestibulo-collic reflex are similar in migraineurs with and without vertigo. Cephalalgia 2008;28: 988–90.

39. Furman JM, Marcus DA, Balaban CD. Vestibular migraine: clinical aspects and pathophysiology. Lancet Neurol 2013;12:706–15.

40. Akerman S, Holland PR, Goadsby PJ. Diencephalic and brainstem mechanisms in migraine. Nat Rev Neurosci 2011;12:570–84.

41. Antilla V, Wessmann M, Kallela M, et al. Genetics of migraine. Handb Clin Neurol 2018;148:493–503.

42. Lee H, Jen JC, Wang H, et al. A genome-wide linkage scan of familial benign recurrent vertigo: linkage to 22q12 with evidence of heterogeneity. Hum Mol Genet 2006;15:251–8.

43. Bahmad F Jr, DePalma SR, Merchant SN, et al. Locus for familial migrainous vertigo disease maps to chromosome 5q35. Ann Otol Rhinol Laryngol 2009; 118:670–6.

44. Balaban CD. Migraine, vertigo and migrainous vertigo: Links between vestibular and pain mechanisms. J Vestib Res 2011;21:315–21.

45. Vass Z, Steyger PS, Hordichok AJ, et al. Capsaicin stimulation of the cochlear and electric stimulation of the trigeminal ganglion mediate vascular permeability in cochlear and vertebro-basilar arteries: a potential cause of inner ear dysfunction in headache. Neuroscience 2001;103:189–201.

46. Koo JW, Balaban CD. Serotonin-induced plasma extravasation in the murine inner ear: possible mechanism of migraine-associated inner ear dysfunction. Cephalalgia 2006;26:1310–9.

47. Marano E, Marcelli V, Di Stasio E, et al. Trigeminal stimulation elicits a peripheral vestibular imbalance in migraine patients. Headache 2005;45:325–31.

48. Kim JS, Yue Q, Jen JC, et al. Familial migraine with vertigo: no mutations found in CACNA1A. Am J Med Genet 1998;79:148–51.

49. von Brevern M, Ta N, Shankar A, et al. Migrainous vertigo: mutation analysis of the candidate genes CACNA1A, ATP1A2, SCN1A, and CACNB4. Headache 2006; 46:1136–41.

50. Nakada T, Yoshida T, Suga K, et al. Endolymphatic space size in patients with vestibular migraine and Ménière's disease. J Neurol 2014;261:2079–84.

51. Sun W, Guo P, Ren T, et al. Magnetic resonance imaging of intratympanic gadolinium helps differentiate vestibular migraine from Ménière's disease. Laryngoscope 2017;127:2382–8.

52. Shin JE, Kim YK, Kim HJ, et al. Altered brain metabolism in vestibular migraine: comparison of interictal and ictal findings. Cephalalgia 2014;34:58–67.

53. Obermann M, Wurthmann S, Schulte B, et al. Central vestibular system modulation in vestibular migraine. Cephalalgia 2014;34:1053–61.

54. Messina R, Rocca MA, Colombo B, et al. Structural brain abnormalities in patients with vestibular migraine. J Neurol 2017;264:295–303.

55. Russo A, Marcelli V, Esposito F, et al. Abnormal thalamic function in patients with vestibular migraine. Neurology 2014;82:2120–6.
56. Lopez-Escamez JA, Carey J, Chung WH, et al. Diagnostic criteria for Menière's disease. J Vestib Res 2015;25:1–7.
57. Huppert D, Strupp M, Brandt T. Long-term course of Menière's disease revisited. Acta Otolaryngol 2010;130:644–51.
58. Radtke A, Lempert T, Gresty MA, et al. Migraine and Meniere's disease: is there a link? Neurology 2002;59:1700–4.
59. Brantberg K, Baloh RW. Similarity of vertigo attacks due to Meniere's disease and benign recurrent vertigo, both with and without migraine. Acta Otolaryngol 2011; 131:722–7.
60. Lopez-Escamez A, Dlugaiczyk J, Jacobs J, et al. Accompanying symptoms overlap during attacks in Menière's disease and vestibular migraine. Front Neurol 2014;5:265.
61. Murofushi T, Tsubota M, Kitao K, et al. Simultaneous presentation of definite vestibular migraine and definite Ménière's disease: overlapping syndrome of two diseases. Front Neurol 2018;9:749.
62. Choi JH, Park MG, Choi SY, et al. Acute transient vestibular syndrome: prevalence of stroke and efficacy of bedside evaluation. Stroke 2017;48:556–62.
63. Lahmann C, Henningsen P, Brandt T, et al. Psychiatric comorbidity and psychosocial impairment among patients with vertigo and dizziness. J Neurol Neurosurg Psychiatry 2015;86:302–8.
64. Kutay Ö, Akdal G, Keskinoglu P, et al. Vestibular migraine patients are more anxious than migraine patients without vestibular symptoms. J Neurol 2017; 264(Suppl 1):37–41.
65. Maldonado-Fernandez M, Birdi JS, Irving GJ, et al. Pharmacological agents for the prevention of vestibular migraine. Cochrane Database Syst Rev 2015;(6):CD010600.
66. Neuhauser H, Radtke A, von Brevern M, et al. Zolmitriptan for treatment of migrainous vertigo: a pilot randomized placebo-controlled trial. Neurology 2003;60:882–3.
67. Prakash S, Shah ND. Migrainous vertigo responsive to intravenous methylprednisolone: case reports. Headache 2009;49:1235–9.
68. Fotuhi M, Glaun B, Quan SY, et al. Vestibular migraine: a critical review of treatment trials. J Neurol 2009;256:711–6.
69. Lepcha A, Amalanathan S, Augustine AM, et al. Flunarizine in the prophylaxis of migrainous vertigo: a randomized controlled trial. Eur Arch Otorhinolaryngol 2014;271:2931–6.
70. Cha YH. Migraine-associated vertigo: diagnosis and treatment. Semin Neurol 2010;30:167–74.
71. Celebisoy N, Gökcay F, Karahan C, et al. Acetazolamide in vestibular migraine prophylaxis: a retrospective study. Eur Arch Otorhinolaryngol 2016;273:2947–51.
72. Liu F, Ma T, Che X, et al. The efficacy of venlafaxine, flunarizine, and valproic acid in the prophylaxis of vestibular migraine. Front Neurol 2017;8:524.
73. Varkey E, Cider A, Carlsson J, et al. Exercise as migraine prophylaxis: a randomized study using relaxation and topiramate as controls. Cephalalgia 2011;31: 1428–38.
74. Lee YY, Yang YP, Huang PI, et al. Exercise suppresses COX-2 pro-inflammatory pathway in vestibular migraine. Brain Res Bull 2015;116:98–105.
75. Alghadir AH, Anwer S. Effects of vestibular rehabilitation in the management of vestibular migraine: a review. Front Neurol 2018;9:440.

76. Wester JL, Ishiyama A, Ishiyama G. Recurrent vestibular migraine vertigo attacks associated with the development of profound bilateral vestibulopathy: a case series. Otol Neurotol 2017;38:1145–8.
77. Salviz M, Yuce T, Acar H, et al. Propranolol and venlafaxine for vestibular migraine prophylaxis: a randomized controlled trial. Laryngoscope 2016;126: 169–74.
78. Baier B, Winkenwerder E, Dieterich M. Vestibular migraine: effects of prophylactic therapy with various drugs. A retrospective study. J Neurol 2009b;256:436–42.
79. Mikulec AA, Faraji F, Kinsella LJ. Evaluation of efficacy of caffeine cessation, nortriptyline, and topiramate therapy in vestibular migraine and complex dizziness of unknown etiology. Am J Otolaryngol 2012;33:121–7.
80. Reploeg MD, Goebel JA. Migraine-associated dizziness: patient characteristics and management options. Otol Neurotol 2002;23:364–71.
81. Power L, Shute W, McOwan B, et al. Clinical characteristics and treatment choice in vestibular migraine. J Clin Neurosci 2018;52:50–3.

Diagnostic Testing for Migraine and Other Primary Headaches

Randolph W. Evans, MD

KEYWORDS

- Headache diagnostic testing • MRI • Computed tomography • Migraine
- Trigeminal autonomic cephalalgias • New daily persistent headache

KEY POINTS

- MRI is usually preferred over computed tomography for the evaluation of headaches.
- Imaging is typically not required for the diagnosis of migraine meeting diagnostic criteria.
- MRI is usually indicated for trigeminal autonomic cephalalgias to exclude secondary causes.

Most primary headaches can be diagnosed without diagnostic testing using a comprehensive history and neurologic and focused general physical examinations.

In some cases, however, diagnostic testing is necessary to distinguish primary from secondary causes that may share similar features. The differential diagnosis of headache is one of the longest in all of medicine, with more than 300 different types and causes. In this article, the reasons for diagnostic testing and the use of neuroimaging, electroencephalography, lumbar puncture, and blood testing are evaluated. The use of diagnostic testing in adults and children who have a normal neurologic examination, migraine, trigeminal autonomic cephalalgias (TACs), and new daily persistent headache (NDPH) is reviewed.

REASONS FOR DIAGNOSTIC TESTING

The indications for diagnostic testing are variable, and neurologists must make decisions on a case-by-case basis when presented with a suspected primary headache if secondary headache is a consideration. Clinical situations whereby neurologists consider diagnostic testing are listed in **Box 1**.

There are many other reasons neurologists recommend diagnostic testing: "our stubborn quest for diagnostic certainty";[1] faulty cognitive reasoning; the medical

This article is adapted from a previously published article in the May 2009 issue of *Neurologic Clinics*, Volume 27, Issue 2; with permission.
Baylor College of Medicine, 1200 Binz #1370, Houston, TX 77004, USA
E-mail address: revansmd@gmail.com

Neurol Clin 37 (2019) 707–725
https://doi.org/10.1016/j.ncl.2019.08.001   neurologic.theclinics.com
0733-8619/19/© 2019 Elsevier Inc. All rights reserved.

Box 1
Reasons to consider neuroimaging for headaches

Temporal and headache features
1. The "first or worst" headache
2. Subacute headaches with increasing frequency or severity
3. A progressive headache or NDPH
4. Chronic daily headache
5. Headaches always on the same side
6. Headaches not responding to treatment
7. New-onset headaches in patients who have cancer or who test positive for HIV infection
8. New-onset headaches after aged 50
9. Patients who have headaches and seizures
10. Headaches associated with symptoms and signs, such as fever, stiff neck, nausea, and vomiting
11. Headaches other than migraine with aura associated with focal neurologic symptoms or signs
12. Headaches associated with papilledema, cognitive impairment, or personality change

From Evans RW. Headaches. In: Evans RW, editor. Diagnostic testing in neurology. Philadelphia: W.B. Saunders; 1999. p. 2; with permission.

---

decision rule that it is better to impute disease than to risk overlooking it; busy practice conditions whereby tests are ordered as a shortcut; patient expectations; financial incentives; professional peer pressure, whereby recommendations for routine and esoteric tests are expected as a demonstration of competence; and medicolegal issues.[2,3] The attitudes and demands of patients and families and the practice of defensive medicine are especially important reasons in the case of headaches. In the era of managed care, equally compelling reasons for not ordering diagnostic studies include physician fears of deselection, at-risk capitation, and economic credentialing.[4] Lack of funds and underinsurance continue to be barriers to appropriate diagnostic testing for many patients.

DIAGNOSTIC TESTING OPTIONS
Computed Tomography Versus MRI

Computed tomography (CT) detects most abnormalities that may cause headaches. CT generally is preferred to MRI for evaluation of acute subarachnoid hemorrhage, acute head trauma, and bony abnormalities. There are several disorders, however, that may be missed on routine CT of the head, including vascular disease, neoplastic disease, cervicomedullary lesions, and infections (**Box 2**). MRI is more sensitive than CT in the detection of posterior fossa and cervicomedullary lesions, ischemia, white matter abnormalities (WMA), cerebral venous thrombosis (CVT), subdural and epidural hematomas, neoplasms (especially in the posterior fossa), meningeal disease (such as carcinomatosis, diffuse meningeal enhancement in low cerebrospinal fluid [CSF] pressure syndrome, and sarcoid), cerebritis, and brain abscess. Pituitary pathologic condition is more likely to be detected on a routine MRI of the brain than a routine CT.

Another concern with CT is exposure to ionizing radiation. The average radiation dose of a CT scan of the head (with or without contrast, both studies double the dose) is an effective dose of 2.0 millisieverts (mSv), which is equivalent to 100 chest radiographs.[5] The most common malignancies associated with radiation exposure include leukemia and breast, thyroid, lung, and stomach cancers. The latency period for solid tumors usually is long, an average of 10 to 20 years, with a

---

Box 2
Causes of headache that can be missed on routine computed tomographic scan of the head

Vascular disease
  Saccular aneurysms
  Arteriovenous malformations (especially posterior fossa)
  Subarachnoid hemorrhage
  Carotid or vertebral artery dissections
  Infarcts
  Cerebral venous thrombosis
  Vasculitis
  White matter abnormalities
  Subdural and epidural hematomas

Neoplastic disease
  Neoplasms (especially in the posterior fossa)
  Meningeal carcinomatosis
  Pituitary tumor and hemorrhage

Cervicomedullary lesions
  Chiari malformations
  Foramen magnum meningioma

Infections
  Paranasal sinusitis
  Meningoencephalitis
  Cerebritis and brain abscess

Other
  Low CSF pressure syndrome
  Neurosarcoid
  Idiopathic hypertrophic pachymeningitis

From Evans RW. Diagnostic testing for migraine and other primary headaches. Neurol Clin. 2009 May;27(2):393-415; with permission.

---

persistent lifelong risk. Leukemia has an earlier latency period with an increased risk 2 to 5 years after radiation exposure. The pediatric population is at increased risk, as a result of increased radiosensitivity and more years of remaining life, for potentially developing cancer. Consider the radiation exposure of some patients who have multiple trips to an emergency department, have migraine and multiple CT scans, and also have multiple CT scans of the head and sinuses in an outpatient setting. For a single CT scan of the head, the estimated lifetime-attributable risk for death from cancer by age is approximately as follows: age 10 years, 0.025%; age 20 years, 0.01%; and age 50 years, 0.003%.[6] Although these are small numbers, are individual studies justified? Up to 2% of all cancer deaths in the United States may be attributable to radiation exposure associated with CT use. The Food and Drug Administration has estimated that exposure to 10 mSv (equivalent to 1 CT of the abdomen) may be associated with an increased risk for developing fatal cancer in one of every 2000 patients.[7]

Thus, MRI generally is preferred over CT for evaluation of headaches. The yield of MRI may vary depending on the field strength of the magnet, the use of paramagnetic contrast, the selection of acquisition sequences, and the use of magnetic resonance (MR) angiography (MRA) and MR venography (MRV). MRI may be contraindicated, however, in the presence of an aneurysm clip or pacemaker. In addition, approximately 8% of patients are claustrophobic, approximately 2% to the point at which they cannot tolerate the study.

Neuroimaging During Pregnancy and Lactation

When there are appropriate indications, neuroimaging should be performed during pregnancy.[8] With the use of lead shielding, a standard CT scan of the head exposes the uterus to less than 1 mrad. The radiation dose for a typical cervical or intracranial arteriogram is less than 1 mrad. The fetus is most susceptible to the teratogenic effects of radiation between the second and 20th weeks of embryonic age[8] with a threshold radiation dose estimated at between 5 and 15 rad.[9] There is no known risk associated with iodinated contrast use during pregnancy or in breastfeeding women, and contrast may be used when indicated.[10]

MRI is more sensitive for rare disorders that may occur during pregnancy, such as pituitary apoplexy, CVT (with the addition of MRV), and metastatic choriocarcinoma.

There is no known risk associated with MRI during pregnancy.[11–13] There may be an increased risk of tissue heating at field strengths more than 1.5 T of uncertain significance.

According to the 2013 American College of Radiology Guidance Document for Safe Practices,[14]

Present data have not conclusively documented any deleterious effects of MR imaging exposure on the developing fetus. Therefore, no special consideration is recommended for the first, versus any other, trimester in pregnancy. Nevertheless, as with all interventions during pregnancy, it is prudent to screen females of reproductive age for pregnancy before permitting them access to MR imaging environments. If pregnancy is established, consideration should be given to reassessing the potential risks versus benefits of the pending study in determining whether the requested MR examination could safely wait to the end of the pregnancy before being performed.

a. *Pregnant patients can be accepted to undergo MR scans at any stage of pregnancy if, in the determination of a level 2 MR personnel-designated attending radiologist, the risk-benefit ratio to the patient warrants that the study be performed. The radiologist should confer with the referring physician and document the following in the radiology report or the patient's medical record:*
   1. *The information requested from the MR study cannot be acquired by means of nonionizing means (eg, ultrasonography).*
   2. *The data are needed to potentially affect the care of the patient or fetus during the pregnancy.*
   3. *The referring physician believes that it is not prudent to wait until the patient is no longer pregnant to obtain this data.*

MR contrast agents should not be routinely provided to pregnant patients.

The decision to administer a gadolinium-based MR contrast agent to pregnant patients should be accompanied by a well-documented and thoughtful risk-benefit analysis.

The American College of Obstetricians and Gynecologists concluded that breastfeeding should not be interrupted after gadolinium administration.[15]

Electroencephalography

The electroencephalogram (EEG) was a standard test for evaluation of headaches in the pre-CT scan era. Gronseth and Greenberg[16] reviewed the literature from 1941 to 1994 on the usefulness of EEG in the evaluation of patients who had headache. Most of the articles had serious methodologic flaws. The only significant abnormality reported in studies with a relatively nonflawed design was prominent driving in response to photic stimulation (the H response) in migraineurs who had a sensitivity ranging from 26%[17] to 100%[18] and a specificity from 80%[19] to 91%.[18] This finding, although interesting, is not necessary for the clinical diagnosis of migraine. If the purpose of the EEG is to exclude an underlying structural lesion, such as a neoplasm, CT or MRI imaging is far superior.

A report of the Quality Standards Subcommittee of the American Academy of Neurology (AAN) suggests the following practice parameter: "The electroencephalogram (EEG) is not useful in the routine evaluation of patients with headache. This does not exclude the use of EEG to evaluate headache patients with associated symptoms suggesting a seizure disorder such as atypical migrainous aura or episodic loss of consciousness. Assuming head imaging capabilities are readily available, EEG is not recommended to exclude a structural cause for headache."[16] The AAN's choosing wisely recommendations include, "Don't perform EEGs for headaches."[17]

A report of the Quality Standards Subcommittee of the AAN and the Practice Committee of the Child Neurology Society[18] makes the following pediatric recommendations: "EEG is not recommended in the routine evaluation of a child with recurrent headaches, as it is unlikely to provide an etiology, improve diagnostic yield, or distinguish migraine from other types of headaches (Level C; class II and class III evidence)."

Lumbar Puncture

MRI or CT scan always is performed before a lumbar puncture for evaluation of headaches except in some cases where acute meningitis is suspected. Lumbar puncture can be diagnostic for meningitis or encephalitis, meningeal carcinomatosis or lymphomatosis, subarachnoid hemorrhage, and high (eg, pseudotumor cerebri) or low CSF pressure. In cases of blood dyscrasias, the platelet count should be 50,000 or greater before safely performing a lumbar puncture. The CSF opening pressure always should be measured when investigating headaches. When measuring the opening pressure, it is important for patients to relax and at least partially extend the head and legs to avoid recording a falsely elevated pressure.

After neuroimaging is performed, lumbar puncture often is indicated in the following circumstances: the first or worst headache, headache with fever or other symptoms or signs suggesting an infectious cause, a subacute or progressive headache (eg, in an human immunodeficiency virus [HIV]-positive patient or a person who has carcinoma), and an atypical chronic headache (eg, to rule out pseudotumor cerebri in an obese woman who does not have papilledema).

There are many potential complications of lumbar puncture, the most common of which is low CSF pressure headache, which occurs approximately 30% of the time using the conventional bevel-tip or Quincke needle.[19] The risk for headache can be reduced dramatically to approximately 5% to 10% by using an atraumatic needle, such as the Sprotte or Whitacre, and replacing the stylet before withdrawing the needle.[20]

Blood Tests

Blood tests generally are not helpful for the diagnosis of headaches. There are many indications, however, such as the following: erythrocyte sedimentation rate or C-reactive protein to consider the possibility of temporal arteritis in a person 50 years or older who has new-onset migraine, because only 2% of migraineurs have an onset at age 50 years or older; erythrocyte sedimentation rate, rheumatoid arthritis factor, and antinuclear antibody test in patients who have headache and arthralgia to evaluate for possible collagen vascular disease, such as lupus[21]; monospot in teenagers who have headaches, sore throat, and cervical adenopathy; complete blood cell count

(CBC), liver function tests, HIV test, or Lyme antibody test in some patients who have a suspected infectious basis; an anticardiolipin antibody and lupus anticoagulant in migraineurs who have extensive WMA on MRI; thyroid-stimulating hormone because headache may be a symptom in 14% of cases of hypothyroidism; CBC because headache may be a symptom when the hemoglobin concentration is reduced by one-half or more; serum urea nitrogen and creatinine to exclude renal failure, which can cause headache; serum calcium because hypercalcemia can be associated with headaches; CBC and platelets because thrombotic thrombocytopenic purpura can cause headaches; and endocrine studies in patients who have headaches and a pituitary tumor.

In addition, blood tests may be indicated as a baseline and for monitoring for certain medications, such as valproic acid for migraine prophylaxis, carbamazepine for trigeminal neuralgia, and lithium for chronic cluster headaches.

HEADACHES AND A NORMAL NEUROLOGIC EXAMINATION
Neuroimaging Studies in Adults

The yield of abnormal neuroimaging studies in studies of patients who have headaches as the only neurologic symptom and normal neurologic examinations depends on several factors, including the duration of the headache, study design (prospective vs retrospective), who orders the scan, and the type of scan performed. The percentage of abnormal scans may be higher when ordered by neurologists or a tertiary care center compared with primary care physicians representing case selection bias. In reported CT scan series, the yield may vary depending on the generation of scanner and whether iodinated contrast was used. The yield of MRI may vary depending on the field strength of the magnet, the use of paramagnetic contrast, the selection of acquisition sequences, and the use of MR angiography.

Frishberg[22] reviewed 8 CT scan studies of 1825 patients who had unspecified headache types and varying durations of headache. The summarized findings from these studies are combined with 4 additional studies of 1566 CT scans in patients who had headache and normal neurologic examinations[21,23–25] for a total of 3389 scans. The overall percentages of various pathologic conditions are as follows: brain tumors, 1%; arteriovenous malformations (AVMs), 0.2%; hydrocephalus, 0.3%; aneurysm, 0.1%; subdural hematoma, 0.2%; and strokes (including chronic ischemic process), 1.1%.

Combining 3 studies of patients who had chronic headaches and a normal neurologic examination with 1282 patients, the only clinically significant pathologic condition was 1 low-grade glioma and 1 saccular aneurysm.[21,23,26]

Weingarten and colleagues[26] extrapolated various types of data from 100,800 adult patients who belonged to a health maintenance organization. The estimated prevalence (in patients who had chronic headache and a normal neurologic examination) of a CT scan demonstrating an abnormality requiring neurosurgical intervention may have been as low as 0.01%. It is not certain whether detection of additional pathologic condition on MRI scan would change this percentage. For example, complaints of headache with a normal neurologic examination may be seen in patients who have Chiari type I malformation, which is easily detected on MRI but not CT scans. Pituitary hemorrhage can produce a migrainelike acute headache with a normal neurologic examination.[27] Pituitary infarction, with severe headache, photophobia, and CSF pleocytosis, initially can be similar to aseptic meningitis or meningoencephaitis.[28] Pituitary pathologic condition is more likely to be detected on a routine MRI than CT scan.

Wang and coworkers[29] retrospectively reviewed the medical records and MRI images of 402 adult patients (286 women and 116 men) who had been evaluated by the neurology service and who had a primary complaint of chronic headache (a duration of 3 months or more) and no other neurologic symptoms or findings. Major abnormalities (a mass, caused mass effect, or was thought the likely cause of patient's headache) were found in 15 patients (3.7%) and included glioma, meningioma, metastases, subdural hematoma, AVM, hydrocephalus (3 patients), and Chiari I malformations (2 patients). They were found in 0.6% of patients who had migraine, 1.4% of those who had tension headaches, 14.1% of those who had atypical headaches, and 3.8% of those who had other types of headaches.

Tsushima and Endo[30] retrospectively reviewed the clinical data and MR studies of 306 adult patients (136 men and 170 women) all of whom were referred for MRI evaluation of chronic or recurrent headache with a duration of 1 month or more, had no other neurologic symptoms or focal findings at physical examination, and had no prior head surgery, head trauma, or seizure: 55.2% had no abnormalities, 44.1% had minor abnormalities, and 0.7% (2) had clinically significant abnormalities (pituitary macroadenoma and subdural hematoma). Neither contrast material enhancement (195) nor repeated MRI (23) contributed to the diagnosis.

Sempere and colleagues[31] reported a study of 1876 consecutive patients (1243 women and 633 men), aged 15 or older, mean age 38 years, who had headaches that had an onset at least 4 weeks previously and who were referred to 2 neurology clinics in Spain. One-third of the headaches were new onset, and two-thirds had been present for more than 1 year. Subjects had the following types: migraine (49%), tension (35.4%), cluster (1.1%), posttraumatic (3.7%), and indeterminate (10.8%). Normal neurologic examinations were found in 99.2% of the patients. CT scan was performed in 1432 patients and MRI in 580; 136 patients underwent both studies.

Neuroimaging studies detected significant lesions in 22 patients (1.2%), of whom 17 had a normal neurologic examination. The only variable or red flag associated with a higher probability of intracranial abnormalities was an abnormal neurologic examination with a likelihood ratio of 42. The diagnoses in these 17 patients were pituitary adenoma (3), large arachnoid cyst (2), meningioma (2), hydrocephalus (2), and Arnold-Chiari type I malformation, ischemic stroke, cavernous angioma, AVM, low-grade astrocytoma, brainstem glioma, colloid cyst, and posterior fossa papilloma (one of each). Of these 17 patients, 8 were treated surgically, including for hydrocephalus (2), and pituitary adenoma, large arachnoid cyst, meningioma, AVM, colloid cyst, and papilloma (one of each).

The rate of significant intracranial abnormalities in patients who had headache and normal neurologic examination was 0.9%. Neuroimaging studies discovered incidental findings in 14 patients (75%): 3 pineal cysts, 3 intracranial lipomas, and 8 arachnoid cysts. The yield of neuroimaging studies was higher in the group with indeterminate headache (3.7%) than in the migraine (0.4%) or tension-type headache (0.8%) groups. The study does not provide information on WMA in migraineurs. MRI performed in patients who had normal CT revealed significant lesions in 2 cases: a small meningioma and an acoustic neurinoma. No saccular aneurysms were detected; MR angiography was not obtained.

Wang and colleagues[32] recruited 1070 health controls and 1070 primary headache patients (including 665 with migraine of all types, 93 with chronic migraine, and 338 with tension-type headaches, 99 with the chronic type) from the Chinese People's Liberation Army General Hospital, who then underwent either CT or MRI scans. Abnormal scans were found in the following: 0.67% in migraine (3/665 with MRI and 0/291 with CT) compared with 0.73% abnormal scans in controls. Abnormalities in migraineurs were 2 with hydrocephalus and 2 with tumors of the throat and nose. They concluded, "The present study found that neuroimaging was unnecessary for the primary headache patients."

The studies do not give information about the detection of paranasal sinus disease, however, which may be the cause of some headaches. For example, sphenoid sinusitis may cause a severe, intractable, new-onset headache that interferes with sleep and is not relieved by simple analgesics. The headache may increase in severity with no specific location. There may be associated pain or paresthesias in the facial distribution of the fifth nerve and photophobia or eye tearing with or without fever or nasal drainage. The headache may mimic other causes, such as migraine or meningitis.[33]

The American College of Radiology Choosing Wisely recommended, "Don't Image for uncomplicated headache."[34]

Headache and a normal neurologic examination neuroimaging in children

Many studies have investigated the findings of neuroimaging in children who had headaches with a normal neurologic examination. The yield of clinically significant abnormalities is low (0.9%–1.2%).[35] A few studies are reviewed.

Chu and Shinnar[36] obtained brain imaging studies in 30 children, aged 7 or younger, who had headaches and were referred to pediatric neurologists. The studies were normal except for 5 that had incidental findings.

Maytal and coworkers[37] obtained MRI or CT scans or both in 78 children, aged 3 to 18, who had headaches. With the exception of 6 patients, the neurologic examinations were normal. The studies were normal except for incidental cerebral abnormalities in 4 and mucoperiosteal thickening of the paranasal sinuses in 7.

Wöber-Bingöl and colleagues[38] prospectively obtained MRI scans in 96 children, aged 5 to 18, who had headaches and normal neurologic examinations and who were referred to an outpatient headache clinic. The studies were normal except for 17 (17.7%) who had incidental findings.

Lewis and Dorbad[39] retrospectively reviewed records of children, aged 6 to 18, who had migraine and chronic daily headache with normal examinations. Of 54 patients who had migraine who underwent CT (42) or MRI (12) scans, the yield of abnormalities was 3.7%, none clinically relevant. Of 25 patients who had chronic daily headache who underwent CT (17) or MRI (8) scans, the yield of abnormalities was 16%, none clinically relevant.

Carlos and colleagues,[40] in a retrospective chart review, identified all pediatric migraine patients who had a CT or MRI to investigate their headaches. Ages ranged from 3 to 18. Of the 93 patients, 35 had CT, 14 had MRI, and 9 had both. Twenty-two had abnormalities, but none was thought related to the patients' headaches.

Alehan[41] prospectively obtained neuroimaging (49 MRI scans and 11 CT scans) in 60 of 72 consecutive children diagnosed with migraine or tension-type headaches. Ten percent had findings related to their headache with no neoplasms, and no patients required surgery.

Occipital headaches in children have been thought to be rare and suggestive of serious intracranial pathologic condition. However, in a retrospective study of 308 children ≤18 years of age referred to a headache clinic for headache with a normal neurologic examination, headaches were solely occipital in 7% and occipital-plus in 14%. Occipital pain alone or with other locations was not significantly associated with clinically significant intracranial pathologic condition on neuroimaging.[42] In children with occipital headaches consistent with migraine or another primary headache disorder with a normal neurologic examination, the yield of neuroimaging is low.[43]

Headaches upon awakening and sleep interruption owing to headache have been commonly regarded as a potential sign of raised intracranial pressure. In a study of 102 children aged between 5 and 17 years, including 77% with headache upon awakening, 19% with sleep interruption owing to headache, and 4% with both, neuroimaging was performed in 101 of the cohort. Imaging was normal in 97 and showed nonsignificant findings in 4.[44] All had primary headaches or medication overuse except for 1 with sinusitis. This symptom alone is not an indication for routine neuroimaging.

Guidelines
A report of the Quality Standards Subcommittee of the AAN and the Practice Committee of the Child Neurology Society[17] makes the following recommendations:

1. Obtaining a neuroimaging study on a routine basis is not indicated in children who have recurrent headaches and a normal neurologic examination (level B; class II and class III evidence).
2. Neuroimaging should be considered in children who have an abnormal neurologic examination (eg, focal findings, signs of increased intracranial pressure, significant alteration of consciousness), the coexistence of seizures, or both (level B; class II and class III evidence).
3. Neuroimaging should be considered in children in whom there are historical features to suggest the recent onset of severe headache or change in the type of headache or if there are associated features that suggest neurologic dysfunction (level B; class II and class III evidence).

The American College of Radiology appropriateness criteria recommend that for children with primary headache, "There is no role for radiography in patients with primary headache."[45]

Risk/Benefit and Cost/Benefit of Neuroimaging

Table 1 summarizes the estimated risks and benefits of neuroimaging in patients who have headaches and normal neurologic examinations (radiation exposure and the increased long-term risk for cancer are discussed previously). Many anxious patients and their family members are not reassured even after a long discussion about the low yield of neuroimaging. Howard and colleagues[46] performed a randomized control trial in a London headache clinic of 150 patients with chronic daily headache (76 were randomized to the offer of a brain scan and 74 were treatment as usual). Patients offered a scan were less worried about a serious cause of the headaches at 3 months, although this was not maintained at 1 year. However, patients with high levels of psychiatric morbidity offered a scan had significantly less costs owing to lower utilization of medical resources.

For other patients, the scan may produce anxiety when nonspecific abnormalities are found, such as incidental findings or anatomic variants[47,48] or white matter lesions. The author suspects that many neurologists have seen patients who have isolated headaches referred by primary care physicians with a request to rule out multiple sclerosis when white matter lesions associated with migraine are detected.

Although the cost of finding significant pathologic condition is high, many payers have significantly reduced the cost of neuroimaging. Cost/benefit estimates should include the cost to physicians of malpractice suits filed when patients who have significant pathologic condition do not have neuroimaging[49] and the cost to patients and society of premature death and disability of undetected treatable lesions.

Table 1
Balance sheet. CT or MRI in patients with headache and normal neurologic examinations. Technology: CT with intravenous contrast or MRI without contrast. Indications: (1) migraine and (2) any headache

	CT, %	MRI, %	No Test
Health outcomes			
Benefits			
Discovery of potentially treatable lesions			
1. Migraine	0.3	0.4	0
2. Any headache	2.4	2.4	0
Relief of anxiety	30	30	0
Harms			
Iodine reaction			
Mild	10	—	—
Moderate	1	—	—
Severe	0.01	—	—
Death	0.002	—	—
Claustrophobia			
Mild	5	15	0
Moderate (needs sedation)	1	5–10	—
Severe (unable to comply)	1–2	—	—
False-positive studies	No data	No data	—
Cost (charges)	Varies widely depending on payer		—

Data from Frishberg BM. The utility of neuroimaging in the evaluation of headache in patients with normal neurologic examinations. Neurology 1994;44:1196.

Following guidelines does not indemnify the physician in a malpractice suit.[2,50] Until physicians are indemnified in malpractice cases when they follow guidelines, one might consider what a jury would consider indications for neuroimaging rather than one's peers.

NEUROIMAGING IN MIGRAINE
Incidence of Pathologic Condition

Combining 16 MRI and CT scan studies for a total of 1625 scans of patients with various types of migraine, the studies found no significant pathologic condition except for 4 brain tumors (3 of which were incidental findings) and 1 AVM (in a patient who had migraine and a seizure disorder).[51] Sempere and colleagues[31] found a similarly low yield of 0.4%.

Mullally and Hall[52] performed a prospective study on 100 subjects with a diagnosis of migraine (45 without aura, 14 with aura, and 41 with chronic migraine) and a normal neurologic examination who had MRI scans of the brain solely at their request. The duration of headaches ranged from 4 months to 40 years. MRI scans were normal in 82 and found clinically insignificant abnormalities in 17. MRI was abnormal in 1 patient (chronic migraine without aura) finding a meningioma requiring surgery and radiotherapy that is similar to the yield of brain tumor in the general asymptomatic population. The investigators conclude, "Brain MRI obtained at the specific request of patients with a diagnosis of migraine in the presence of normal neurologic examination results has a yield that is equivalent to that of the general asymptomatic population. Patients do not seem to have more insight than the examining clinician with regard to detecting underlying structural abnormalities, and brain MRI should not performed as part of the routine evaluation of migraine without a clear clinical indication."

A meningioma is not necessarily an incidental finding in a migraineur. Evans and colleagues[53] reported a 47-year-old woman with a left frontal secretory meningioma that mimicked transformed migraine with and without aura. As discussed above, there is potential harm to the patient and physician's medicolegal liability if these rare cases are not detected.

Wang and colleagues[32] recruited 1070 health controls and 1070 primary headache patients (including 665 with migraine) from the Chinese People's Liberation Army General Hospital who then underwent either CT or MRI scans. Abnormal scans were found in the following: 0.67% in migraine (3/665 with MRI and 0/291 with CT) compared with 0.73% abnormal scans in controls. Abnormalities in migraineurs were 2 with hydrocephalus and 2 with tumors of the throat and nose. They conclude, "The present study found that neuroimaging was unnecessary for the primary headache patients."

White Matter Hyperintensities and Subclinical Infarcts

WMA are foci of hyperintensity on proton density, fluid attenuation inversion recovery, and T2-weighted images in the deep and periventricular white matter resulting from interstitial edema or perivascular demyelination. WMA are easily detected on MRI but are not seen on CT scan. The percentages of WMA for all types of migraine range from 4% to 59% and in controls from 0% to 31%.[54]

The clinical significance of WMA is not known. There might be microvascular damage because of gliosis, demyelination, and loss of axons.[55]

WMA are not specific to migraine and can be present in nonmigraine headaches and older age. Depending on the number, distribution, and location, there may be a secondary cause, such as multiple sclerosis, cerebral autosomal dominant arteriopathy with subclinical infarcts and leukoencephalopathy, or mitochondrial myopathy, encephalopathy, lactic acidosis, and strokelike episodes.

In the general population-based MRI study in the Norwegian county of Nord-Trondelag (HUNT MRI),[56] having tension-type headache or developing headache in middle age was linked to extensive WMA. Migraine did not increase the odds of having extensive WMA.

Silent infarctlike lesions (ILLs) have been reported in migraineurs typically located in the cerebellum, subcortex, and deep gray matter. The cause, nature, and clinical significance are not clear.[57] Evaluation for stroke risk factors is appropriate.

In a metaanalysis of WMA and ILLs,[54] there was an association for migraine with aura (odds ratio 1.68) but not for migraine without aura. The association of ILLs was greater for migraine with aura than without, but there was no association for either type of migraine compared with controls.

In a study of female twins aged 30 to 60 years in the population-based Danish Twin Registry,[58] there was no evidence of an association between silent brain infarcts, WMA, and migraine with aura. A prospective study found no association of WMA and cognitive changes in migraineurs.[59]

Practice Parameters

A report of the Quality Standards Subcommittee of the AAN[54] makes the following recommendation: "Neuroimaging is not usually warranted in patients with migraine and a normal neurologic examination (Grade B)." The American Headache Society

Choosing Wisely[60] recommendation is the following: do not perform neuroimaging studies in patients with stable headaches that meet criteria for migraine.

Although the yield is low, **Box 3** lists some reasons to consider neuroimaging in migraineurs. There are numerous migraine mimics.[61]

Trigeminal Autonomic Cephalalgias

TACs are primary headache syndromes characterized by severe unilateral headaches typically associated with ipsilateral cranial autonomic features, such as lacrimation, conjunctival injection, nasal congestion, and rhinorrhea. TACs include cluster headache, paroxysmal hemicrania, hemicrania continua (HC), and short-lasting unilateral neuralgiform headache with conjunctival injection and tearing (SUNCT), with cluster headache the most common.[62] **Table 2** provides the clinical features.

There are many secondary causes of TACs. It can be difficult in some cases to determine causality with a lesion that can be incidental. de Coo and colleagues[63] propose the following categories: probably secondary (when there was a dramatic improvement of the headache after treatment of the underlying lesion); possibly secondary (when the patient was treated but did not become headache free, or was not treated, but where a causal relation was possible based on previous experience with other patients); and unknown (patients in which a causal relation between the phenotype and the lesion was less likely or at least unclear).

Secondary cluster headaches

There are numerous causes of secondary cluster headaches or clusterlike headaches.[64,65] Vascular causes include the following: carotid and vertebral artery dissection, pseudoaneurysm of intracavernous carotid artery, anterior communicating artery aneurysm, AVMs (occipital lobe, middle cerebral artery territory, in soft tissue above ear, frontal lobe, and corpus callosum), infarction (cervical cord and lateral medullary),

---

Box 3
Reasons to consider neuroimaging in migraineurs

Unusual, prolonged, or persistent aura

Increasing frequency, severity, or change in clinical features

First or worst migraine

Migraine with brainstem aura

Confusional

Hemiplegic

Late-life migraine accompaniments

First onset ≥50 years of age

Aura without headache

Headaches always on the same side?

Posttraumatic

Patient or family and friend request

From Evans RW. Diagnosis of headaches and medico-legal aspects. In: Evans RW, Mathew NT, editors. Handbook of headache. 2nd edition. Philadelphia: Lippincott-Williams & Wilkins; 2005. p. 21; modified, with permission.

Table 2
Comparison of the trigeminal autonomic cephalalgias

	Cluster Headache[1]	Paroxysmal Hemicrania[2]	SUNCT/SUNA[3]	HC[4]
Ratio of female to male	1:3	Slightly more women	1:1.5	2:1
Pain				
Quality	Sharp, stabbing, throbbing	Sharp, stabbing, throbbing	Sharp, stabbing, throbbing	Baseline: aching; exacerbations: sharp, stabbing, throbbing
Severity	Very severe	Very severe	Severe	Baseline: mild to moderate; exacerbations: moderate to severe
Attacks				
Frequency (per day)	1–8[a]	5–50	1 to hundreds	Constant
Duration (min)	15–180	2–30	0.01–10[b]	Baseline: 3 mo or more; exacerbations: 30 min to 3 d
Ratio of episodic to chronic	90:10	35:65	10:90	15:85[c]
Associated features				
Restlessness	90%	80%	65%	70%
Circadian periodicity	82%[5]	Rare	Rare	Rare
Triggers				
Alcohol	Yes	Yes	No	Yes
Nitroglycerin	Yes	Yes	No	Rare
Neck movements	No	Yes	Yes	No
Cutaneous	No	No	Yes	No
Treatment response				
Oxygen	70%	No effect	No effect	No effect
Sumatriptan 6 mg subcutaneous	90%	20%	Rare effect	No effect
Indomethacin	Rare effect	100%	No effect	100%

Abbreviation: SUNA, short-lasting unilateral neuralgiform headache attacks with cranial autonomic symptoms.
[a] Cluster headache frequency is officially 1 headache every other day up to 8 per day.[6]
[b] SUNCT and SUNA duration is 1 to 600 s.
[c] For HC, the ratio of episodic to chronic refers to the ratio of remitting to unremitting attacks.
From Burish M. Cluster Headache and Other Trigeminal Autonomic Cephalalgias. Continuum (Minneap Minn). 2018 Aug;24(4,Headache):1137-1156, with permission.

frontotemporal subdural hematoma, trigeminal root compression, pontine cavernous angioma, external jugular vein thrombosis, petrosal venous compression of trigeminal nerve, segmental cavernous carotid ectasia, and indirect carotid-cavernous fistula. Tumors include the following: pituitary, hypothalamic, meningiomas (parasellar, sphenoidal, tentorial, and high cervical), epidermoid tumor (behind the dorsum sella turcica and clivus), nasopharyngeal carcinoma, C3 root fibrosis, lipoma at C1-2, and glioblastoma multiforme involving the cingulate gyrus. Infective causes include maxillary sinusitis, orbitosphenoidal aspergillosis, and herpes zoster ophthalmicus. Posttraumatic or surgery include facial trauma, following enucleation of eye, and cataract surgery. Dental are impacted wisdom tooth and following dental extraction. Miscellaneous causes are cervical syringomyelia, Chiari malformation, idiopathic intracranial hypertension, and multiple sclerosis.

Levy and colleagues[66] reported a series of 84 consecutive patients who had pituitary tumors (65% macroadenomas). Using International Headache Society (IHS) classification, 4 met criteria for SUNCT, 3 for cluster, and 1 for HC. Cavernous sinus invasion was present in 2 of the 3 cluster cases. Of the 4 SUNCT cases, 2 were prolactinomas and 2 were growth hormone–secreting tumors. Although information is provided on response of all headaches to treatment, response to treatment of the TACs is not provided.

Pituitary adenomas account for up to 17% of all primary brain tumors with a prevalence as high as 115 per 100,000. With the exception of pituitary hemorrhage or infarction, there is likely only a small subset of patients with headaches directly caused by pituitary disease.[67]

Secondary paroxysmal hemicrania
Secondary causes or associations include the following: head trauma; thrombocytopenia; temporal arteritis; pituitary and parasellar lesions; cerebral hemorrhage; cerebral metastasis; AVM, meningioma (cavernous sinus and anterior clinoid; aneurysm (cavernous segment); cavernous sinus dural fistula after carotid artery aneurysm embolization; with use of phosphodiesterase inhibitors; clinically isolated syndrome; and orbital metastaic leiomyosarcoma.[65,68]

Secondary short-lasting unilateral neuralgiform headache attacks with conjunctival injection and tearing/short-lasting unilateral headache attacks with autonomic features
Secondary causes or associations include the following: pituitary tumors; posterior fossa tumors; frontotemporal meningioma; compression of trigeminal nerve by superior cerebellar artery; vertebral artery dissection with dorsolateral medullary infarct, right pontine capillary telangiectasia, and developmental venous anomaly; multiple sclerosis, lung adenocarcinoma, acute and previous infection with herpes zoster in the first trigeminal distribution; viral meningitis; and postradiation to a pituitary adenoma.[63,65]

Secondary hemicrania continua
Rarely, HC may have a secondary cause, which includes the following[65,69]: vascular (cervical internal carotid and vertebral artery dissection, unruptured cavernous internal artery aneurysm, venous malformation of the right masseter, and pontine stroke); neoplasms (nasopharyngeal carcinoma of the nasopharynx, mesenchymal tumor of the sphenoid, adenocarcinoma or small cell carcinoma of the lung, prolactinoma, osteoid osteoma of the ethmoid sinus, benign pineal cyst, and cerebellopontine angle epidermoid); infection (sphenoid sinusitis, HIV, dental disease, and leprosy); and miscellaneous (head trauma, hypertrophic pachymeningitis, transdermal nitroglycerin patch,

following cranial surgery, C7 root irritation owing to disc herniation, inflammatory orbital pseudotumor, and scleritis).

Patients meeting IHS criteria for a TAC rarely have a secondary cause for their headache detected on neuroimaging. Appropriate testing is indicated, however, especially if atypical symptoms and/or signs or risk factors for secondary causes are present. MRI of the brain and MRA of the neck may be indicated. CT of the chest may be considered in smokers.

Secondary new daily persistent headache

NDPH is described by the *International Classification of Headache Disorders, 3rd edition (ICHD-3)*[70]: "Persistent headache, daily from its onset, which is clearly remembered. The pain lacks characteristic features, and may be migraine-like or tension-type-like, or have elements of both." The diagnostic criteria are the following:

A. Persistent headache fulfilling criteria B and C
B. Distinct and clearly remembered onset, with pain becoming continuous and unremitting within 24 hours
C. Present for longer than 3 months
D. Not better accounted for by another *ICHD-3* diagnosis

Box 4 lists some primary and secondary causes of new daily headache present for more than 3 months that may have a normal neurologic examination. Some of these secondary disorders may have a thunderclap or sudden onset of severe headache (primary NDPH can have a thunderclap onset[71]), whereas others may develop gradually over 1 to 3 months. Chronic migraine and chronic tension-type headaches increase in frequency over time and are not daily from onset, whereas HC can be daily from onset.

Tests to be considered depending on the case include blood tests (such as CBC, serum chemistries, thyroid function, erythrocyte sedimentation rate and C-reactive

---

Box 4
Differential diagnosis of new daily headaches present for more than 3 months

Primary headaches
 New daily persistent headache
 Chronic migraine
 Chronic tension-type
 Hemicrania continua

Secondary headaches (NDPH mimics)
 Primary with medication overuse
 Infection (chronic meningitis, Lyme disease, infectious mononucleosis, postmeningitis headache, sphenoid sinusitis, post-Dengue)
 Neoplasms (primary and metastatic)
 Vascular (chronic subdural hematoma, cervical artery dissection, reversible cerebral vasoconstriction syndrome, subarachnoid hemorrhage, dural arteriovenous fistula, hypertension, cerebral venous thrombosis, arteriovenous malformation)
 Posttraumatic headaches
 High and low cerebrospinal fluid pressure (pseudotumor cerebri, postlumbar puncture, spontaneous intracranial hypotension)
 Inflammatory (temporal arteritis and Behçet syndrome[73])
 Miscellaneous (temporal arteritis, Chiari malformation, a single Valsalva event,[74] intranasal contact point, multinodular goiter,[75] cervicogenic, temporomandibular joint dysfunction)

From Evans RW. Diagnostic testing for migraine and other primary headaches. Neurol Clin. 2009 May;27(2):393-415; with permission.

protein in patients 50 years of age and older, Lyme antibodies, and heterophile antibodies), MRI of the brain with and without contrast, MRV of the brain, and MRA of the head and neck (if there is a thunderclap or severe sudden onset).[72]

Guideline
The European Headache Federation[76] has the following recommendations: "Brain MRI with detailed study of the pituitary area and cavernous sinus, is recommended for all TACs. When three consecutive preventive treatments fail additional MRA brain and carotid/vertebral arteries may be required and in the presence of a (partial) Horner's syndrome, additional imaging of the apex of the lung may be warranted, especially in smokers. Pituitary function testing should be considered in refractory TAC patients in addition." Evaluation for lung cancer is a consideration in HC especially in smokers.

For NDPH, "A gadolinium-enhanced brain MRI with MRV and a lumbar puncture with CSF manometry can be indicated in selected patients."

REFERENCES

1. Kassirer JP. Our stubborn quest for diagnostic certainty. A cause of excessive testing. N Engl J Med 1989;320:1489–91.
2. Evans RW, Johnston JC. Migraine and medical malpractice. Headache 2011; 51(3):434–40.
3. Woolf SH, Kamerow DB. Testing for uncommon conditions. The heroic search for positive test results. Arch Intern Med 1990;15:2451–8.
4. Black SB, Evans RW. Economic credentialing of physicians by insurance companies and headache medicine. Headache 2012;52(6):1037–40.
5. Costello JE, Cecava ND, Tucker JE, et al. CT radiation dose: current controversies and dose reduction strategies. AJR Am J Roentgenol 2013;201(6):1283–90.
6. Brenner DJ, Hall EJ. Computed tomography—an increasing source of radiation exposure. N Engl J Med 2007;357:2277–84.
7. U.S. Food and Drug Administration. What are the radiation risks from CT?. 2017. Available at: https://www.fda.gov/radiation-emittingproducts/radiationemitting productsandprocedures/medicalimaging/medicalx-rays/ucm115329.htm. Accessed November 25, 2018.
8. Gao G, Zucconi RL, Zucconi WB. Emergent neuroimaging during pregnancy and the postpartum period. Neuroimaging Clin N Am 2018;28(3):419–33.
9. Berlin L. Radiation exposure and the pregnant patient. AJR Am J Roentgenol 1996;167:1377–9.
10. American College of Radiology Committee on Drugs and Contrast Media. ACR manual on contrast media, version 10.3 2018. Available at: https://www.acr.org/-/media/ACR/Files/Clinical-Resources/Contrast_Media.pdf. Accessed December 1, 2018.
11. Kruskal JB. Diagnostic imaging in pregnant and nursing women. In: Post TW, editor. UpToDate. Waltham (MA): UpToDate; 2019.
12. Strizek B, Jani JC, Mucyo E, et al. Safety of MR imaging at 1.5 T in fetuses: a retrospective case-control study of birth weights and the effects of acoustic noise. Radiology 2015;275:530–7.
13. Ray JG, Vermeulen MJ, Bharatha A, et al. Association between MRI exposure during pregnancy and fetal and childhood outcomes. JAMA 2016;316:952–61.
14. Expert panel on MR Safety. ACR guidance document on MR safe practices: 2013. J Magn Reson Imaging 2013;37:501–30.
15. Committee on Obstetric Practice. Committee opinion no. 723: guidelines for diagnostic imaging during pregnancy and lactation. Obstet Gynecol 2017;130:e210.

16. Gronseth GS, Greenberg MK. The utility of the electroencephalogram in the evaluation of patients presenting with headache: a review of the literature. Neurology 1995;45(7):1263–7.
17. Langer-Gould AM, Anderson WE, Armstrong MJ, et al. The American Academy of Neurology's top five choosing wisely recommendations. Neurology 2013;81(11): 1004–11.
18. Lewis DW, Ashwal S, Dahl G, et al, Quality Standards Subcommittee of the American Academy of Neurology, Practice Committee of the Child Neurology Society. Practice parameter: evaluation of children and adolescents with recurrent headaches: report of the Quality Standards Subcommittee of the American Academy of Neurology and the Practice Committee of the Child Neurology Society. Neurology 2002;59:490–8.
19. Evans RW. Complications of lumbar puncture. In: Evans RW, editor. Neurology and trauma. 2nd edition. New York: Oxford University Press; 2006. p. 697–715.
20. Armon C, Evans RW. Addendum to assessment: prevention of post-lumbar puncture headaches: report of the therapeutics and technology assessment subcommittee of the American Academy of Neurology. Neurology 2005;65:510–2.
21. Dumas MD, Pexman W, Kreeft JH. Computed tomography evaluation of patients with chronic headache. Can Med Assoc J 1994;151:1447–52.
22. Frishberg BM. The utility of neuroimaging in the evaluation of headache in patients with normal neurologic examination. Neurology 1994;44:1191–7.
23. Akpek S, Arac M, Atilla S, et al. Cost effectiveness of computed tomography in the evaluation of patients with headache. Headache 1995;35:228–30.
24. Demaerel P, Boelaert I, Wilms G, et al. The role of cranial computed tomography in the diagnostic work-up of headache. Headache 1996;36:347–8.
25. Sotaniemi KA, Rantala M, Pyhtinen J, et al. Clinical and CT correlates in the diagnosis of intracranial tumours. J Neurol Neurosurg Psychiatry 1991;54:645–7.
26. Weingarten S, Kleinman M, Elperin L, et al. The effectiveness of cerebral imaging in the diagnosis of chronic headache: a reappraisal. Arch Intern Med 1992;152: 2457–62.
27. Evans RW. Migrainelike headaches in pituitary apoplexy. Headache 1997;37: 455–6.
28. Embil JM, Kramer M, Kinnear S, et al. A blinding headache. Lancet 1997; 349:182.
29. Wang HZ, Simonson TM, Greco WR, et al. Brain MR imaging in the evaluation of chronic headache in patients without other neurologic symptoms. Acad Radiol 2001;8:405–8.
30. Tsushima Y, Endo K. MR imaging in the evaluation of chronic or recurrent headache. Radiology 2005;235:575–9.
31. Sempere AP, Porta-Etessam J, Medrano V, et al. Neuroimaging in the evaluation of patients with non-acute headache. Cephalalgia 2005;25:30–5.
32. Wang R, Liu R, Dong Z, et al. Unnecessary neuroimaging for patients with primary headaches. Headache 2018. https://doi.org/10.1111/head.13397.
33. Marmura MJ, Silberstein SD. Headaches caused by nasal and paranasal sinus disease. Neurol Clin 2014;32(2):507–23.
34. American College of Radiology. Choosing wisely: ten things physicians and patients should question. 2017. Available at: http://www.choosingwisely.org/societies/american-college-of-radiology/. Accessed December 1, 2018.
35. Bonthius DJ, Lee AG, Hershey AD. Headaches in children: approach to evaluation and general management strategies. In: Post TW, editor. UpToDate. Waltham (MA): UpToDate; 2019.

36. Chu ML, Shinnar S. Headaches in children younger than 7 years of age. Arch Neurol 1992;49:79–82.
37. Maytal J, Bienkowski RS, Patel M, et al. The value of brain imaging in children with headaches. Pediatrics 1996;96:413–6.
38. Wöber-Bingöl C, WöberC, Prayer D, et al. Magnetic resonance imaging for recurrent headache in childhood and adolescence. Headache 1996;36:83–90.
39. Lewis DW, Dorbad D. The utility of neuroimaging in the evaluation of children with migraine or chronic daily headache who have normal neurological examinations. Headache 2000;40:629–32.
40. Carlos RA, Santos CS, Kumar S, et al. Neuroimaging studies in pediatric migraine headaches. Headache 2000;40:404.
41. Alehan FK. Value of neuroimaging in the evaluation of neurologically normal children with recurrent headache. J Child Neurol 2002;17:807–9.
42. Bear JJ, Gelfand AA, Goadsby PJ, et al. Occipital headaches and neuroimaging in children. Neurology 2017;89(5):469–74.
43. Irwin SL, Gelfand AA. Occipital headaches and neuroimaging in children. Curr Pain Headache Rep 2018;22(9):59.
44. Ahmed MAS, Ramseyer-Bache E, Taylor K. Yield of brain imaging among neurologically normal children with headache on wakening or headache waking the patient from sleep. Eur J Paediatr Neurol 2018;22(5):797–802.
45. Expert Panel on Pediatric Imaging, Hayes LL, Palasis S, Bartel TB, et al. ACR appropriateness criteria(®) headache-child. J Am Coll Radiol 2018;15(5S):S78–90.
46. Howard L, Wessely S, Leese M, et al. Are investigations anxiolytic or anxiogenic? A randomised controlled trial of neuroimaging to provide reassurance in chronic daily headache. J Neurol Neurosurg Psychiatry 2005;76(11):1558–64.
47. Evans RW. Incidental findings and normal anatomical variants on MRI of the brain in adults for primary headaches. Headache 2017;57(5):780–91.
48. Strauss LD, Cavanaugh BA, Yun ES, et al. Incidental findings and normal anatomical variants on brain MRI in children for primary headaches. Headache 2017;57(10):1601–9.
49. Evans RW. Headaches and neuroimaging. JAMA Intern Med 2015;175(2):312.
50. Evans RW, Henry PC. Medico-legal aspects of headache medicine. Case 4: the migraine that wasn't. Headache 2008;48:870–5.
51. Evans RW. Diagnostic testing for migraine and other primary headaches. Neurol Clin 2009;27(2):393–415.
52. Mullally WJ, Hall KE. Value of patient-directed brain magnetic resonance imaging scan with a diagnosis of migraine. Am J Med 2018;131(4):438–41.
53. Evans RW, Timm JS, Baskin DS. A left frontal secretory meningioma can mimic transformed migraine with and without aura. Headache 2015;55:849–52.
54. Bashir A, Lipton RB, Ashina S, et al. Migraine and structural changes in the brain: a systematic review and meta-analysis. Neurology 2013;81(14):1260–8.
55. Young VG, Halliday GM, Kril JJ. Neuropathologic correlates of white matter hyperintensities. Neurology 2008;71:804–11.
56. Honningsvåg LM, Håberg AK, Hagen K, et al. White matter hyperintensities and headache: a population-based imaging study (HUNT MRI). Cephalalgia 2018;38(13):1927–39.
57. Ramzan M, Fisher M. Headache, migraine, and stroke. In: Post TW, editor. UpToDate. Waltham (MA): UpToDate; 2019.

58. Gaist D, Garde E, Blaabjerg M, et al. Migraine with aura and risk of silent brain infarcts and white matter hyperintensities: an MRI study. Brain 2016;139(Pt 7): 2015–23.
59. Rist PM, Dufouil C, Glymour MM, et al. Migraine and cognitive decline in the population-based EVA study. Cephalalgia 2011;31:1291–300.
60. Loder E, Weizenbaum E, Frishberg B, et al, American Headache Society Choosing Wisely Task Force. Choosing wisely in headache medicine: the American Headache Society's list of five things physicians and patients should question. Headache 2013;53(10):1651–9.
61. Evans RW. Migraine mimics. Headache 2015;55(2):313–22.
62. Burish M. Cluster headache and other trigeminal autonomic cephalalgias. Continuum (Minneap Minn) 2018;24(4, Headache):1137–56.
63. de Coo IF, Wilbrink LA, Haan J. Symptomatic trigeminal autonomic cephalalgias. Curr Pain Headache Rep 2015;19:39.
64. Goadsby PJ. Cluster headache. In: Roos RP, editor. MedLink neurology. San Diego (CA): MedLink Corporation; 2018. Available at: www.medlink.com.
65. Chowdhury D. Secondary (symptomatic) trigeminal autonomic cephalalgia. Ann Indian Acad Neurol 2018;21(Suppl S1):57–69.
66. Levy MJ, Matharu MS, Meeran K, et al. The clinical characteristics of headache in patients with pituitary tumours. Brain 2005;128:1921–30.
67. Donovan LE, Welch MR. Headaches in patients with pituitary tumors: a clinical conundrum. Curr Pain Headache Rep 2018;22:57.
68. Goadsby PJ. Paroxysmal hemicrania. In: Roos RP, editor. MedLink neurology. San Diego (CA): MedLink Corporation; 2017. Available at: www.medlink.com.
69. Dougherty C. Hemicrania continua. In: Roos RP, editor. MedLink neurology. San Diego (CA): MedLink Corporation; 2018. Available at: www.medlink.com.
70. Headache Classification Committee of the International Headache Society (IHS). The international classification of headache disorders, 3rd edition. Cephalalgia 2018;38:1–211.
71. Robbins MS, Evans RW. The heterogeneity of new daily persistent headache. Headache 2012;52(10):1579–89.
72. Nierenburg H, Newman LC. Update on new daily persistent headache. Curr Treat Options Neurol 2016;18(6):25.
73. Vishwanath V, Wong E, Crystal SC, et al. Headache in Behçet's syndrome: review of literature and NYU Behçet's syndrome center experience. Curr Pain Headache Rep 2014;18(9):445.
74. Rozen TD. New daily persistent headache (NDPH) triggered by a single Valsalva event: a case series. Cephalalgia 2019;39(6):785–91.
75. Evans RW, Timm JS. New daily persistent headache caused by a multinodular goiter and headaches associated with thyroid disease. Headache 2017;57(2): 285–9.
76. Mitsikostas DD, Ashina M, Craven A, et al. European Headache Federation consensus on technical investigation for primary headache disorders. J Headache Pain 2015;17:5.

Acute Treatment of Migraine

Stewart J. Tepper, MD[a,b,c,*]

KEYWORDS

- Acute migraine treatment • Migraine • Triptans • Ergots • Gepants • Ditans
- NSAIDs • Neuroleptics

KEY POINTS

- All patients with migraine need acute treatment provided.
- The goal of acute treatment of migraine is a sustained pain-free response, one and done.
- The efficacy of acute treatments for migraine can be monitored by 2 validated patient-reported outcome measures, the Migraine-Assessment of Current Therapy and the Migraine Treatment Optimization Questionnaire.
- Overuse of acute migraine treatment is associated with transformation from episodic migraine to chronic migraine.
- Optimal acute migraine treatment is linked to reduced risk of transformation from episodic migraine to chronic migraine.

INTRODUCTION

All migraine patients need acute treatment provided. Selection of acute medication is best based on disability as a surrogate marker of disease severity, although other measures of the migraine attack can be used to tailor treatments.

The standard of care for acute therapy is a sustained pain-free response, one and done. Achieving this result reduces disability, optimally restoring function with minimal adverse events and cost. The overall efficacy of acute treatments for migraine can be monitored by 2 validated patient-reported outcome measures, the

Disclosures: Grants for research (no personal compensation): Alder, Allergan, Amgen, ATI, Dr. Reddy's, ElectroCore, eNeura, Neurolief, Scion Neurostim, Teva, Zosano. Consultant and/or Advisory Boards: Acorda, Alder, Alexsa, Allergan, Alphasights, Amgen, ATI, Axsome Therapeutics, Cefaly, Charleston Labs, DeepBench, Dr. Reddy's, ElectroCore, Eli Lilly, eNeura, GLG, Guidepoint Global, Magellan Rx Management, Neurolief, Nordic BioTech, Pfizer, Scion Neurostim, Slingshot Insights, Sorrento Therapeutics, Supernus, Teva, Zosano. Stock Options: ATI. Royalties: Springer. Salary: Dartmouth-Hitchcock Medical Center, American Headache Society.

[a] Geisel School of Medicine at Dartmouth, Hanover, NH, USA; [b] Dartmouth Headache Center, Lebanon, NH, USA; [c] Neurology Department, Dartmouth-Hitchcock Medical Center, 1 Medical Center Drive, Lebanon, NH 03748, USA
* Neurology Department, Dartmouth-Hitchcock Medical Center, 1 Medical Center Drive, Lebanon, NH 03748.
E-mail address: Stewart.J.Tepper@Dartmouth.edu

Neurol Clin 37 (2019) 727–742
https://doi.org/10.1016/j.ncl.2019.07.006
0733-8619/19/© 2019 Elsevier Inc. All rights reserved.

neurologic.theclinics.com

Migraine–Assessment of Current Therapy (Migraine-ACT) and the Migraine Treatment Optimization Questionnaire (MTOQ). There is a natural history consequence in selecting the best acute treatment of migraine, because optimal acute treatment is associated with a reduced risk of progression of episodic migraine to chronic migraine.

The American Headache Society (AHS) published an evidence assessment of acute treatments for migraine in 2015. The authors stated, "The specific medications—triptans (almotriptan, eletriptan, frovatriptan, naratriptan, rizatriptan, sumatriptan [oral, nasal spray, injectable, transcutaneous patch], zolmitriptan [oral and nasal spray]) and dihydroergotamine (nasal spray, inhaler) are effective (level A)", whereas "effective nonspecific medications include acetaminophen, nonsteroidal anti-inflammatory drugs (aspirin, diclofenac, ibuprofen, and naproxen), opioids (butorphanol nasal spray) [not recommended], sumatriptan/naproxen, and the combination of acetaminophen/ aspirin/caffeine" also have level A evidence. "Ergotamine and other forms of dihydroergotamine…ketoprofen, intravenous and intramuscular ketorolac, flurbiprofen, intravenous magnesium (in migraine with aura), and the combination of isometheptene compounds, codeine/acetaminophen, tramadol/acetaminophen… prochlorperazine, droperidol, chlorpromazine, and metoclopramide are probably effective (level B)." Again, opioids are not recommended. Furthermore, "[t]here is inadequate evidence for butalbital and butalbital combinations, phenazone, intravenous tramadol, methadone, butorphanol or meperidine injections, intranasal lidocaine, and corticosteroids, including dexamethasone (level C).[1]

Finally, 3 noninvasive neuromodulation devices are Food and Drug Administration (FDA) approved for acute treatment of migraine as of early 2019, with at least 2 more in development. These devices offer an alternative method for treating migraine acutely without significant adverse events and likely without risk of overuse and the transformation of episodic to chronic migraine.

PRINCIPLES OF ACUTE TREATMENT OF MIGRAINE

All patients with migraine need acute treatment provided. The usual patient complaining of headache as either a primary or a secondary complaint in a primary care provider or Neurology office has disabling migraine.[2] Thus, because the impact or disability of migraine for the average patient is severe, the need for the provider to help select the best acute treatment is manifest which should ideally be the right treatment the first time.

Optimal acute treatment yields both a pain-free response and a sustained pain-free response. The International Headache Society (IHS) 2012 Third Edition Guidelines for Controlled Trials of Drugs in Migraine ranked the percentage of patients pain free at 2 hours the recommended outcome measure for randomized controlled trials (RCTs) of acute migraine medications.[3] This is also the outcome patients have selected in multiple evaluations, including 2 validated patient-reported outcome (PRO) tools, in which patients were give options for outcomes from long lists of potential choices.[4–6]

However, the IHS Guidelines go on to describe a second, even more ideal goal for acute treatment, as follows, "The sustained pain freedom rate is defined as the percentage of study participants who are pain-free at 2 h[ours] with no use of rescue medication or relapse (recurrence) within the subsequent 46 h[hours]. Sustained pain freedom is a recommended secondary efficacy measure…Sustained pain freedom is the ideal migraine treatment response and should be the ultimate goal in drug development."[3] Sustained pain freedom is a "one and done" response to treatment.

Historically, acute migraine treatment trials used multiple endpoints; regulatory authorities adopted these endpoints, and both gradually changed over time. The triptan development programs implemented a categorical pain scale for migraine severity of 0 to 3: no or zero pain, mild or 1-, moderate or 2-, and severe or 3-level pain. During the era of triptan clinical trials, the goal of treatment was the movement of pain by active treatment compared with placebo from moderate to severe pain to zero or mild pain. This change from pain at 2 to 3 to 0 to 1 continues to be variably named in the literature, and all of these terms mean the same: headache response, headache relief, pain response, and pain relief.

The FDA currently requires that in pivotal placebo-controlled RCTs of acute medication treatments for migraine that subjects be instructed to wait until moderate to severe levels of pain to treat. This is ostensibly to make extra sure that a given treated attack is a migraine, but is not the way that providers should be instructing patients to take acute medications in real life, because they clearly work better when taken earlier. Thus, the pivotal trials routinely underestimate the efficacy of acute medications.

The IHS Guidelines address this issue by stating, "Either early in the attack or after an attack is fully developed is acceptable as the timing for test drug intervention …In principle, study drug administration should be started as early as possible during the headache phase in order to mimic clinical practice."[3]

IMPACT OF OPTIMAL ACUTE TREATMENT

Examining the consequences of sustained pain freedom by an acute medication leads to a greater understanding of the potential salutary result of a successful intervention. The natural history of migraine involves the potential for transformation from episodic to chronic migraine. This undesirable outcome is linked to the frequency of migraine days. That is, those with high-frequency episodic migraine, from 10 to 14 headache days per month, are most likely to progress to chronic migraine across time.[7–9]

In addition, there is a link between type and frequency of acute migraine treatment days. The hierarchy of association suggests that use of butalbital more than once weekly, of opioids more than twice weekly, and of triptans and combination analgesics more than 10 days per month is associated with transformation from episodic to chronic migraine.[9]

The relationship of risk, if there is one, for nonsteroidal anti-inflammatory drugs (NSAIDs) is more complex. With NSAID use less than 5 days per month, NSAIDs appear to be protective against migraine chronification. At use approaching 15 days per month, the statistical interaction between the risk from the high frequency of migraine days and the high frequency of NSAID intake becomes difficult to untangle, and the results are either that NSAIDs are not associated with transformation or the findings are inconclusive.[9]

It is intuitive that a sustained pain-free response should be optimal for acute treatment of a migraine attack. The use of a single dose resulting in pain freedom within 2 hours without recurrence or further medication would be the most cost-effective treatment as well as satisfying the most requested outcome by patients of 2-hour pain freedom. However, in pushing the consequences of this outcome further, it may be useful to hypothesize a typical patient with 4 migraine attacks per week of 3 days' duration each.

If this patient takes a suboptimal acute treatment, with resultant migraine recurrence and multiple dosing, she takes her acute medicine 12 days per month, which puts her above the threshold for the association of acute medication use days and transformation from episodic to chronic migraine. In addition, 12 days of migraine per month puts her in the highest-risk group for chronification based on her having high-frequency episodic migraine.

If, on the other hand, she takes her acute medication and gets a 2-hour sustained pain-free response, then instead of 12 days of migraine per month, she gets 4 days of migraine per month, and really, less than 2 hours for each of those 4 days, so 8 hours of migraine per month. This puts her in the lowest-risk group for transformation from episodic to chronic migraine, and this outcome was accomplished with the best acute treatment without the need for migraine preventive treatment.

The hypothesis that suboptimal acute treatment is linked to a higher risk of transformation from episodic to chronic migraine was demonstrated in the American Migraine Prevalence and Prevention (AMPP) trial and published in 2015. In the data analysis of this large, prospective, population-based study, 5681 with episodic migraine in 2006 were followed prospectively for 1 year, and 3.1% progressed to chronic migraine in 2007.[10,11]

The efficacy of acute treatment was evaluated using the MTOQ-4, which will be described subsequently. Treatment efficacy was assigned as maximum, moderate, poor, and very poor. Only 1.9% of the maximum acute treatment episodic migraine group developed chronic migraine across the year. New onset chronic migraine was seen in 2.7% of the moderate treatment efficacy group, 4.4% of the poor treatment efficacy group, and 6.8% of the very poor acute treatment efficacy patients.[10,11]

The very poor acute treatment efficacy group had more than twice the increased risk of new onset chronic migraine (odds ratio = 2.55) compared with the optimal treatment efficacy group. Inadequate acute treatment efficacy was clearly associated with an increased risk of new onset chronic migraine over the course of 1 year, confirming the hypothesis.[10,11] The hope is that maximum acute treatment might prevent progression of episodic to chronic migraine, which is not yet proven. However, the AMPP findings strikingly show the potential worth of seeking optimal acute treatment for migraine patients, and of using evaluations of acute treatment efficacy to assess progress.

PATIENT-REPORTED OUTCOME TOOLS FOR ACUTE MIGRAINE TREATMENT ASSESSMENT

As noted, 2 validated PRO tools are available for assessment of acute treatment efficacy, the Migraine-ACT and the MTOQ. Migraine-ACT was a compilation of the 4 top choices from 27 tested in 4 domains and consists of the domains and their questions in **Box 1**. Each "yes" response is scored "1." A Migraine-ACT score of ≤2 is the score associated with a clinical indication to switch acute medications.[5,12,13]

The MTOQ questionnaire can be administered in entirety (19 items) or in truncated forms (MTOQ-4, MTOQ-6). The investigators commented that they "modified the response options to 4 frequency-based response options (never, rarely, < half the time, and ≥ half the time) and selected 6 key questions. The ordinal 6-item version (MTOQ-6) was included in the AMPP Study survey in 2006 and 2007. Additional validation work has been done on this version of the questionnaire. From the 6 items, the author selected the 4 that best assessed treatment efficacy (for example, MTOQ-4).[6,10,14] The 4 questions of MTOQ-4 are very similar to Migraine-ACT, confirming the validity of the independent assessments of items for assessment of acute treatment of migraine, and are listed in **Box 2**:

SELECTING THE CORRECT ACUTE TREATMENT

Selection of acute treatment of migraine requires stratification, that is, matching acute treatment to characteristics of the attack or the patient. Migraine attacks vary

> **Box 1**
> **Migraine assessment of current therapy**
>
> Consistency of response: *Does your migraine medication work consistently in the majority of your attacks?*
>
> Global assessment of relief: *Does the headache pain disappear within 2 hours?*
>
> Impact: *Are you able to function normally within 2 hours?*
>
> Emotional response: *Are you comfortable enough with your medication to be able to plan your daily activities?*
>
> *From* Dowson AJ, Tepper SJ, Baos V, et al. Identifying patients who require a change in their current acute migraine treatment: the Migraine Assessment of Current Therapy (Migraine-ACT) questionnaire. Curr Med Res Opin. 2004;20(7):1125-35; with permission.

interpatient and intrapatient. Attack characteristics to consider for treatment choice include the following:

- Time of attack onset. Close to half of migraine attacks occur in the morning,[15] and progression of an attack from moderate to severe during sleep, with the attendant migraine-associated symptoms, make morning attacks more difficult to treat.
- Time to peak intensity and associated features. If the time to peak is ≤30 minutes, nonoral alternatives should be considered.
- Severe nausea and vomiting. The presence of difficult-to-treat nausea in attacks increases the risk of transformation to chronic migraine[16] and therefore also increases the need for aggressive acute therapies, usually nonoral.
- Long-duration attacks with multiple recurrence. This problem is frequently seen in menstrually related migraine and merits acute treatment with higher sustained pain response efficacy.
- Status migrainosus. The International Classification of Headache Disorders, 3rd Edition defines status migrainosus as "a debilitating migraine attack lasting for more than 72 hours."[17] This type of attack may require special acute rescue treatments.

A significant problem for picking the right treatment is variability of attacks in the same patient across time. Stratifying attacks by the above features and working

> **Box 2**
> **Migraine treatment optimization questionnaire-4**
>
> 1. After taking your migraine medication, are you pain free within 2 hours for most attacks?
> 2. Does 1 dose of your migraine medication usually relieve your headache and keep it away for at least 24 hours?
> 3. Are you comfortable enough with your migraine medication to be able to plan your daily activities?
> 4. After taking your migraine medication, do you feel in control of your migraines enough so that you feel there will be no disruption to your daily activities?
>
> *From* Lipton RB, Fanning KM, Serrano D, et al. Ineffective acute treatment of episodic migraine is associated with new-onset chronic migraine. Neurology. 2015;84(7):688-95; with permission.

with patients to provide matching treatments to various attacks, evaluated by a diary, is important to achieving sustained pain freedom consistently.

Another method of stratifying care is matching treatment to degree of disability. Lipton and colleagues[18] performed a seminal study in which they compared strategies for selecting acute treatments. This study was the Disabilities in Strategies of Care study or the DISC study. The investigators compared outcomes for 3 approaches to selecting acute treatment rather than comparing the treatments themselves:

1. Step care across attacks, prescribing a low-level, nonspecific treatment first (aspirin plus metoclopramide), and if they failed after 3 attacks, stepping up to a triptan for the fourth attack (zolmitriptan)
2. Step care within attacks, prescribing a low-level, nonspecific treatment (aspirin plus metoclopramide) to be taken at the beginning of a migraine and stepping up to zolmitriptan in 2 hours if the nonspecific treatment failed
3. Stratified care, administering the Migraine Disability Assessment scale (and giving aspirin-metoclopramide to low-level migraine-associated disability and zolmitriptan to higher levels of disability

The results of the DISC study clearly showed better outcomes for patients if they had significant migraine-related disability and were given a triptan at the beginning, rather than stepping through other treatments first.[18] A follow-on pharmacoeconomic study of the DISC data confirmed that stratified care by disability was also more cost-effective than step care.[19]

Furthermore, it is established that the average patient coming into the average primary care office or Neurology office complaining of headache as a primary or secondary complaint has disabling migraine as measured by a validated impact scale.[2] This finding makes triptans the first-line treatment choice in patients without vascular disease and with disabling migraine.

Stratifying acute treatment by attack characteristics and by disability represents the key to selecting the right treatment the first time. Matching these clinical characteristics to treatments with the highest levels of evidence (see the following section) is most likely to yield the best results most quickly.

HOW DO ACUTE MIGRAINE MEDICATIONS WORK?

Migraine pain is, for the most part, generated by release of calcitonin gene-related peptide (CGRP) in the dura mater, with resultant vasodilation and neurogenic inflammation. Triptans and ergots are agonists at some serotonin (5-HT) subreceptors. Activation of 5-HT_{1D} receptors prevents the release of CGRP and prevents nociceptive afferents from carrying the signals back to the brainstem for transduction. Agonism at 5-HT_{1B} receptors results in vasoconstriction of blood vessels dilated by CGRP. NSAIDs inhibit neurogenic inflammation and work centrally to reverse central sensitization.

ACUTE PHARMACOLOGIC TREATMENTS

The AHS published an evidence assessment of acute treatments for migraine in 2015.[1] The investigators performed a detailed assessment of the literature, including the previous US guidelines of 2000.[20] The 2015 findings are contained in **Table 1**:

TRIPTANS

All 7 triptans have level A evidence for acute treatment of episodic migraine. However, not all triptans are the same in efficacy or formulation. Furthermore, patients may be

Table 1
American Headache Society 2015 acute migraine treatment evidence assessment

Level A	Level B	Level C	Level U	Others
Analgesic Acetaminophen 1000 mg (for nonincapacitating attacks)	Antiemetics Chlorpromazine IV 12.5 mg[a] Droperidol IV 2.75 mg Metoclopramide IV 10 mg[a] Prochlorperazine IV/IM 10 mg; PR 25 mg[a]	Antiepileptic Valproate IV 400–1000 mg	NSAIDs Celecoxib 400 mg	Level B negative other Octreotide SC 100 µg
Ergots DHE Nasal spray 2 mg Pulmonary inhaler 1 mg[a]	Ergots DHE[a] IV, IM, SC 1 mg Ergotamine/caffeine 1/100 mg[a]	Ergots Ergotamine 1–2 mg[a]	Others Lidocaine IV[a] Hydrocortisone IV 50 mg[a]	Level C negative antiemetics Chlorpromazine IM 1 mg/kg[a] Granisetron IV 40–80 µg/kg[a]
NSAIDs Aspirin 500 mg[a] Diclofenac 50, 100 mg Ibuprofen 200, 400 mg Naproxen 500, 550 mg[a]	NSAIDs Flurbiprofen 100 mg[a] Ketoprofen 100 mg Ketorolac IV/IM 30–60 mg	NSAIDs Phenazone 1000 mg		NSAIDs Ketorolac tromethamine nasal spray
Opioids Butorphanol nasal spray 1 mg[a]		Opioids Butorphanol IM 2 mg[a] Codeine 30 mg PO[a] Meperidine IM 75 mg[a] Methadone IM 10 mg[a] Tramadol IV 100 mg[a]		Analgesic Acetaminophen IV 1000 mg

(continued on next page)

Table 1
(continued)

Level A	Level B	Level C	Level U	Others

Triptans
Almotriptan 12.5 mg
Eletriptan 20, 40, 80 mg
Frovatriptan 2.5 mg
Naratriptan 1, 2.5 mg[a]
Rizatriptan 5, 10 mg[a]
Sumatriptan
  Oral 25, 50, 100 mg[a]
  Nasal spray 10, 20 mg[a]
  Patch 6.5 mg
  SC 4, 6 mg[a]
Zolmitriptan nasal spray
  2.5, 5 mg
  Oral 2.5, 5 mg[a]
 	
Combinations
AAC 500/500/130 mg[a]
Sumatriptan/naproxen 85/500 mg
	Others
	MgSO$_4$ IV (migraine with aura) 1–2 g
	Isometheptene 65 mg[a]
	
	Combinations
	Codeine/acetaminophen 25/400 mg[a]
	Tramadol/acetaminophen 75/650 mg
		Steroid
		Dexamethasone IV 4–16 mg
		
		Others
		Butalbital 50 mg[a]
		Lidocaine intranasal[a]
		
		Combinations
		Butalbital/acetaminophen/ caffeine/codeine 50/325/ 40/30 mg[a]
		Butalbital/acetaminophen/ caffeine 50/325/40 mg[a]		

Level A: Medications are established as effective for acute migraine treatment based on available evidence.

Level B: Medications are probably effective for acute migraine treatment based on available evidence.

Level C: Medications are possibly effective for acute migraine treatment based on available evidence.

Level U: Evidence is conflicting or inadequate to support or refute the efficacy of the following medications for acute migraine.

Level B negative: Medication is probably ineffective for acute migraine.

Level C negative: Medication is possibly ineffective for acute migraine.

Abbreviations: IM, intramuscular; IV, intravenous; PO, oral; SC, subcutaneous.

[a] Based on 2000 American Academy of Neurology evidence review.

From Marmura MJ, Silberstein SD, Schwedt TJ. The acute treatment of migraine in adults: the American Headache Society evidence assessment of migraine pharmacotherapies. Headache. 2015;55(1):3–20.; with permission.

more different than triptans, and several clinical tries on several attacks may be necessary to find the correct triptan for the patient. All of the oral triptan formulations are available in generic form. Certain injectable sumatriptan doses and certain nasal triptan formulations are only available as branded products.

Triptans can be divided into 2 groups: group 1, those with fast onset, high potency, and likely greater chance of migraine recurrence, and group 2, those with slower onset, lower potency, and lower chance of recurrence (**Table 2**). Short time to peak intensity requires choosing from group 1.

Prominent vomiting necessitates nonoral formulations. Only 2 triptans come in nonoral formulations, sumatriptan and zolmitriptan. The triptan orally dissolvable tablets have no buccal or sublingual absorption; they are merely oral pills that taste better and do not require water.

Frequent recurrence may suggest a trial with naratriptan. Treating early with naratriptan and achieving a pain-free response seem to predict better sustained response with lower recurrence.[21]

Table 2
Triptan by groups[22]

Group 1: Fast Onset, Higher Potency	Group 2: Slower Onset, Lower Potency
Sumatriptan • Subcutaneous 3, 4, 6 mg • Oral 25, 50, **100 mg** • Nasal 5, **20 mg** • Breath powered dry powder **22 mg**	Naratriptan • Oral 1.25, **2.5 mg**
Zolmitriptan • Oral and ODT 2.5, 5 mg • Nasal 2.5, **5 mg**	Frovatriptan • Oral **2.5 mg**
Rizatriptan • Oral and ODT 5, **10 mg**	
Almotriptan • Oral 6.25, **12.5 mg**	
Eletriptan • Oral 20, **40 mg**	
Sumatriptan/naproxen sodium • Oral **85/500 mg**	

Optimal dose, when known, is in bold.
Abbreviation: ODT, orally dissolvable tablet.
Adapted from Rapoport AM, Tepper SJ, Bigal ME, Sheftell FD. The triptan formulations: how to match patients and products. CNS Drugs. 2003;17(6):431-47; with permission.

ERGOTS

Both dihydroergotamine (DHE) and ergotamine tartrate have level A evidence for effectiveness in acute treatment of migraine. Both are difficult to use; neither currently has a consistently effective patient friendly formulation.

DHE is the more useful of the 2 ergots clinically. DHE is effective at reversing central sensitization deep in attacks, and it can be used parenterally repetitively to terminate status migrainosus and to aid in wean from overuse of other acute medications.

Currently, there are only 2 formulations of DHE, parenteral and nasal. The parenteral DHE can be self-injected subcutaneously or intramuscularly, but there is no commercial autoinjector. DHE can be given intravenously as well. The self-injected dose may need to be titrated to reduce nausea.

Liquid nasal DHE is currently extremely expensive. Use requires patients to construct and prime a nasal device and administer 4 sprays over 15 minutes without sniffing. Nasal stuffiness, low efficacy, and inconsistency of clinical effect limit its use, in addition to its difficult access owing to cost.

Ergotamine tartrate tablets in the currently available form do not allow for pill-cutting to reduce adverse events. As a result, for many patients, nausea prevents this from being a useful treatment. In addition, ergotamine is very habituating and can lead to both medication/ergot overuse headache and fibrotic complications.[23]

NONSPECIFIC MIGRAINE TREATMENTS

The list of nonspecific treatments for migraine with level A or B evidence includes NSAIDs, combination analgesics, neuroleptics, and opioids alone or in combination. The best evidence is for aspirin, acetaminophen, diclofenac, ibuprofen, and naproxen as well as the aspirin-acetaminophen-caffeine combination (AAC), and the sumatriptan-naproxen sodium combination. Some of these medications (acetaminophen, AAC, ibuprofen) were specifically studied in trials that restricted participation to less severe migraine attacks.[24,25]

The high-level evidence for opioids (butorphanol, codeine, and tramadol combinations) should be discounted because of evidence for the high risk of habituation and medication overuse headache, and because opioids interfere with the effectiveness of migraine-specific treatment.[26,27] In the AMPP population-based study, any opioid use in migraine was associated with a wide variety of terrible patient outcomes, including increased headache days per month, severe headache-related disability, moderate to severe depression, anxiety, cardiovascular events, and increased health care utilization.[28] Opioids should not be used in acute treatment of migraine.

Diclofenac is effective in migraine treatment with level A evidence, in both the oral 50-mg tablet form and the much faster diclofenac potassium for oral solution.[29,30] The latter was superior to the conventional tablet in a pivotal RCT.[30] Time to maximal serum concentration for the liquid form is 15 minutes. The major problem with this formulation is access, because it is only available in a brand name product in the United States. A second problem with its use is that of NSAIDs studied and currently available, because diclofenac has among the highest risk for cardiovascular complications.[29–31]

Naproxen sodium has a superior safety profile with respect to cardiovascular risk and is an excellent NSAID for acute treatment of migraine. Its combination with sumatriptan showed benefit over the individual components in 2 pivotal modified factorial studies.[32,33]

Neuroleptics are underutilized in terminating migraine acutely. Five of the top 8 acute medications for migraine ranked in a detailed structured review were neuroleptics (**Fig. 1**). They can be used alone, in conjunction with triptans and/or NSAIDs, and are effective in terminating status migrainosus.[34]

NONINVASIVE NEUROMODULATION

Noninvasive neuromodulation devices were not included in the AHS evidence assessment of acute therapies. Three noninvasive neuromodulation devices are FDA approved for acute treatment of migraine.

The FDA sets different standards for approval of noninvasive neuromodulation for headache treatment than for medications. The devices do need to be safe and

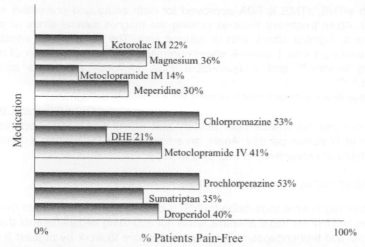

Fig. 1. Ranking of acute migraine medications by RCT result. Weighted averages of the percentages of pain free for all medications for which there were ≥2 randomized trials with the medication used as a single agent. (*From* Kelley NE, Tepper DE. Rescue therapy for acute migraine, part 3: opioids, NSAIDs, steroids, and post-discharge medications. Headache. 2012;52(3):467-82; with permission.)

effective for approval, but they do not necessarily need to achieve the study primary endpoint if other endpoints are positive. The devices do not necessarily need to have a sham-controlled trial to obtain an indication either.

All 3 approved neuromodulations are classified as having nonsignificant risk, meaning that they have minimal, no, or trivial adverse events of no consequence. The risk-benefit because of the absence of side effects shifts, and these devices should therefore be considered for patients with sensitivity to acute medications, multiple acute medication contraindications, overuse of acute medications, or inadequate benefit from standard acute migraine medications. They can be used alone or adjunctively. Many patients want to use them before medications.

EXTERNAL TRIGEMINAL NEUROSTIMULATION; TRANSCUTANEOUS SUPRAORBITAL NEUROSTIMULATION

The external trigeminal neurostimulator (e-TNS) or transcutaneous supraorbital neurostimulator stimulates the supraorbital and supratrochlear nerves and likely modulates central trigeminocervical pathways. The FDA-approved device now has an acute setting, in which the e-TNS is activated for 60 minutes to eliminate or reduce acute migraine pain. An RCT of acute benefit was the basis for FDA approval.[35]

The Dual e-TNS device also has a prevention mode, which is FDA approved for migraine prophylaxis. The prevent mode is set for 20 minutes as a nightly dose, with benefits manifested in migraine prevention by the third month of steady usage. An advantage of e-TNS is that it can be used both acutely and preventively in migraine therapy.

SINGLE-PULSE TRANSCRANIAL STIMULATION

Single-pulse transcranial stimulation (sTMS) delivers magnetic pulses to the occiput. Effectiveness is likely multifactorial. First, activation of the device terminates cortical spreading depolarization, the basis of migraine aura. Second, pulsing the magnet posteriorly modulates and inhibits thalamocortical pain pathways.

As with e-TNS, sTMS is FDA approved for both acute and preventive migraine treatment. Acute treatment involves pulsing the magnet several times at onset of an aura or a migraine attack with or without aura. The evidence for effectiveness in acute treatment was 1 positive sham-controlled RCT for termination of migraine with aura attacks,[36] and 2 open-label trials for both preventive and acute treatment.[37,38]

The preventive treatment protocol calls for 4 pulses to be administered twice daily as prophylaxis, with benefits seen in reduction of migraine days by 3 months. Because patients can use the device both acutely and preventively, FDA approval set a maximum of 17 pulses per day. Again, an advantage of sTMS is that it can be used both acutely and preventively in migraine therapy.

NONINVASIVE VAGAL NERVE STIMULATION

Noninvasive vagal nerve stimulation (nVNS) is delivered with a hand-held device that modulates and inhibits vagal afferents while not activating vagal efferents that cause bradycardia and bronchospasm. This device appears to work by at least 3 mechanisms, suppression of cortical spreading depolarization, inhibition of thalamocortical pathways, and modulation of central trigeminovascular and trigeminocervical pathways.

nVNS is administered for acute treatment of migraine with the FDA-approved protocol of 2 cycles of 2 minutes each and the option of 2 more 2-minute cycles 15 minutes later if pain has not yet resolved. This protocol was found effective for numerous outcome measures in an Italian RCT.[39] nVNS is also approved for acute treatment of episodic cluster headache and adjunctive prevention of cluster headache.

ACUTE TREATMENT OF MIGRAINE IN THE FUTURE

There are 3 areas of development for acute treatment of migraine in the future, new devices and formulations of existing medications, new classes of acute migraine drugs, and new noninvasive neuromodulation devices. Each of these areas has therapies that have completed pivotal trials, and new acute treatments are likely to be available by late 2019 or 2020.

New devices for delivering existing medications include microneedle array skin patches. One of these has already reported a positive pivotal trial for a zolmitriptan patch.[40] Another microneedle array patch of sumatriptan is planned for study as well.

A new form of sumatriptan nasal spray with a permeation enhancer has also reported a positive regulatory trial.[41] A liquid formulation of celecoxib is in development.[42] There are also studies underway of 2 new nasal sprays of DHE, one using a hydrofluoroalkane propellant and one using a dry powder.

The 2 new classes of acute migraine medications are the ditans and the gepants. Lasmiditan is a 5-HT$_{1F}$ agonist that primarily works centrally to terminate acute migraine attacks.

The 2-hour pain-free responses reported in pivotal trials of lasmiditan are similar to triptans at 28% to 38%.[43] 5-HT$_{1F}$ agonist action does not cause vasoconstriction, unlike triptans and ergots, which is an advantage for this new class of acute medication. There are central adverse events of dizziness and drowsiness, the rates of which do not exceed those seen with rizatriptan, and which appear related to its central mechanism of action. Lasmiditan was submitted to the FDA for the indication of treating migraine acutely in late 2018.

The second new class of acute migraine medications is the gepants. These are small molecule CGRP receptor antagonists, and two, ubrogepant and rimegepant, have completed positive regulatory trials for acute migraine treatment and await FDA submission.

Neither has published pivotal RCTs as of January 2019, but abstract presentations suggest 2-hour pain freedom in the 20% range and excellent tolerability. These medications block the CGRP receptor and prevent CGRP-induced vasodilation, but do not cause vasoconstriction. So far, there has been no significant safety concern with the liver metabolism of these medications.

Two additional noninvasive nonsignificant risk neuromodulation devices are in development for acute treatment of migraine. Remote nonpainful skin stimulation was effective in a proof of concept study published in 2017,[44,45] and the pivotal trial was reported in late 2018 as meeting all primary and secondary outcome measures.

This device is applied to the arm and stimulates for up to an hour to terminate migraine. It is thought to work via a conditioned pain modulation effect.

A combined occipital and supraorbital transcutaneous nerve stimulator delivered positive results in a proof of concept study for acute treatment of migraine in 2017.[44] This device is in a pivotal trial as of late 2018.

The number and variety of acute migraine therapies in development are very encouraging and suggest considerable extension of the acute armamentarium to come in the next several years.

SUMMARY

Acute treatment of migraine is important for all migraine patients and requires matching attack and patient characteristics to current therapeutic options. This matching is called stratified care and is the basis of all acute migraine treatment management.

The efficacy of acute migraine medications can be assessed with 2 PRO tools, Migraine-ACT and MTOQ. Suboptimal acute treatment is linked to increased likelihood of progression from episodic to chronic migraine, whereas maximum acute treatment was associated with lower risk of chronification. The best acute treatment results in a sustained pain-free response, one and done, for patients.

The AHS published an evidence assessment of acute migraine pharmacotherapies in 2015. They noted level A evidence for triptans, DHE, and sumatriptan/naproxen. Level A evidence is also available for medications tested specifically in less severe migraine, including acetaminophen, aspirin, AAC, and ibuprofen. Neuroleptics and most NSAIDs had level B evidence. Inadequate evidence for efficacy was noted for butalbital and most opioids, with both classes highly associated with transformation of episodic to chronic migraine, and neither class recommended for acute treatment.

Three noninvasive neuromodulation devices have FDA approval for acute treatment of migraine, external trigeminal neurostimulation, single-pulse transcranial magnetic stimulation, and nVNS. All 3 devices have nonsignificant risks and offer alternatives to medication for patients with excellent safety and tolerability.

The future for acute treatment includes new devices and formulations of existing medications, new classes of acute medications, and new noninvasive nonsignificant risk neuromodulation devices. These new therapies are anticipated over the next several years.

REFERENCES

1. Marmura MJ, Silberstein SD, Schwedt TJ. The acute treatment of migraine in adults: the American Headache Society evidence assessment of migraine pharmacotherapies. Headache 2015;55(1):3–20.

2. Tepper SJ, Dahlöf CG, Dowson A, et al. Prevalence and diagnosis of migraine in patients consulting their physician with a complaint of headache: data from the Landmark Study. Headache 2004;44(9):856–64.
3. Tfelt-Hansen P, Pascual J, Ramadan N, et al. Guidelines for controlled trials of drugs in migraine: third edition. A guide for investigators. Cephalalgia 2012; 32(1):6–38.
4. Lipton RB, Stewart WF. Acute migraine therapy: do doctors understand what patients with migraine want from therapy? Headache 1999;39(supplement 2): S20–6.
5. Dowson AJ, Tepper SJ, Baos V, et al. Identifying patients who require a change in their current acute migraine treatment: the migraine assessment of current therapy (migraine-ACT) questionnaire. Curr Med Res Opin 2004;20(7):1125–35.
6. Lipton RB, Kolodner K, Bigal ME, et al. Validity and reliability of the migraine-treatment optimization questionnaire. Cephalalgia 2009;29(7):751–9.
7. Scher AI, Stewart WF, Ricci JA, et al. Factors associated with the onset and remission of chronic daily headache in a population-based study. Pain 2003; 106(1–2):81–9.
8. Katsarava Z, Schneeweiss S, Kurth T, et al. Incidence and predictors for chronicity of headache in patients with episodic migraine. Neurology 2004;62(5): 788–90.
9. Bigal ME, Serrano D, Buse D, et al. Acute migraine medications and evolution from episodic to chronic migraine: a longitudinal population-based study. Headache 2008;48(8):1157–68.
10. Lipton RB, Fanning KM, Serrano D, et al. Ineffective acute treatment of episodic migraine is associated with new-onset chronic migraine. Neurology 2015;84(7): 688–95.
11. Serrano D, Buse DC, Manack Adams A, et al. Acute treatment optimization in episodic and chronic migraine: results of the American Migraine Prevalence and Prevention (AMPP) Study. Headache 2015;55(4):502–18.
12. Kilminster SG, Dowson AJ, Tepper SJ, et al. Reliability, validity, and clinical utility of the Migraine-ACT questionnaire. Headache 2006;46(4):553–62.
13. Tepper SJ, Baos V, Dowson AJ, et al. The migraine assessment of current therapy (migraine-ACT) questionnaire: further investigation of study results. Headache Care 2005;2:27–31.
14. Lipton RB, Manack AN, Serrano D, et al. Acute treatment optimization for migraine: results of the American Migraine Prevalence & Prevention (AMPP) Study. Headache 2012;52(5):873 (abstract).
15. Fox AW, Davis RL. Migraine chronobiology. Headache 1998;38(6):436–41.
16. Reed ML, Fanning KM, Serrano D, et al. Persistent frequent nausea is associated with progression to chronic migraine: AMPP study results. Headache 2015;55(1): 76–87.
17. Headache Classification Committee of the International Headache Society (IHS). The international classification of headache disorders, 3rd edition. Cephalalgia 2018;38(1):1–211.
18. Lipton RB, Stewart WF, Stone AM, et al. Stratified care vs step care strategies for migraine: the Disability in Strategies of Care (DISC) study: a randomized trial. JAMA 2000;284(20):2599–605.
19. Sculpher M, Millson D, Meddis D, et al. Cost-effectiveness analysis of stratified versus stepped care strategies for acute treatment of migraine: the Disability In Strategies for Care (DISC) Study. Pharmacoeconomics 2002;20(2):91–100.

20. Silberstein SD. Practice parameter—evidence-based guidelines for migraine headache (an evidence-based review): report of the quality standards Subcommittee of the American Academy of Neurology for the United States Headache Consortium. Neurology 2000;55(6):754–62.
21. Sheftell F, O'Quinn S, Watson C, et al. Low migraine headache recurrence with naratriptan: clinical parameters related to recurrence. Headache 2000;40(2): 103–10.
22. Rapoport AM, Tepper SJ, Bigal ME, et al. The triptan formulations: how to match patients and products. CNS Drugs 2003;17(6):431–47.
23. Bigal ME, Tepper SJ. Ergotamine and dihydroergotamine: a review. Curr Pain Headache Rep 2003;7(1):55–62.
24. Lipton RB, Stewart WF, Ryan RE Jr, et al. Efficacy and safety of the nonprescription combination of acetaminophen, aspirin and caffeine in alleviating headache pain of an acute migraine attack. Three double-blind, placebo-controlled trials. Arch Neurol 1998;55(2):210–7.
25. Goldstein J, Hoffman HD, Armellino JJ, et al. Treatment of severe, disabling migraine attacks in an over-the-counter population of migraine sufferers: results from three randomized, placebo-controlled studies of the combination of acetaminophen, aspirin, and caffeine. Cephalalgia 1999;19(7):684–91.
26. Jakubowski M, Levy D, Goor-Aryeh I, et al. Terminating migraine with allodynia and ongoing central sensitization using parenteral administration of COX1/COX2 inhibitors. Headache 2005;45(7):850–61.
27. Ho TW, Rodgers A, Bigal ME. Impact of recent prior opioid use on rizatriptan efficacy. A post hoc pooled analysis. Headache 2009;49(3):395–403.
28. Buse DC, Pearlman SH, Reed ML, et al. Opioid use and dependence among persons with migraine: results of the AMPP study. Headache 2012;52(1):18–36.
29. Dahlöf C, Björkman R. Diclofenac-K (50 and 100 mg) and placebo in the acute treatment of migraine. Cephalalgia 1993;13(2):117–23.
30. Diener HC, Montagna P, Gács G, et al. Efficacy and tolerability of diclofenac potassium sachets in migraine: a randomized, double-blind, cross-over study in comparison with diclofenac potassium tablets and placebo. Cephalalgia 2006; 26(5):537–47.
31. Schmidt M, Sørensen HT, Pedersen L. Diclofenac use and cardiovascular risks: series of nationwide cohort studies. BMJ 2018;362:k3426.
32. Limmroth V, Przywara S. Analgesics. Monogr Clin Neurosci. In: Diener HC, editor. Drug treatment of migraine and other headaches, vol. 17. Basel (Switzerland): Karger; 2000. p. 30–43.
33. Brandes JL, Kudrow D, Stark SR, et al. Sumatriptan-naproxen for acute treatment of migraine: a randomized trial. JAMA 2007;297(13):1443–54.
34. Kelley NE, Tepper DE. Rescue therapy for acute migraine, part 3: opioids, NSAIDs, steroids, and post-discharge medications. Headache 2012;52(3): 467–82.
35. Chou DE, Yugrakh MS, Gross G, et al. Acute treatment of migraine with e-TNS: a multi-center, double-blind, randomized, sham-controlled trial. IHC Late Breaking Abstracts, Supplement to Cephalalgia 2017;37(Supplement 1):320 (abstract).
36. Lipton RB, Dodick DW, Silberstein SD, et al. Single-pulse transcranial magnetic stimulation for acute treatment of migraine with aura: a randomised, double-blind, parallel-group, sham-controlled trial. Lancet Neurol 2010;9(4):373–80.
37. Bhola R, Kinsella E, Giffin N, et al. Single-pulse transcranial magnetic stimulation (sTMS) for the acute treatment of migraine: evaluation of outcome data for the UK post market pilot program. J Headache Pain 2015;16:535.

38. Starling AJ, Tepper SJ, Marmura MJ, et al. A multicenter, prospective, single arm, open label, observational study of sTMS for migraine prevention (ESPOUSE Study). Cephalalgia 2018;38(6):1038–48.
39. Tassorelli C, Grazzi L, de Tommaso M, et al. Noninvasive vagus nerve stimulation as acute therapy for migraine: the randomized PRESTO study. Neurology 2018; 91(4):e364–73.
40. Spierings ELH, Brandes JL, Kudrow DB, et al. Randomized, double-blind, placebo-controlled, parallel-group, multi-center study of the safety and efficacy of ADAM zolmitriptan for the acute treatment of migraine. Cephalalgia 2018;38(2): 215–24.
41. Lipton RB, Munjal S, Brand-Schieber E, et al. DFN-02 (sumatriptan 10 mg with a permeation enhancer) nasal spray vs placebo in the acute treatment of migraine: a double-blind, placebo-controlled study. Headache 2018;58(5):676–87.
42. Munjal S, Bennett A. Efficacy and safety of DFN-15, an oral liquid formulation of celecoxib, in adults with migraine: a multicenter, randomized,placebo-controlled, double-blind, crossover study. Neuropsychiatr Dis Treat 2017;13:2797–802.
43. Kuca B, Silberstein SD, Wietecha L, et al. Lasmiditan is an effective acute treatment for migraine: a phase 3 randomized study. Neurology 2018;91(24): e2222–32.
44. Hering-Hanit R. A prospective, randomized, single blind, parallel-group, placebo controlled clinical study to evaluate the short-term effectiveness of combined occipital and supraorbital transcutaneous nerve stimulation (OS-TNS) in treating migraine. Cephalalgia 2017;37(Suppl 1):73 (abstract).
45. Yarnitsky D, Volokh L, Ironi A, et al. Nonpainful remote electrical stimulation alleviates episodic migraine pain. Neurology 2017;88(13):1250–5.

Migraine in the Emergency Department

Benjamin W. Friedman, MD, MS[a,b,]*

KEYWORDS

- Migraine • Emergency department • Neuroimaging • Medication

KEY POINTS

- Diagnostic testing is of limited value among patients with migraine who present to an emergency department.
- Various nonopioid, disease-specific treatments are available for patients who present to an emergency department with migraine headache and associated features.
- Emergency physicians should recognize that the acute migraine presentation is part of an underlying disorder; care should be geared to the underlying headache disorder in addition to the acute attack.

OVERVIEW

Use of an emergency department (ED) for management of migraine is common.[1] When considered on a national level, many ED visits for migraine result in suboptimal care, with overexposure to unnecessary neuroimaging[2] and medication choices that are not evidence-based.[1] On the other hand, various effective parenteral therapies are available for use in the ED and are being used increasingly.[1] When care is optimized, EDs can deliver fast and effective headache relief expeditiously 24 hours of the day. This article will serve as a guide for emergency practitioners seeking to optimize their care of patients with migraine and for those health care providers from other specialties who wish to communicate more effectively with their EDs to improve the experience of patients with migraine who need emergency care.

EPIDEMIOLOGY

Headache is the fifth most common chief complaint among patients visiting US EDs, accounting for nearly 4 million patient visits annually.[3] Of these headache visits, most are attributable to a primary headache disorder. Migraine is the most common

a Department of Emergency Medicine, Albert Einstein College of Medicine, 1300 Morris Park Avenue, New York, NY 10461, USA; b Montefiore Medical Center, Bronx, NY, USA
* Department of Emergency Medicine, Albert Einstein College of Medicine, 1300 Morris Park Avenue, New York, NY 10461.
E-mail address: bwfriedmanmd@gmail.com

Neurol Clin 37 (2019) 743–752
https://doi.org/10.1016/j.ncl.2019.07.005
0733-8619/19/© 2019 Elsevier Inc. All rights reserved.
neurologic.theclinics.com

identifiable headache diagnosis, and, because it is frequently underdiagnosed in the ED, probably accounts for a substantial percentage of all ED headaches.

For many patients with migraine, the ED is the destination of choice when the migraine is severe, persistent, or refractory to usual medications. Some patients, particularly those with worsening or intensifying headache, present to the ED because of concern for a secondary cause of headache. For some patients, the ED is the primary source of headache care. Ease of access to alternative health care settings or providers can, for many patients, influence the necessity of the ED visit.

When considering the high population prevalence of migraine, use of the ED for management of migraine is relatively uncommon. Fewer than 10% of all Americans with migraine report a headache visit to an ED or an urgent care within a 12-month period.[4] Risk factors for an ED visit for migraine are analogous to other chronic diseases: lower socioeconomic status, worse underlying disease, and psychiatric comorbidities (**Box 1**). Although socioeconomic status is beyond the skill of a physician to improve, optimizing the care of the underlying migraine disorder and treating psychiatric comorbidities may lower the risk of an ED visit.

The role of the ED for the delivery of migraine care depends on the community it serves. Ideally, migraine patients would be medically optimized in the outpatient setting, and require emergent visits only rarely. Invariably, some patients with migraine will experience headache and associated symptoms refractory to the treatments available in their medicine cabinet. In some communities, effective parenteral therapy for migraine may be available in a nonemergent setting. In these communities, the ED would only be necessary during nights and weekends.

An ED visit is an expensive alternative to outpatient care, although in closed or capitated health care systems, an ED visit may make the most economic sense, because of relatively low marginal costs to see 1 additional patient. Often, an ED visit may be associated with long wait times to be seen, a chaotic, noisy environment, and suboptimal care; this may be the most compelling reason to avoid unnecessary ED visits.

Health care providers who care for migraine patients should minimize their risk of an ED visit by optimizing the medical care of their patient and discussing contingencies for when abortive medication is ineffective. Health care providers who treat many patients with migraine should discuss how best to coordinate care with their local emergency providers.

APPROACH TO DIAGNOSTIC WORKUP

For many patients with migraine who arrive in an ED, the diagnosis is apparent, because the patient reports they are having their typical migraine attack, or an

---

Box 1
Risk factors associated with emergency department use

History of ED use

Lower socioeconomic strata

Worse underlying migraine disorder

Depression

Headache managed by headache specialist

Data from Friedman BW, Serrano D, Reed M, Diamond M, Lipton RB. Use of the emergency department for severe headache. A population-based study. Headache 2009;49(1):21-30.

exacerbation of a recurrent headache disorder that clearly meets established migraine criteria.

More challenging are those patients who present atypically, or with a headache that in someway differs from their usual pattern. For these patients, the appropriate diagnostic pathway is uncertain. The mere fact that the patient is in an ED connotes a higher risk of a pathologic process, a fact of which emergency physicians are cognizant. Well-validated clinical decision rules are available to identify which patients need a diagnostic workup among those who present with a nontraumatic headache that rapidly peaked in intensity[5] or a headache in the setting of head trauma[6] (**Boxes 2 and 3**). It is unclear when to perform a diagnostic workup when the patient presents with a headache that does not fit a pattern or for whom the clinical decision rules are not applicable. Some examples of these difficult-to-categorize headaches are the following: a headache that meets probable migraine criteria, although without an established headache history, or when the headache seems like previous migraine attacks, but it did not respond to usual medication, or lasted longer that usual, or was more intense than usual, or differed in laterality or associated symptoms. For these headaches, it is often unclear whether diagnostic workup is indicated. Although the risk of a pathologic process in younger patients is low, it is clear that pathologic processes occasionally present subtly.

Over the past few decades, there has been a trend in US EDs to order more and more diagnostic neuroimaging.[2] Because the number of pathologic findings remained constant, the number of normal scans has increased markedly, a problematic finding because of increased costs to the health care system, increased throughput time in already overcrowded EDs, and the small but plausible increased risk associated with radiation dose. In the absence of evidence, the author recommends treating headaches that seem like migraine as migraine. Response to treatment does not exclude pathologic diagnoses, but re-evaluating patients after treatment allows one to put the headache into better perspective. After treatment, headaches often seem more in keeping with previous attacks.

Once the diagnosis of migraine has been established, emergent diagnostic testing is of little value. With the exception of a pregnancy test, which may help guide treatment, laboratory analyses do not add appreciably to treatment of a migraine patient. Patients with profound nausea and vomiting may present with marked dehydration and electrolyte abnormalities, but these patients are usually apparent after conclusion of the history and physical examination.

Box 2
Clinical features associated with pathologic intracranial pathologies

Risk factors for intracranial hemorrhage following head trauma.[6] The absence of these features effectively excludes the diagnosis of intracranial hemorrhage among nonelderly adults who are not using coagulation inhibitors.

Seizure
GCS less than 15 2 hours after injury
Suspected open or depressed skull fracture
Any sign of basilar skull fracture
$\geq$2 episodes of vomiting
Retrograde amnesia $\geq$30 minutes to the event
Dangerous mechanism (pedestrian struck, ejected from vehicle, fall >3 feet or >5 stairs)

Data from Stiell IG, Wells GA, Vandemheen K, Clement C, Lesiuk H, Laupacis A, et al. The Canadian CT Head Rule for patients with minor head injury. Lancet 2001;357(9266):1391-6.

Box 3
Clinical features associated with pathologic intracranial pathologies

Risk factors for nontraumatic subarachnoid hemorrhage among adults with a headache that peaks in intensity within 60 minutes.[5] The absence of these features effectively excludes the diagnosis of subarachnoid hemorrhage.
    Symptom of neck pain or stiffness
    Age greater than 40 years
    Witnessed loss of consciousness
    Onset during exertion
    Thunderclap headache
    Limited neck flexion on examination

Data from Perry JJ, Sivilotti MLA, Sutherland J, Hohl CM, Emond M, Calder LA, et al. Validation of the Ottawa Subarachnoid Hemorrhage Rule in patients with acute headache. CMAJ 2017;189(45):E1379-E85.

Some have argued that a precise diagnosis does not help an emergency health care provider manage patients with acute headache. Once malignant secondary causes of headache have been excluded from the differential diagnosis, the most important question is: to which medication is this patient most likely to respond, not, what is this patient's most likely diagnosis. Because of the high prevalence of migraine and probable migraine among ED cohorts, it is not surprising that this approach has gained traction; the reason that migraine therapy often works among ED headache patients is that many of these patients have migraine. Additionally, it has become increasingly clear that nonmigraine primary headaches, including tension-type headache[7] and cluster,[8] are likely to respond to commonly used parenteral migraine therapies. Finally, less common primary headaches often do not have specific evidence-based treatment regimens. Therefore, there is some truth to the argument against assigning a precise primary headache diagnosis in the ED. However, optimized therapy does require assigning a diagnosis, particularly among headaches that prove more difficult to treat, because subtleties in treatment depend on this diagnosis. As will be discussed in the next section, corticosteroids are an example of a medication that should be administered to most ED patients with migraine, but should not be administered to patients without migraine.

TREATMENT

A 1 size fits all approach to treatment is generally not appropriate. ED patients with migraine have a variety of needs and experiences, which can help the emergency provider tailor the approach to treatment.

Some migraine patients may be adequately treated with oral medication. In urban EDs, up to one-third of headache patients report that they have not taken any medication at all, not even acetaminophen or ibuprofen, before presenting to the ED.[9] For some of these patients, treatment with an oral nonsteroidal anti-inflammatory drug (NSAID) may be appropriate, both to alleviate the pain, and to demonstrate to the patient how to alleviate similar pain in the future. Patients may report a history of good response to an oral triptan; for these patients, treating them with what has worked before is likely to work again.

Emergency providers tend to have a low threshold for insertion of an intravenous (IV) catheter and administration of IV fluids to migraine patients. This strategy is intuitively sensible for a disease in which nausea, vomiting, and anorexia are exceedingly common. However, thoughtless administration of IV fluids may not result in better outcomes.[10] IV fluids should be reserved for those patients with clinical signs or laboratory values indicative of dehydration. It is unknown whether isotonic solutions are better for migraine patients than normal saline solution.

Various parenteral medications are available for treatment of acute migraine (**Table 1**). Although few of these parenteral treatments are US Food and Drug Administration (FDA) approved specifically for migraine, evidence from randomized trials and lower-quality evidence from case series and retrospective reviews have resulted in clinical experience with dozens of parenteral medications from a surprisingly wide array of medication classes. When choosing among these medications, the provider should use patient experience as a guide, with the additional goal of improving that individual patient's long-term migraine outcomes. Some medications, such as opioids and barbiturates, may have helped the patient previously, but are far more likely to worsen migraine disease trajectory.[11]

The next several sections will discuss the many medications that are commonly used, or mentioned, for patients with migraine, and the evidence supporting efficacy.

Antidopaminergic Medications

Commonly used in US EDs and elsewhere, the antidopaminergic medications are highly efficacious and are considered first-line treatment.[12] Multiple different antidopaminergic medications have been shown to be efficacious for acute migraine.

When treating patients with migraine, emergency physicians often combine parenteral medications, sometimes with the goal of increasing efficacy and sometimes to minimize medication adverse effects. Well-described extrapyramidal adverse effects may occur after administration of these antidopaminergic medications and should cause the clinician to consider use of anticholinergic medication such as diphenhydramine to prevent these symptoms.[13] Irreversible motor symptoms have not been reported after isolated doses of antidopaminergic medications for acute headache. Akathisia on the other hand is exceedingly common, having been reported in up to one-third of patients who receive IV prochlorperazine.[14]

Table 1 Parenteral migraine treatment	
Medication	**Dose**
Antidopaminergic medications	
Metoclopramide	10 mg intravenously
Prochlorperazine	10 mg intravenously
Droperidol	2.5 mg intravenously
Haloperidol	5 mg intravenously
Chlorpromazine	10 mg intravenously
Migraine-specific medication	
Sumatriptan	6 mg subcutaneously
Dihydroergotamine	1 mg intravenously
COX inhibitors	
Ketorolac	15 mg intravenously
Acetylsalicylic acid	1000 mg
Other	
Dexamethasone	10 mg intravenously
Magnesium	1–2 mg intravenously
Propofol	30–40 mg bolus, followed by 10–20 mg bolus

Migraine-Specific Medication

Subcutaneous sumatriptan is highly efficacious for acute migraine, with a number needed to treat of 2 for headache relief and 3.2 for sustained headache freedom when compared with placebo.[15] When compared head to head with IV antidopaminergic medications, subcutaneous sumatriptan is generally less efficacious than the antidopaminergic medications, and thus has not been used with much frequency in the ED setting.[12] On average, patients with migraine wait several days before presenting to the ED for management of their headache; for this reason too, sumatriptan is usually not a first-choice medication, as efficacy of sumatriptan is inversely associated with headache duration.[16] Unpleasant adverse effects, including chest pain, may also complicate administration in the ED.[17] Use of subcutaneous sumatriptan should be limited to those patients who have reported good results with it previously.

Oral second-generation triptans can play a role for certain patients who can tolerate oral medication and who do not need IV access for hydration. Although not tested specifically in the ED setting, highly effective oral medications can save nursing resources and may improve throughput times.

IV dihydroergotamine should not be used in patients with cardiovascular risk factors, and it interacts poorly with a variety of medications. However, when administered intravenously and in conjunction with an antiemetic antidopaminergic agent, this medication is also useful, particularly for patients who do not respond to first- or second-line therapies.

Cyclooxygenase Inhibitors

Parenteral NSAIDs are highly efficacious for migraine and may be used as monotherapy or in conjunction with one of the other classes of medication discussed previously.[12] Similarly, acetyl salicylic acid may be used as either monotherapy or in combination with other treatments.[12]

Magnesium

More than any other medication discussed in this article, there is still a tremendous amount of uncertainty as to whether magnesium is of benefit for patients with acute migraine.[12] Widely varying results from clinical trials make summary statements difficult. Existing evidence does not support the use of magnesium as a first- or second-line treatment. If it does have a role for acute migraine, this is most likely to be in migraine patients with aura.[12]

Antiepileptic Medications

Although mechanistically appealing and useful for preventive therapy, antiepileptic medications do not yet have a role to play in the acute management of migraine.[12]

Intranasal Lidocaine

Targeting the sphenopalatine ganglion with intranasal application of lidocaine is an appealing concept but one that has not consistently demonstrated benefit.[18] This may be related to technical difficulties, as the sphenopalatine ganglion is not easily accessible. Proprietary devices designed to facilitate the application do not achieve the desired outcome.[19]

Anesthetic Agents

Ketamine, used at subanesthetic analgesic doses, does not appear to be effective for acute migraine.[20] Some data suggest propofol may be effective in the short term.[21] Whether that relief can be sustained is not yet known. Because safety for this indication has not yet been established, and because of increased monitoring requirements, propofol should not yet be used as a first- or second-line treatment for acute migraine.[12] It should be reserved for patients who have failed to improve with more standard medication and who are being considered for admission to the hospital.

Nerve Blocks

Increasingly, nerve blocks are playing a role in the management of acute migraine as evidence demonstrating efficacy increases and clinicians become more familiar with these techniques (**Fig. 1**). Greater occipital nerve block is more efficacious than sham therapy, and may play a role in selected ED patients.[22] Optimal technique is not yet known; it may be that numbing the greater occipital nerve ipsilateral to the headache may be sufficient. Alternatively, a bilateral approach, or an around-the-skull approach that targets all scalp innervation, may provide superior analgesia.

Corticosteroids

Administering corticosteroids in the ED will decrease the frequency and intensity of headache relapse in the days after ED discharge.[23] Unfortunately, the benefit is modest, with a number needed to treat of nearly 10, and relapse is difficult to predict. Available data also do not indicate the optimal dose, route, or duration of therapy.

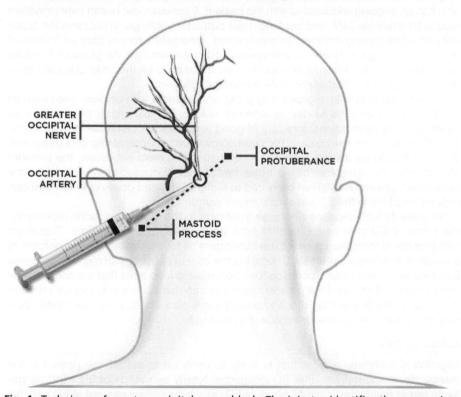

Fig. 1. Technique of greater occipital nerve block. The injector identifies the appropriate location using landmarks on the patient's head. The medial landmark is the occipital protuberance. The lateral landmark is the mastoid process. Using these landmarks to form a line, the injector identifies the correct location, which is one-third of the distance from the occipital protuberance along this line (two-thirds of the distance away from the mastoid process).

Some data suggest that IV dexamethasone, administered at the same time as the initial abortive treatment, may begin to improve outcomes within a few hours.[24] Clinicians should weigh the potential benefit versus known adverse effects and make the decision to administer on a patient-by-patient basis.

Opioids

Opioids play an important role in the management of acute, severe pain and are unparalleled in their ability to bridge patients with acute painful processes to definitive care. Opioids are less useful in chronic recurrent pain syndromes, where bridging therapy is less applicable. In previous decades, opioids were commonly used as first-line therapy for acute migraine.[1] More recently, as evidence supporting alternate therapies has burgeoned, use of opioids as first-line therapy is beginning to diminish. It is now clear that use of opioids for treatment of acute migraine is associated with less headache relief, more adverse effects, longer throughput times, and less overall satisfaction with care.[25] When being considered for patients with migraine, opioids should be reserved for patients with persistent severe pain despite several other appropriate treatments.

The Difficult Migraine Patient

As a chronic recurrent ailment, migraine is best managed by a health care provider who has an ongoing relationship with the patient. Because most health care providers cannot be available 24/7, and because most outpatient settings do not have the capability of administering intravenous medication, emergency rooms play an important role to fill these gaps. However, emergency rooms cannot take the place of a regular health care provider. Patients who exclusively use the ED for their migraine care must be encouraged to obtain appropriate outpatient follow-up.

At times, patients with migraine may insist on treatment with opioids. The rationale for the request may be related to adverse reactions experienced previously after receiving other medications, a history of good response to opioids, or to a nontherapeutic euphoria from the opioids. Because opioids are suboptimal migraine treatment, their use should be discouraged. For most patients in most situations, the provider should insist on using one of the other treatments discussed previously, with the caveat that patients should not be forced to suffer. Repeated doses of parenteral opioids for migraine in the ED are almost never warranted.

For patients with migraine who seek treatment in the ED for headache repeatedly, the focus of ED care needs to shift from acute relief to ongoing care. Treatment with parenteral therapeutics should be contingent on follow-up care with an outpatient provider with relevant expertise. Optimizing the care of patients with migraine who visit EDs frequently may require coordination of care using resources that are not available during a busy shift: developing patient-specific treatment plans may require an interdisciplinary efforts involving those knowledgeable about social and psychiatric barriers to care as well as relevant medical specialists.

Follow-up Care

Migraine is a chronic ailment that is likely to continue to plague the patient in the weeks, days, and months after ED discharge. Nearly two-thirds of ED migraine patients report headache within 48 hours of ED discharge.[26] Fifty percent of ED patients report functional impairment within 48 hours of ED discharge.[26] Patients frequently suffer after-shock headaches during the week after ED discharge. On average, patients report 3 headache days during this week.[24] Often, these headache are as severe as the original headache that brought the patient into the ED. Patients should understand that their risk of short- and long-term headache recurrence, be provided with the tools to manage their headache, and assisted with access to ongoing care. In some health care systems, outpatient appointments may be more difficult to obtain; in these situations, emergency physicians may need to prescribe abortive therapies that will serve patients until they can access definitive care.

SUMMARY

The ED is a valuable resource that can provide expeditious migraine care at all hours of the day and night. In the ED, a variety of highly effective therapies can be provided in a monitored setting. Health care providers who work in the ED, and those who have patients who use the ED, should coordinate efforts to optimize the experience of the many migraine patients who are forced to visit an ED with headache.

REFERENCES

1. Friedman BW, West J, Vinson DR, et al. Current management of migraine in US emergency departments: an analysis of the National Hospital Ambulatory Medical Care Survey. Cephalalgia 2015;35(4):301–9.
2. Gilbert JW, Johnson KM, Larkin GL, et al. Atraumatic headache in US emergency departments: recent trends in CT/MRI utilisation and factors associated with severe intracranial pathology. Emerg Med J 2012;29(7):576–81.
3. Rui P, Kang K. National Hospital Ambulatory Medical Care Survey: 2015 Emergency Department Summary Tables. Available at: http://www.cdc.gov/nchs/data/ahcd/nhamcs_emergency/2015_ed_web_tables.pdf. Accessed July 26.
4. Friedman BW, Serrano D, Reed M, et al. Use of the emergency department for severe headache. A population-based study. Headache 2009;49(1):21–30.
5. Perry JJ, Sivilotti MLA, Sutherland J, et al. Validation of the Ottawa subarachnoid hemorrhage rule in patients with acute headache. CMAJ 2017;189(45):E1379–85.
6. Stiell IG, Wells GA, Vandemheen K, et al. The Canadian CT head rule for patients with minor head injury. Lancet 2001;357(9266):1391–6.
7. Friedman BW, Adewunmi V, Campbell C, et al. A randomized trial of intravenous ketorolac versus intravenous metoclopramide plus diphenhydramine for tension-type and all nonmigraine, noncluster recurrent headaches. Ann Emerg Med 2013;62(4):311–8.e4.
8. Rozen TD. Olanzapine as an abortive agent for cluster headache. Headache 2001;41(8):813–6.
9. Friedman BW, Greenwald P, Bania TC, et al. Randomized trial of IV dexamethasone for acute migraine in the emergency department. Neurology 2007;69(22):2038–44.
10. Balbin JE, Nerenberg R, Baratloo A, et al. Intravenous fluids for migraine: a post hoc analysis of clinical trial data. Am J Emerg Med 2016;34(4):713–6.
11. Bigal ME, Serrano D, Buse D, et al. Acute migraine medications and evolution from episodic to chronic migraine: a longitudinal population-based study. Headache 2008;48(8):1157–68.
12. Orr SL, Friedman BW, Christie S, et al. Management of adults with acute migraine in the emergency department: the American Headache Society evidence assessment of parenteral pharmacotherapies. Headache 2016;56(6):911–40.
13. D'Souza RS, Mercogliano C, Ojukwu E, et al. Effects of prophylactic anticholinergic medications to decrease extrapyramidal side effects in patients taking acute antiemetic drugs: a systematic review and meta-analysis. Emerg Med J 2018;35(5):325–31.

14. Vinson DR, Migala AF, Quesenberry CP Jr. Slow infusion for the prevention of akathisia induced by prochlorperazine: a randomized controlled trial. J Emerg Med 2001;20(2):113–9.
15. Oldman AD, Smith LA, McQuay HJ, et al. Pharmacological treatments for acute migraine: quantitative systematic review. Pain 2002;97(3):247–57.
16. Burstein R, Collins B, Jakubowski M. Defeating migraine pain with triptans: a race against the development of cutaneous allodynia. Ann Neurol 2004;55(1):19–26.
17. Akpunonu BE, Mutgi AB, Federman DJ, et al. Subcutaneous sumatriptan for treatment of acute migraine in patients admitted to the emergency department: a multicenter study. Ann Emerg Med 1995;25(4):464–9.
18. Avcu N, Dogan NO, Pekdemir M, et al. Intranasal lidocaine in acute treatment of migraine: a randomized controlled trial. Ann Emerg Med 2017;69(6):743–51.
19. Schaffer JT, Hunter BR, Ball KM, et al. Noninvasive sphenopalatine ganglion block for acute headache in the emergency department: a randomized placebo-controlled trial. Ann Emerg Med 2015;65(5):503–10.
20. Zitek T, Gates M, Pitotti C, et al. A comparison of headache treatment in the emergency department: prochlorperazine versus ketamine. Ann Emerg Med 2018; 71(3):369–377 e1.
21. Moshtaghion H, Heiranizadeh N, Rahimdel A, et al. The efficacy of propofol vs. subcutaneous sumatriptan for treatment of acute migraine headaches in the emergency department: a double-blinded clinical trial. Pain Pract 2015;15(8): 701–5.
22. Friedman BW, Mohamed S, Robbins MS, et al. A randomized, sham-controlled trial of bilateral greater occipital nerve blocks with bupivacaine for acute migraine patients refractory to standard emergency department treatment with metoclopramide. Headache 2018;58(9):1427–34.
23. Colman I, Friedman BW, Brown MD, et al. Parenteral dexamethasone for acute severe migraine headache: meta-analysis of randomised controlled trials for preventing recurrence. BMJ 2008;336(7657):1359–61.
24. Latev A, Friedman BW, Irizarry E, et al. A randomized trial of a long-acting depot corticosteroid versus dexamethasone to prevent headache recurrence among patients with acute migraine who are discharged from an emergency department. Ann Emerg Med 2019;73(2):141–9.
25. Friedman BW, Irizarry E, Solorzano C, et al. Randomized study of IV prochlorperazine plus diphenhydramine vs IV hydromorphone for migraine. Neurology 2017; 89(20):2075–82.
26. Friedman BW, Hochberg ML, Esses D, et al. Recurrence of primary headache disorders after emergency department discharge: frequency and predictors of poor pain and functional outcomes. Ann Emerg Med 2008;52(6):696–704.

Preventive Treatment for Episodic Migraine

Simy K. Parikh, MD, Stephen D. Silberstein, MD*

KEYWORDS

- Headache • Episodic migraine • Diagnosis • Prevention • Treatment
- CGRP monoclonal antibodies • Transcutaneous electrical nerve stimulation
- Single-pulse transcranial magnetic stimulator

KEY POINTS

- Episodic migraine is a debilitating condition that requires the use of preventive (prophylactic) management to reduce the frequency, duration, or severity of attacks.
- There is evidence for the efficacy and use of calcitonin gene-related peptide monoclonal antibodies, a transcutaneous electrical nerve stimulation device (Cefaly), and a single-pulse transcranial magnetic stimulator (SpringTMS), for preventive treatment of episodic migraine.
- In 2012, guideline updates were made to the major medication classes recommended for preventive episodic migraine treatment.

INTRODUCTION

Migraine is a disabling central nervous system disorder characterized by moderate or severe head pain. Migraine is prevalent; it is the third most common disorder in the world.[1] It is the third leading cause of worldwide disability of males and females younger than age 50 years[2] and it incurs substantial resource utilization, health care costs, and indirect costs from reduced work productivity.[3,4] The prevalence of migraine is 12% in the general population. One to 2% of the population have chronic migraine, or migraine occurring more than 15 d/mo for more than 3 months.[5,6] About

Financial Disclosure Information: S.K. Parikh has received research support from Groten Family Fund. S.D. Silberstein has the following financial disclosures: As a consultant and/or advisory panel member, Dr S.D. Silberstein receives, or has received, honoraria from Abide Therapeutics; Alder Biopharmaceuticals; Allergan, Inc; Amgen; Avanir Pharmaceuticals, Inc; Biohaven Pharmaceuticals; Cefaly; Curelator, Inc; Dr Reddy's Laboratories; Egalet Corporation; GlaxoSmithKline Consumer Health Holdings, LLC; eNeura, Inc; electroCore Medical, LLC; Lilly USA, LLC; Medscape, LLC; NINDS; Satsuma Pharmaceuticals; Supernus Pharmaceuticals, Inc; Teva Pharmaceuticals; Theranica; and Trigemina, Inc.
Jefferson Headache Center, Thomas Jefferson University Hospital, Thomas Jefferson University, 900 Walnut Street, Suite #200, Philadelphia, PA 19107, USA
* Corresponding author.

E-mail address: stephen.silberstein@jefferson.edu

10% of the population have episodic migraine, or migraine occurring less than 15 d/mo. Episodic migraine is debilitating. Nearly a third of patients with episodic migraine have migraine occurring more than once a week, whereas 8% experience "high-frequency" episodic migraine with attacks occurring 10 to 14 d/mo.[3,7] The frequency of episodic migraine can decrease, remain unchanged, or escalate; every year, about 2.5% of patients with episodic migraine develop chronic migraine (previously known as transformed migraine).[8–10] Counseling to treat obesity (body mass index >30) and snoring, mitigate stress, and avoid acute medication overuse (especially opioids and barbiturates) should be given to all patients with episodic migraine to help reduce risk of chronic migraine.[8,9] It is unclear whether preventive therapy for episodic migraine can modify one's risk for transformed migraine[11]; however, it can help manage symptoms. This review discusses principles of migraine preventive treatment and then focuses on evidence-based preventive treatment options for people with episodic migraine.

Pharmacologic treatment of migraine may be acute (abortive) or preventive (prophylactic), and patients with frequent or severe migraine often require both approaches. Preventive therapy is used to reduce the frequency, duration, or severity of attacks. Additional benefits include enhancing the response to acute treatments and improving a patient's socioeconomic function.[12] US, Canadian, and European Guidelines have established circumstances in which preventive treatment is warranted (**Box 1**).[13–18] Because a migraine preventive drug is considered successful if it reduces migraine attack frequency by at least 50% within 3 months, a migraine diary is highly recommended for treatment evaluation.[13,15]

If preventive therapy is indicated, the agent should be chosen based on the drug's relative efficacy in randomized double-blind, placebo-controlled trials; its side effect (SE) profile; and the patient's preference, and coexistent and comorbid conditions.[19] For sustained benefit, preventive therapy should be used for 6 months, with the option to continue to 12 months.[20]

UPDATES IN PREVENTIVE THERAPY FOR EPISODIC MIGRAINE

Migraine-specific treatment options are now available for the preventive treatment of episodic migraine. Three calcitonin gene-related peptide monoclonal antibodies (CGRP mAbs) were approved in 2018 for the preventive treatment of episodic migraine. A noninvasive transcutaneous electrical nerve stimulation device, Cefaly

---

Box 1
Summary of criteria for starting migraine preventive treatment

1. Recurring migraine that significantly interferes with the patient's daily routine despite acute treatment. For example, two or more migraine attacks/month impairing function for ≥3 days or infrequent migraine attacks that produce profound disability during each attack.

2. Failure of, contraindication to, or intolerable side effects to acute medications.

3. Acute medication overuse or the risk of developing acute medication overuse.

4. Special circumstances, such as hemiplegic migraine or migraine attacks with a risk of permanent neurologic injury.

5. High-frequency episodic migraine or a pattern of increasing migraine attacks over time.

6. Patient preference, or patient desire to have as few acute attacks as possible.

(CEFALY-Technology, Seraing, Belgium), was approved for preventive episodic migraine treatment in 2014. A noninvasive single-pulse transcranial magnetic stimulator (sTMS), SpringTMS (eNeura, Inc, Baltimore, MD, USA), was approved for preventive migraine treatment in 2017. In 2012, the American Academy of Neurology (AAN) and the American Headache Society (AHS) provided evidence-based updates to the major medication classes recommended for preventive episodic migraine treatment, which include ß-adrenergic blockers, antidepressants, anticonvulsants, angiotensin receptor blockers, and angiotensin-converting enzyme inhibitors.

SPECIFIC EPISODIC MIGRAINE PREVENTIVE AGENTS
Calcitonin Gene-Related Peptide Monoclonal Antibodies

CGRP is a 37–amino acid neuropeptide. It was first described in 1983; the name "calcitonin gene-related peptide" derives from the discovery that CGRP is produced in neural tissue via alternate processing of the same gene that produces a precursor to calcitonin in the thyroid.[21] CGRP is involved in nociception, which is transmitted by the Aδ and C peripheral nerve fibers.[22–24] Thinly myelinated, medium diameter Aδ fibers are responsible for the transmission of acute pain, whereas unmyelinated small-diameter C fibers are responsible for lingering or burning pain.[22] In migraine, CGRP-independent activation of meningeal C fibers cause C fibers to release CGRP into the dura; CGRP then binds to receptors on nearby trigeminovascular Aδ fibers, stimulating transmission of acute pain.[23–29] CGRP mAbs are thought to selectively inhibit Aδ afferents, specifically inhibiting Aδ input to high-threshold neurons that transduce mechanical stimuli into nociceptive signals.[28,29] However, they do not act on wide dynamic-range dorsal horn neurons, which are thought to have a role in central sensitization, and do not directly act on C fibers.[28,29] From this reasoning, CGRP mAbs would be effective in people with episodic migraine whose pain is dependent on acute pain signals from high-threshold neurons activated by meningeal Aδ fibers nociceptors, but may not be effective in people whose migraine pain is independent of these signals.[28,29]

Three CGRP mAbs were approved in 2018 for the preventive treatment of episodic migraine (Table 1): erenumab-aooe (Aimovig; AMG334), fremanezumab-vfrm (Ajovy; TEV-48125), and galcanezumab-gnlm (Emgality; LY2951742), which are subsequently referred to as erenumab, fremanezumab, and galcanezumab in this review. Another CGRP mAb, eptinizumab (ALD403), is an intravenous formulation that is currently in phase 3 trials.

Table 1		
CGRP mAbs for the preventive treatment of episodic migraine		
CGRP mAb	**Administration**	**Dose**
Erenumab-aooe (Aimovig; AMG334)	Subcutaneous prefilled autoinjections	140 mg, or 70 mg every 28 d
Fremanezumab-vfrm (Ajovy; TEV-48125)	Subcutaneous prefilled syringe at either the 225-mg monthly dose or 675-mg quarterly dose	225 mg every 28 d, or 675 mg every 3 mo
Galcanezumab-gnlm (Emgality; LY2951742)	Subcutaneous prefilled autoinjector or prefilled syringe	Initial loading dose of 240 mg followed by a maintenance 120-mg dose every 28 d
Eptinizumab (ALD4030)	Intravenous infusion	To be determined; ongoing phase 3 trial

Erenumab

Erenumab is a human mAb that binds to and antagonizes the functioning of the CGRP receptor. It is delivered subcutaneously with a prefilled autoinjector. It was approved on May 17, 2018, by the US Food and Drug Administration (FDA) for the preventive treatment of episodic and chronic migraine.

The 6-month phase 3 STRIVE trial and the 3-month phase 3 ARISE trial assessed erenumab's efficacy in patients with episodic migraine (4–14 migraine d/mo).[30,31] In the ARISE trial patients received monthly doses of subcutaneous placebo or 70-mg erenumab, whereas in the STRIVE trial patients received monthly doses of subcutaneous placebo, 70 mg or 140 mg of erenumab.[30,31] Both trials showed a significant difference in migraine frequency reduction with erenumab 70 mg compared with placebo.[30,31] The STRIVE trial showed a significant difference in migraine frequency reduction with erenumab 140 mg compared with placebo; whereas patients treated with 140 mg compared with 70 mg had more numerical improvement in migraine frequency, there was no statistically significant difference.[31] In addition, both trials showed that erenumab resulted in a significant reduction in the number of days of acute migraine-specific medication (ergots or triptan) use.[30,31] The overall safety profile of erenumab was similar to that of placebo, with injection-site pain and constipation noted as the most prevalent SEs.[30,31] One-year efficacy and 3-year safety and tolerability interim data analysis of a 5-year open-label extension study (OLE) were collected.[32,33] At 1 year, efficacy at 70 mg was sustained without the development of tachyphylaxis.[32] Three-year safety and tolerability data, including 235 patients who received 140-mg erenumab for greater than or equal to 1 year, showed a safety profile of the 70-mg and 140-mg doses consistent with the ARISE and STRIVE trials, with common SEs in the OLE reported as respiratory tract infections and back pain, and no increase in cardiovascular events.[33]

Erenumab is also effective in patients who have failed multiple preventive treatments because of lack of efficacy or intolerable SEs. The 12-week phase 3b LIBERTY study assessed the efficacy of erenumab 140 mg as compared with placebo in patients with episodic migraine who had failed two to four preventive treatments; results showed a statistically significant reduction in monthly migraine days (MMD) and number of days of migraine-specific acute medication intake.[34]

In summary, erenumab can be prescribed as monthly subcutaneous prefilled auto-injections at either the 140-mg or 70-mg dose for the preventive treatment of episodic migraine. The 140-mg dose is effective in patients who have failed multiple preventive medications. Three-year data from a 5-year OLE have shown its continued safety.

Fremanezumab

Fremanezumab is a humanized mAb that selectively binds to both isoforms of the ligand on the CGRP molecule itself and prevents CGRP binding to the CGRP receptor. It is delivered subcutaneously with a prefilled syringe. It was approved on September 14, 2018, by the FDA for the preventive treatment of episodic and chronic migraine.

The 12-week phase 3 HALO-EM trial assessed fremanezumab's efficacy in patients with episodic migraine (6–14 headache days, with at least 4 migraine days during a 28-day pretreatment period).[35] The trial assessed the mean change in mean number of MMD for the 225-mg monthly dose and 675-mg quarterly dose regimen as compared with placebo. There was a significant difference in migraine frequency reduction with both dosing regimens compared with placebo. The most common SE was injection site pain. Fremanezumab was also studied in patients with high-frequency episodic migraine (8–14 migraine d/mo) in a phase 2 clinical trial measuring efficacy outcomes at Weeks 9 to 12. Patients received placebo, monthly doses of

225 mg, or quarterly (once every 3 months) doses of 675 mg of fremanezumab.[36] Similar to the HALO-EM trial, the results at Week 12 showed a significant difference in migraine frequency reduction with both dosing regimens compared with placebo, although there was not a statistically significant difference in efficacy between the 225-mg monthly or quarterly dosing regimens. The most common SE was injection site reaction.[36] A 1-year OLE showed a safety-profile consistent with the HALO-EM 12-week data.[37] Six-month efficacy data from the OLE showed an increase in greater than 50% responder rate from Week 12 to Month 6; however, among responders, there were no further significant reductions in mean MMD.[38] The OLE also showed a decrease in migraine-specific acute medication intake.[38]

In summary, fremanzumab can be prescribed as a subcutaneous prefilled syringe at either the 225-mg monthly dose or 675-mg quarterly dose for the preventive treatment of episodic migraine. Six-month data from a 1-year OLE have shown an increase in responder rate over time and its continued safety.

Galcanezumab

Galcanezumab is a humanized mAb that binds to the CGRP ligand and thereby inhibits CGRP binding to the CGRP receptor. It is delivered subcutaneously with either a prefilled autoinjector or prefilled syringe. It was approved by the FDA on September 26, 2018. Galcanezumab was studied for episodic migraine prevention (4–14 migraine d/mo) in two 6-month double-blind, placebo-controlled studies: the North American EVOLVE-1 and global EVOLVE-2 studies.[39,40] The 6-month EVOLVE-1 and EVOLVE-2 tested the efficacy of 120-mg monthly after an initial 240-mg loading dose or 240-mg monthly dosing regimens as compared with placebo.[39,40] Results from both studies at 6 months showed a statistically significant difference in migraine frequency reduction with both dosing regimens compared with placebo, although there was no significant difference in efficacy between the dosing regimens.[39,40] The primary SE was injection site pain.[39,40] In addition, acute medication use for migraine treatment (not just limited to migraine-specific abortives) was significantly reduced.[39,40] Post hoc analyses of EVOLVE-1 and EVOLVE-2 pooled data showed that an increase in greater than 50% responder rate after Months 1 or and 2 was likely, with the highest likelihood being in patients who had at least a modest response in Months 1 or 2.[41] It also showed more than a third of patients treated with 120-mg or 240-mg doses achieved 100% response for greater than or equal to 1 month, typically in the last 3 months of the 6-month double-blind period.[42]

In summary, galcanezumab is prescribed as a subcutaneous prefilled autoinjector or prefilled syringe, given as a loading dose of 240 mg followed by subsequent monthly doses of 120 mg. Safety has been established for the 6 months of the study. The medication also reduced use of general acute migraine treatment medications. Post hoc analysis shows that an increase in greater than 50% responder rate over time is likely in patients who had an initial modest response.

Eptinezumab

Eptinezumab is a humanized mAb that selectively binds to the CGRP ligand and blocks its binding to CGRP receptors. In contrast to other CGRP antibodies, eptinezumab is in late-phase development as an intravenous formulation designed to produce a more immediate therapeutic response. The phase 3 PROMISE-1 trial tested an intravenous infusion of eptinezumab 30, 100, and 300 mg for patients with episodic migraine (<14 migraine d/mo) every 12 weeks.[43–45] Early results have shown that after a single infusion with either the 100-mg or 300-mg dose, the likelihood of migraine was significantly reduced on the first day following treatment with sustained benefits maintained across at least two infusions for 24 weeks.[43] SEs to eptinezumab were consistent with placebo.[43] Additionally, greater than 50%, greater than 75%, and greater than 100% responder rates and migraine-free intervals increased following a second infusion of either the 100-mg or 300-mg dose at 12 weeks.[45] PROMISE-1 is still ongoing and eptinezumab is still pending FDA approval for use.

External Trigeminal Nerve Stimulation Device (Cefaly)

External trigeminal nerve stimulation may be used for episodic migraine prevention. Cefaly is a noninvasive device placed on a self-adhesive electrode over the forehead that transcutaneously delivers electrical impulses to stimulate action potentials in the supratrochlear and supraorbital branches of the ophthalmic nerve. It was FDA approved for use in episodic migraine in 2014. Studies assessing mechanism of action at a single simulation program (frequency of 60 Hz, and maximal intensity of 16 mA) have shown that over time, Cefaly may cause neuromodulation in central pain-controlling areas, specifically the rostral anterior cingulate cortices (ACC).[46,47] One study using 18-fluorodeoxyglucose PET showed that pretreatment hypometabolism in the orbitofrontal and rostral ACC in patients with episodic migraine (4–14 migraine d/mo) was more normalized 3 months after Cefaly use.[46] The device was used for at least a third of the recommended preventive treatment time of 20 min/d.[46] Another study used BOLD-fMRI to assess the functional response to trigeminal heat stimulation in patients with low-frequency migraine (≤5 attacks/mo) who used Cefaly for at least 800 minutes over a 6-month period.[47] The study found excessive activation of the ACC by noxious trigeminal heat simulation in patients with episodic migraine as assessed by an increased BOLD response on the fMRI; use of Cefaly normalized this response.[47] These findings suggest that Cefaly slowly neuromodulates activity in brain regions, such as the ACC, which provide descending pain regulation to the trigeminovascular nociceptors involved in initiating migraine attacks.[46–48]

The PREMICE trial, a multicenter, prospective, randomized, sham-controlled study, showed that patients with episodic migraine (at least two migraine attacks/mo) who used Cefaly at a single simulation program for 20 minutes daily for 3 months had significantly decreased MMD, monthly headache days, and use of migraine-specific acute medications, as compared with sham.[49] In addition, the greater than 50% responder rate was greater in those who used Cefaly as compared with sham.[49] Additional statistical analysis on the difference in migraine day reduction between verum and sham groups suggested that Cefaly use may be more beneficial for patients with more frequent migraine days.[50] A small open-label study of 20 patients with low-frequency episodic migraine (<5 migraine attacks/mo) provided further support for use.[51] Patients used Cefaly for at 800 minutes over 60 days.[51] Results showed a significant decrease in number of MMD, and reduction in pain severity and acute medication use.[51] A large prospective registry of 2313 patients assessed safety and satisfaction with Cefaly, finding that it was overall safe and well-tolerated.[52] Only 4.3% of patients reported SEs, which were minor and reversible.[52] The most frequent SE was intolerance to focal device-induced paresthesia.[52]

In summary, Cefaly is prescribed as an external trigeminal nerve stimulation device that uses a self-adhering electrode over the forehead to transcutaneously stimulate the upper branches of the trigeminal nerve. There is evidence supporting efficacy, safety, and tolerability in the use and tolerability of Cefaly for migraine prevention for patients with low-frequency episodic migraine.

Invasive Single-Pulse Transcranial Magnetic Stimulator Device (SpringTMS)

SpringTMS, initially approved only for acute treatment in patients with migraine with aura,[53] was approved by the FDA for preventive treatment in migraine with and without aura in 2017. It is a portable device that a patient places on the occiput to deliver a pulse. Electromagnetic induction stimulates delivery of an electrical current from the scalp and into the superficial layers of the cortex.[54] In some animal models, sTMS has been shown to inhibit mechanical and chemically induced cortical spreading depression.[55] In addition, it exhibits a thalamocortical modulatory effect by inhibiting evoked and spontaneous firing of third-order thalamocortical projection neurons.[55] The ESPOUSE study was a multicenter, prospective, open-label, observational study that assessed SpringTMS as a preventive treatment in 132 patients with 4 to 25 head-ache d/mo; 90% had episodic migraine.[54] For prevention, subjects administered four pulses twice a day. Subjects were also allowed to use the device for acute treatment (up to three deliveries of three consecutive pulses with 15-minute intervals) as needed 30 minutes after preventive treatment use. Overall, 46% of the subjects had greater than 50% response with decrease in headache frequency.[54] There was also a significant reduction in disability and in the days of acute medication use.[54] The device was generally well-tolerated; the most common SEs included lightheadedness, tingling, tinnitus, dizziness, headache, scalp discomfort, or bothersome sound.[54] In summary, twice daily use of the sTMS device, SpringTMS, has been shown to have efficacy in the reduction of headache days in an open-label observational study with overall good tolerability.

2012 REVISIONS IN PREVENTIVE TREATMENT GUIDELINES

In 2012 the AAN and AHS provided evidence-based guidelines for the preventive treatment of episodic migraine in the United States based on an analysis of randomized controlled trials published between 1999 and 2007.[15] These guidelines updated recommendations from the year 2000, and categorized medications as the following: having established efficacy (level A), probably effective (level B), possibly effective (level C), inadequate data (level U), or not effective/probably not effective/possibly not effective (other).[15] The following discussion is organized by medication class, and highlights medications with level A, level, B, and level C evidence. No new evidence was found for the guidelines update regarding clonidine, guanfacine, and carbamazepine (all level C), and they are not discussed in detail in this review.[15]

β-Adrenergic Blockers

β-Blockers is a widely used class of drugs in prophylactic migraine treatment (Table 2). According to the 2012 AAN and AHS guidelines, propranolol, timolol, and metoprolol have been categorized as medications with established efficacy (level A).[15] Probably effective (level B) β-blockers include atenolol and nadolol. β-blockers categorized as possibly effective (level C) are nebivolol and pindolol.[15] Notably, inadequate data (level U) were available for bisoprolol and acebutolol was established as possibly not effective.[15] No new evidence was found for timolol, atenolol, nadolol, pindolol, bisoprolol, and acebutolol.[15]

β-blockers likely exhibit a preventive effect for episodic migraine through centrally mediated processes.[56,57] These include reduction of neuronal firing of noradrenergic neurons in vigilance-enhancing pathways[56,57] and γ-aminobutyric acid (GABA)-mediated regulation of neuronal firing in the periaqueductal gray matter.[57,58] Some effective β-blockers interact with the serotonergic system by affecting serotonin synthesis and blocking 5-HT2c and 5-HT2b receptors.[57,59] Studies on propranolol specifically show

Table 2
β-Blockers and antidepressants with level A or B evidence in the preventive treatment of episodic migraine

Agent	Effective Range of Daily Dose	Comment
β-Blockers		
Level A evidence (established efficacy)		
Propranolol	40–240 mg	Use the short-acting form BID or TID Use the long-acting form QID or BID
Metoprolol	100–200 mg	Use the short-acting form BID Use the long-acting form QID
Timolol	20–60 mg	Divide the dose Short half-life
Level B evidence (probably effective)		
Atenolol	50–200 mg	Use QID Fewer side effects than propranolol
Nadolol	20–160 mg	Use QID Fewer side effects than propranolol
Antidepressants		
Level B evidence (probably effective)		
Amitriptyline (tertiary amine, tricyclic antidepressant)	10–200 mg	Start at 10 mg in evening 8–10 h before waking
Venlafaxine (selective serotonin norepinephrine reuptake inhibitor)	75–225 mg	Start at 37.5 mg in AM

that it does not impact cerebral vessels directly; rather, it may centrally modulate autonomic vessel tone sensitivity to the sensory stimuli during the migraine.[60] Propranolol inhibits nitric oxide production by blocking inducible nitric oxide synthase. Propranolol also inhibits kainate-induced currents and is synergistic with N-methyl-D-aspartate blockers, which reduce neuronal activity and have membrane-stabilizing properties.[61]

Contraindications to the use of ß-blockers include asthma, cardiac insufficiency, and Raynaud disease.[62] ß-blockers can also cause fatigue, dizziness, and exacerbate depression. β_2-Blockers can also lead to poor response to hypoglycemia and should be used with caution in patients with diabetes. Other potential SEs include gastrointestinal complaints, decreased exercise tolerance, orthostatic hypotension, bradycardia, and impotence. Abrupt cessation of ß-blockers can lead to rebound hypertension and increased migraine.[57]

Antidepressants

Antidepressants consist of several different drug classes with different mechanisms of action. Evidence exists (level B) to support the use of amitriptyline, a tricyclic antidepressant (TCA), and venlafaxine, a selective serotonin norepinephrine reuptake inhibitor (SSNRI), as probably effective for episodic migraine prevention (see **Table 2**).[15] Meanwhile, TCA protriptilyine, and selective serotonin reuptake inhibitor fluoxetine, and SSNRI fluvoxamine have inadequate or conflicting data supporting their use (level U).[15]

Migraine preventive effects of TCAs are likely related to the inhibition of norepinephrine and serotonin reuptake and 5-HT2 receptor antagonism. Similarly, SSNRIs potentiate serotonergic and noradrenergic transmission.[57] Evidence also suggests antidepressants may also modulate dopamine production[57] and that it enhances the body's own pain-modulating pathways and opioid effect at the opioid receptors.[63] The prophylactic effect of antidepressants does not result from treating masked depression.[64,65]

The TCA dose range for episodic migraine prevention is wide and must be individualized. Of note, patients with comorbid depression may require higher doses of TCAs to treat underlying depression. Amitriptyline, a tertiary amine, is sedating and therefore should be started in the evening, ideally 8 to 10 hours before waking. The starting dose of amitriptyline is 10 to 25 mg. The usual effective dosage for migraine ranges from 25 to 200 mg. Nortriptyline, a major metabolite of amitriptyline, is a secondary amine that is less sedating than amitriptyline. The starting dose is 10 to 25 mg at bedtime. The dose ranges from 10 to 150 mg a day.

SEs are common with TCA use. Anticholinergic SEs include dry mouth, a metallic taste, epigastric distress, constipation, dizziness, mental confusion, tachycardia, blurred vision, and urinary retention. Other SEs include weight gain, orthostatic hypotension, and reflex tachycardia. TCAs should be avoided in patients with bipolar disorder because they can transform depression into hypomania or frank mania, and they can exacerbate glaucoma. Older patients may develop confusion or delirium.[66] The anticholinergics and antiadrenergic SEs of these agents may pose increased risks for cardiac conduction abnormalities, especially in the elderly. Patients at high risk for SEs should be carefully monitored or other agents considered.

Patients who are not able to tolerate TCAs may benefit from an SSNRI. Venlafaxine has been shown to be effective in a double-blind, placebo-controlled trial[67] and a separate placebo and amitriptyline controlled trial.[68] The usual effective dose of venlafaxine is 150 mg a day. Duloxetine, another SSNRI, was shown to be effective at the dose range of 60 to 120 mg in patients with episodic migraine (4–10 migraine attacks/mo) in a prospective, open-label study published in 2013.[69] For preventive treatment, duloxetine is typically initiated at 20 mg or 30 mg daily, and titrated by either 20 mg or 30 mg daily dose each week until a range dose of 60 to 120 mg daily is reached (see **Table 4**). Treatment with doses at or higher than the typical antidepressant dose of 60 mg is thought to be more efficacious for pain treatment.[70]

Compared with TCAs, SSNRIs have fewer anticholinergic SEs, and less α-blockade, resulting in a reduced risk of orthostatic hypotension and falls. Common SEs include insomnia, nervousness, mydriasis, and seizures.

Antiepileptic Drugs

Antiepileptic drugs are widely used for episodic migraine prevention and have efficacy established through well-conducted placebo-controlled trials (**Table 3**). Topiramate and divalproex sodium/sodium valproate (VPA) have established evidence (level A) and FDA approval for treatment in migraine prevention. Carbamazepine was categorized as possibly effective (level C), and inadequate data (level U) were provided for the use of gabapentin and acetazolamide in the preventive treatment of migraine.[15] Lamotrigine was established as not effective and oxcarbazepine as possibly not effective.[15]

Table 3
Antiepileptic drugs with level A or B evidence in the preventive treatment of episodic migraine

Agent	Effective Range of Daily Dose	Comment
Level A evidence (established efficacy)		
Topiramate	50–200 mg	Start 15–25 bedtime Increase 15–25 mg/wk Attempt to reach 50–100 mg Increase further if necessary Associated with weight loss, not weight gain
Valproate/divalproex	500–1500 mg/d	Start 250–500 mg/d Monitor levels if compliance is an issue Max dose is 60 mg/kg/d

Topiramate

The mechanism of action of topiramate in migraine prevention is thought to be secondary to its modulation of voltage-gated sodium channels, high voltage-gated calcium channels, $GABA_A$ receptors, and AMPA/kainate receptors. The efficacy of topiramate in treating episodic migraine has been widely studied.[11,71–84] Topiramate, given in doses ranging from 50 to 200 mg/d, is effective in migraine prevention, although studies have suggested that doses of 200 mg/d are no more effective and have more SEs than 100 mg/d in patients without intractable migraine.[71,72,84,85] Of note, the INTREPID trial studied patients with episodic migraine using topiramate 100 mg/d for 6 months.[11] In patients with high-frequency episodic migraine, topiramate was effective in reducing headache and migraine days, but did not prevent the development of chronic daily headache.[11]

Topiramate can have dose-dependent neurocognitive SEs, which include fatigue, mood changes including suicidal ideation, dizziness, word-finding problems, slowed thinking/mental processing, and concentration/attention and memory difficulty.[80,84,86] In addition, because of its inhibition of carbonic anhydrase, topiramate may cause paraesthesias, which may be relieved with potassium supplementation.[84] SEs from this action also include taste disturbances, an increased risk for renal calculi, metabolic acidosis, and hypokalemia.[84] Like other sulfonamide medications, topiramate may lead to an increased, but rare, risk of ophthalmic SEs, including acute angle closure glaucoma and visual problems without increase intraocular pressure.[84] Other adverse effects include decreased appetite and dose-dependent weight loss.[84] Topiramate at doses greater than 200 mg/d may substantially interfere with the efficacy of oral contraceptives; topiramate is teratogenic during pregnancy.

Topiramate is started at a dose of 15 to 25 mg at bedtime; the dose can then be increased by 15 to 25 mg/wk. Titration should be halted if troublesome SEs develop, and resumed when they resolve. If SEs do not resolve, the dose should be decreased to the last tolerated dose, then increased by a lower dose more slowly. The goal is to reach a dose of 50 to 100 mg/d given twice a day. It is our experience that patients who tolerate the lower doses with only partial improvement often have increased benefit with higher doses.

Divalproex sodium/sodium valproate

The mechanism of VPA in migraine prevention is not completely understood; however, it does increase neuroinhibitory GABA activity. VPA also inhibits N-methyl-D-aspartate-evoked neuroexcitatory signals and at high doses may also increase extracellular serotonin and dopamine and their active metabolites.[87] Several randomized, placebo-controlled studies have confirmed sodium VPA efficacy in preventing migraine or reducing the frequency, severity, and duration of attacks[88–96] with dosages ranging from 500 to 1500 mg per day. Extended-release divalproex sodium has also been shown to be effective for migraine prevention; this formulation may have a more favorable compliance and SE profile.[89]

Nausea, vomiting, and gastrointestinal distress are the most common SEs; their incidence decreases, however, particularly after 6 months.[97] Later, tremor and alopecia can occur. VPA has little effect on neurocognitive function and rarely causes sedation. Rare, severe SEs include hepatitis and pancreatitis. The frequency varies with the number of concomitant medications used, the patient's age, the presence of genetic and metabolic disorders, and the patient's general state of health. These idiosyncratic reactions are unpredictable.[98] Hyperandrogenism, ovarian cysts, and obesity are of concern in young women with epilepsy using VPA.[99] Absolute contraindications are pregnancy because of teratogenicity and a history of pancreatitis or a hepatic disorder.[97] Other contraindications are thrombocytopenia, pancytopenia, and bleeding disorders.

Valproic acid/sodium VPA is available as 250-mg capsules and as syrup (250 mg/5 mL). Divalproex sodium is available as 125-, 250-, and 500-mg capsules and a sprinkle formulation. Start with 250 to 500 mg/d in divided doses and slowly increase the dose. Monitor serum levels if there is a question of toxicity or compliance. The maximum recommended dose is 60 mg/kg/d.

Zonisamide

Zonisamide is an anticonvulsant similar in mechanism of action to topiramate with the additional inhibition of T-type calcium channels (**Table 4**). Recently, a 3-month double-blind randomized controlled trial of 80 patients with episodic migraine (4–15 migraine d/mo) compared the efficacy of zonisamide 200 mg/d with topiramate 100 mg/d.[100] There was equal improvement in migraine frequency and no significant differences between the two groups.[100] These results suggest that zonisamide could be as effective as topiramate in migraine prevention, whereas other open-label studies suggest its efficacy in patients who cannot tolerate topiramate.[100–104] SEs include appetite and weight reduction, memory and concentration impairment, paraesthesias, drowsiness, and anemia; there is also a risk of Stevens-Johnson syndrome. Zonisamide is teratogenic and should not be used during pregnancy. Zonisamide is typically started at a dose of 50 or 100 mg/d and titrated by 50 or 100 mg weekly up to 400 mg/d with titration schedule and dosages adjusted based on tolerability.[100–103]

Table 4		
Miscellaneous medications in the preventive treatment of migraine		
Agent	**Effective Range of Daily Dose**	**Comment**
Angiotensin-converting enzyme and angiotensin receptor antagonists		
Lisinopril	10–40 mg	Positive small controlled trial
Candesartan	16 mg	Positive small controlled trial
Others		
Duloxetine	60–120 mg	Positive small open-label prospective study
Zonisamide	100–400 mg	Positive small controlled study

Angiotensin-Converting Enzyme Inhibitors and Angiotensin II Receptor Blocker

Lisinopril, an angiotensin-converting enzyme inhibitor, and candesartan, an angiotensin receptor blocker, were categorized as possibly effective (level C) for episodic migraine prevention (see **Table 4**).[15] A double-blind, placebo-controlled, crossover study studied lisinopril 10 mg for 1 week followed by 20 mg for 11 weeks versus placebo in patients who experienced 2 to 6 migraine d/mo.[105] Results showed a significant decrease in migraine frequency compared with placebo.[105] A randomized, double-blind, placebo-controlled, crossover study of candesartan at 16 mg in patients with a median migraine attack frequency of 4 d/mo showed a significant decrease in mean frequency and greater than 50% responder rate over 12 weeks compared with placebo.[106] Candesartan 16 mg daily was later found to be comparable with propranolol 160 mg daily.[107] Significant SEs for candesartan include dizziness, tiredness, and paraesthesias.[107]

SUMMARY

Preventive therapy plays an important role in episodic migraine management. There are inconclusive data whether preventive therapy can impact the natural course of migraine to prevent episodic migraine from transforming into chronic migraine. However, with the addition of a preventive medication, patients may experience reduced attack frequency and improved response to acute treatment, which can result in reduced health care resource utilization and improved quality of life. Migraine-specific preventive medications and nonpharmacologic treatment options are now available and could increase use and tolerability of preventive treatment of episodic migraine.

REFERENCES

1. Vos T, Flaxman AD, Naghavi M, et al. Years lived with disability (YLDs) for 1160 sequelae of 289 diseases and injuries 1990-2010: a systematic analysis for the Global Burden of Disease Study 2010. Lancet 2012;380(9859):2163–96.

2. Vos T, Allen C, Arora M. Global, regional, and national incidence, prevalence, and years lived with disability for 310 diseases and injuries, 1990-2015: a systematic analysis for the Global Burden of Disease Study 2015. Lancet 2016; 388(10053):1545–602.

3. Lipton RB, Bigal ME, Diamond M, et al. Migraine prevalence, disease burden, and the need for preventive therapy. Neurology 2007;68(5):343–9.

4. Stokes M, Becker WJ, Lipton RB, et al. Cost of health care among patients with chronic and episodic migraine in Canada and the USA: results from the International Burden of Migraine Study (IBMS). Headache 2011;51(7):1058–77.

5. Lipton RB. Chronic migraine, classification, differential diagnosis, and epidemiology. Headache 2011;51(Suppl 2):77–83.

6. Manack AN, Buse DC, Lipton RB. Chronic migraine: epidemiology and disease burden. Curr Pain Headache Rep 2011;15(1):70–8.

7. Buse DC, Scher AI, Dodick DW, et al. Impact of migraine on the family: perspectives of people with migraine and their spouse/domestic partner in the cameo study. Mayo Clin Proc 2016. https://doi.org/10.1016/j.mayocp.2016.02.013.

8. Bigal ME, Serrano D, Buse D, et al. Acute migraine medications and evolution from episodic to chronic migraine: a longitudinal population-based study. Headache 2008;48(8):1157–68.

9. Lipton RB. Tracing transformation: chronic migraine classification, progression, and epidemiology. Neurology 2009;72(5 Suppl):S3–7.
10. Katsarava Z, Buse DC, Manack AN, et al. Defining the differences between episodic migraine and chronic migraine. Curr Pain Headache Rep 2012;16(1): 86–92.
11. Lipton RB, Silberstein S, Dodick D, et al. Topiramate intervention to prevent transformation of episodic migraine: the topiramate INTREPID study. Cephalalgia 2011;31(1):18–30.
12. Silberstein SD, Winner PK, Chmiel JJ. Migraine preventive medication reduces resource utilization. Headache 2003;43(3):171–8.
13. Silberstein SD. Headaches in pregnancy. Neurol Clin 2004;22(4):727–56.
14. Diamond S, Bigal ME, Silberstein S, et al. Patterns of diagnosis and acute and preventive treatment for migraine in the United States: results from the American Migraine Prevalence and Prevention study. Headache 2007;47(3): 355–63.
15. Silberstein SD, Holland S, Freitag F, et al. Evidence-based guideline update: pharmacologic treatment for episodic migraine prevention in adults: report of the Quality Standards Subcommittee of the American Academy of Neurology and the American Headache Society. Neurology 2012;78(17):1337–45.
16. Holland S, Silberstein SD, Freitag F, et al. Evidence-based guideline update: NSAIDs and other complementary treatments for episodic migraine prevention in adults: report of the Quality Standards Subcommittee of the American Academy of Neurology and the American Headache Society. Neurology 2012;78(17): 1346–53.
17. Pringsheim T, Davenport WJ, Mackie G, et al. Canadian Headache Society guideline for migraine prophylaxis. Can J Neurol Sci 2012;39(2 Suppl 2):S1–59.
18. Carville S, Padhi S, Reason T, et al, Guideline Development Group. Diagnosis and management of headaches in young people and adults: summary of NICE guidance. BMJ 2012;345:e5765.
19. Silberstein SD. Preventive treatment of migraine: an overview. Cephalalgia 1997; 17(2):67–72.
20. Diener H-C, Agosti R, Allais G, et al. Cessation versus continuation of 6-month migraine preventive therapy with topiramate (PROMPT): a randomised, double-blind, placebo-controlled trial. Lancet Neurol 2007;6(12):1054–62.
21. Rosenfeld MG, Mermod JJ, Amara SG, et al. Production of a novel neuropeptide encoded by the calcitonin gene via tissue-specific RNA processing. Nature 1983;304(5922):129–35.
22. Basbaum AI, Bautista DM, Scherrer G, et al. Cellular and molecular mechanisms of pain. Cell 2009;139(2):267–84.
23. Eftekhari S, Edvinsson L. Possible sites of action of the new calcitonin gene-related peptide receptor antagonists. Ther Adv Neurol Disord 2010;3(6):369–78.
24. Eftekhari S, Warfvinge K, Blixt FW, et al. Differentiation of nerve fibers storing CGRP and CGRP receptors in the peripheral trigeminovascular system. J Pain 2013;14(11):1289–303.
25. Edvinsson L, Warfvinge K. Recognizing the role of CGRP and CGRP receptors in migraine and its treatment. Cephalalgia 2017. https://doi.org/10.1177/0333102417736900. 333102417736900.
26. Iyengar S, Ossipov MH, Johnson KW. The role of calcitonin gene-related peptide in peripheral and central pain mechanisms including migraine. Pain 2017; 158(4):543–59.

27. Hansen JM, Hauge AW, Olesen J, et al. Calcitonin gene-related peptide triggers migraine-like attacks in patients with migraine with aura. Cephalalgia 2010; 30(10):1179–86.

28. Melo-Carrillo A, Strassman AM, Nir R-R, et al. Fremanezumab-A humanized monoclonal anti-CGRP antibody-inhibits thinly myelinated (Aδ) but not unmyelinated (C) meningeal nociceptors. J Neurosci 2017;37(44):10587–96.

29. Melo-Carrillo A, Noseda R, Nir R-R, et al. Selective inhibition of trigeminovascular neurons by fremanezumab: a humanized monoclonal anti-CGRP antibody. J Neurosci 2017;37(30):7149–63.

30. Dodick DW, Ashina M, Brandes JL, et al. ARISE: a phase 3 randomized trial of erenumab for episodic migraine. Cephalalgia 2018;38(6):1026–37.

31. Goadsby PJ, Reuter U, Hallström Y, et al. A controlled trial of erenumab for episodic migraine. N Engl J Med 2017;377(22):2123–32.

32. Ashina M, Dodick D, Goadsby PJ, et al. Erenumab (AMG 334) in episodic migraine: interim analysis of an ongoing open-label study. Neurology 2017; 89(12):1237–43.

33. Ashina M, Goadsby PJ, Reuter U, et al. Long-term safety and tolerability of erenumab: three-plus year results from an ongoing open-label extension study in episodic migraine. In: 60th Annual Scientific Meeting of the American Headache Society. San Francisco, 2018.

34. Reuter U, Goadsby PJ, Lanteri-Minet M, et al. Efficacy and tolerability of erenumab in patients with episodic migraine in whom two-to-four previous preventive treatments were unsuccessful: a randomised, double-blind, placebo-controlled, phase 3b study. Lancet 2018;392(10161):2280–7.

35. Dodick DW, Silberstein SD, Bigal ME, et al. Effect of fremanezumab compared with placebo for prevention of episodic migraine: a randomized clinical trial. JAMA 2018;319(19):1999–2008.

36. Bigal ME, Dodick DW, Rapoport AM, et al. Safety, tolerability, and efficacy of TEV-48125 for preventive treatment of high-frequency episodic migraine: a multicentre, randomised, double-blind, placebo-controlled, phase 2b study. Lancet Neurol 2015;14(11):1081–90.

37. Goadsby P, Yeung PP, Blankenbiller T, et al. Fremanezumab long-term efficacy and safety: interim results of a one-year study. Presented at the: 60th Annual Scientific Meeting American Headache Society. San Francisco Marriott Marquis San Francisco, CA, June 28, 2018.

38. Brandes J, Yeung PP, Cohen JM, et al. Long-term impact of fremanezumab on response rates, acute headache medication use, and disability in patients with episodic migraine: interim results of a one-year study. Presented at the: 60th Annual Scientific Meeting American Headache Society. San Francisco Marriott Marquis San Francisco, CA, June 28, 2018.

39. Stauffer VL, Dodick DW, Zhang Q, et al. Evaluation of galcanezumab for the prevention of episodic migraine: the EVOLVE-1 randomized clinical trial. JAMA Neurol 2018;75(9):1080–8.

40. Skljarevski V, Matharu M, Millen BA, et al. Efficacy and safety of galcanezumab for the prevention of episodic migraine: results of the EVOLVE-2 Phase 3 randomized controlled clinical trial. Cephalalgia 2018;38(8):1442–54.

41. Nichols R, Doty E, Sacco S, et al. Analysis of initial nonresponders to galcanezumab in patients with episodic or chronic migraine: results from the EVOLVE-1, EVOLVE-2, and REGAIN randomized, double-blind, placebo-controlled studies. Headache 2018. https://doi.org/10.1111/head.13443.

42. Rosen N, Pearlman E, Ruff D, et al. 100% response rate to galcanezumab in patients with episodic migraine: a post hoc analysis of the results from phase 3, randomized, double-blind, placebo-controlled EVOLVE-1 and EVOLVE-2 Studies. Headache 2018;58(9):1347–57.

43. Saper J, Lipton R, Kudrow D, et al. Primary results of PROMISE-1 (Prevention Of Migraine via Intravenous eptinezumab Safety and Efficacy–1) trial: a phase 3, randomized, double-blind, placebo-controlled study to evaluate the efficacy and safety of eptinezumab for prevention of frequent episodic migraines (S20.001). Neurology 2018;90(15 Supplement):S20.001.

44. Silberstein SD, McAllister P, Berman G, et al. Eptinezumab reduced migraine frequency, duration, and pain intensity through week 24: results from the Phase 3 PROMISE-1 Trial (P4.091). Neurology 2018;90(15 Supplement):P4.091.

45. Egilius LH, Spierings TS, Cady R, et al. Repeat infusions of eptinezumab associated with greater migraine reductions and longer migraine-free intervals: results from the phase 3 PROMISE-1 trial (P4.108). Neurology 2018;90(15 Supplement):P4.108.

46. Magis D, D'Ostilio K, Thibaut A, et al. Cerebral metabolism before and after external trigeminal nerve stimulation in episodic migraine. Cephalalgia 2017; 37(9):881–91.

47. Russo A, Tessitore A, Esposito F, et al. Functional changes of the perigenual part of the anterior cingulate cortex after external trigeminal neurostimulation in migraine patients. Front Neurol 2017;8:282.

48. Ambrosini A, D'Alessio C, Magis D, et al. Targeting pericranial nerve branches to treat migraine: current approaches and perspectives. Cephalalgia 2015; 35(14):1308–22.

49. Schoenen J, Vandersmissen B, Jeangette S, et al. Migraine prevention with a supraorbital transcutaneous stimulator: a randomized controlled trial. Neurology 2013;80(8):697–704.

50. Schoenen JE. Migraine prevention with a supraorbital transcutaneous stimulator: a randomized controlled trial. Neurology 2016;86(2):201–2.

51. Russo A, Tessitore A, Conte F, et al. Transcutaneous supraorbital neurostimulation in "de novo" patients with migraine without aura: the first Italian experience. J Headache Pain 2015;16:69.

52. Magis D, Sava S, d Elia TS, et al. Safety and patients' satisfaction of transcutaneous supraorbital neurostimulation (tSNS) with the Cefaly device in headache treatment: a survey of 2,313 headache sufferers in the general population. J Headache Pain 2013;14:95.

53. Lipton RB, Dodick DW, Silberstein SD, et al. Single-pulse transcranial magnetic stimulation for acute treatment of migraine with aura: a randomised, double-blind, parallel-group, sham-controlled trial. Lancet Neurol 2010;9(4):373–80.

54. Starling AJ, Tepper SJ, Marmura MJ, et al. A multicenter, prospective, single arm, open label, observational study of sTMS for migraine prevention (ESPOUSE Study). Cephalalgia 2018;38(6):1038–48.

55. Andreou AP, Holland PR, Akerman S, et al. Transcranial magnetic stimulation and potential cortical and trigeminothalamic mechanisms in migraine. Brain 2016;139(Pt 7):2002–14.

56. Hieble JP. Adrenoceptor subclassification: an approach to improved cardiovascular therapeutics. Pharm Acta Helv 2000;74(2–3):163–71.

57. Galletti F, Cupini LM, Corbelli I, et al. Pathophysiological basis of migraine prophylaxis. Prog Neurobiol 2009;89(2):176–92.

58. Xiao C, Zhou C, Atlas G, et al. Labetalol facilitates GABAergic transmission to rat periaqueductal gray neurons via antagonizing beta1-adrenergic receptors–a possible mechanism underlying labetalol-induced analgesia. Brain Res 2008;1198:34–43.

59. Chugani DC, Niimura K, Chaturvedi S, et al. Increased brain serotonin synthesis in migraine. Neurology 1999;53(7):1473–9.

60. Min J-H, Kwon H-M, Nam H. The effect of propranolol on cerebrovascular reactivity to visual stimulation in migraine. J Neurol Sci 2011;305(1–2):136–8.

61. Ramadan NM. Prophylactic migraine therapy: mechanisms and evidence. Curr Pain Headache Rep 2004;8(2):91–5.

62. Morey SS. Guidelines on migraine: part 5. Recommendations for specific prophylactic drugs. Am Fam Physician 2000;62(11):2535–9.

63. Feinmann C. Pain relief by antidepressants: possible modes of action. Pain 1985;23(1):1–8.

64. Panerai AE, Monza G, Movilia P, et al. A randomized, within-patient, cross-over, placebo-controlled trial on the efficacy and tolerability of the tricyclic antidepressants chlorimipramine and nortriptyline in central pain. Acta Neurol Scand 1990; 82(1):34–8.

65. Kishore-Kumar R, Max MB, Schafer SC, et al. Desipramine relieves postherpetic neuralgia. Clin Pharmacol Ther 1990;47(3):305–12.

66. Clegg A, Young JB. Which medications to avoid in people at risk of delirium: a systematic review. Age Ageing 2011;40(1):23–9.

67. Ozyalcin SN, Talu GK, Kiziltan E, et al. The efficacy and safety of venlafaxine in the prophylaxis of migraine. Headache 2005;45(2):144–52.

68. Bulut S, Berilgen MS, Baran A, et al. Venlafaxine versus amitriptyline in the prophylactic treatment of migraine: randomized, double-blind, crossover study. Clin Neurol Neurosurg 2004;107(1):44–8.

69. Young WB, Bradley KC, Anjum MW, et al. Duloxetine prophylaxis for episodic migraine in persons without depression: a prospective study. Headache 2013; 53(9):1430–7.

70. Lunn MPT, Hughes RAC, Wiffen PJ. Duloxetine for treating painful neuropathy, chronic pain or fibromyalgia. Cochrane Database Syst Rev 2014;(1):CD007115.

71. Silberstein SD, Neto W, Schmitt J, et al, MIGR-001 Study Group. Topiramate in migraine prevention: results of a large controlled trial. Arch Neurol 2004;61(4): 490–5.

72. Brandes JL, Saper JR, Diamond M, et al. Topiramate for migraine prevention: a randomized controlled trial. JAMA 2004;291(8):965–73.

73. Diener H-C, Tfelt-Hansen P, Dahlöf C, et al. Topiramate in migraine prophylaxis: results from a placebo-controlled trial with propranolol as an active control. J Neurol 2004;251(8):943–50.

74. Dodick DW, Freitag F, Banks J, et al. Topiramate versus amitriptyline in migraine prevention: a 26-week, multicenter, randomized, double-blind, double-dummy, parallel-group noninferiority trial in adult migraineurs. Clin Ther 2009;31(3): 542–59.

75. Storey JR, Calder CS, Hart DE, et al. Topiramate in migraine prevention: a double-blind, placebo-controlled study. Headache 2001;41(10):968–75.

76. Shaygannejad V, Janghorbani M, Ghorbani A, et al. Comparison of the effect of topiramate and sodium valporate in migraine prevention: a randomized blinded crossover study. Headache 2006;46(4):642–8.

77. Gupta P, Singh S, Goyal V, et al. Low-dose topiramate versus lamotrigine in migraine prophylaxis (the Lotolamp study). Headache 2007;47(3):402–12.

78. Rapoport A, Mauskop A, Diener H-C, et al. Long-term migraine prevention with topiramate: open-label extension of pivotal trials. Headache 2006;46(7): 1151–60.
79. Ashtari F, Shaygannejad V, Akbari M. A double-blind, randomized trial of low-dose topiramate vs propranolol in migraine prophylaxis. Acta Neurol Scand 2008;118(5):301–5.
80. Adelman J, Freitag FG, Lainez M, et al. Analysis of safety and tolerability data obtained from over 1,500 patients receiving topiramate for migraine prevention in controlled trials. Pain Med 2008;9(2):175–85.
81. Afshari D, Rafizadeh S, Rezaei M. A comparative study of the effects of low-dose topiramate versus sodium valproate in migraine prophylaxis. Int J Neurosci 2012;122(2):60–8.
82. Keskinbora K, Aydinli I. A double-blind randomized controlled trial of topiramate and amitriptyline either alone or in combination for the prevention of migraine. Clin Neurol Neurosurg 2008;110(10):979–84.
83. Silberstein SD. Topiramate in migraine prevention: evidence-based medicine from clinical trials. Neurol Sci 2004;25(Suppl 3):S244–5.
84. Silberstein SD. Topiramate in migraine prevention: a 2016 perspective. Headache 2017;57(1):165–78.
85. Diener HC, Bussone G, Van Oene JC, et al. Topiramate reduces headache days in chronic migraine: a randomized, double-blind, placebo-controlled study. Cephalalgia 2007;27(7):814–23.
86. Shank RP, Maryanoff BE. Molecular pharmacodynamics, clinical therapeutics, and pharmacokinetics of topiramate. CNS Neurosci Ther 2008;14(2):120–42.
87. Cutrer FM, Limmroth V, Moskowitz MA. Possible mechanisms of valproate in migraine prophylaxis. Cephalalgia 1997;17(2):93–100.
88. Klapper J. Divalproex sodium in migraine prophylaxis: a dose-controlled study. Cephalalgia 1997;17(2):103–8.
89. Freitag FG, Collins SD, Carlson HA, et al. A randomized trial of divalproex sodium extended-release tablets in migraine prophylaxis. Neurology 2002; 58(11):1652–9.
90. Hering R, Kuritzky A. Sodium valproate in the prophylactic treatment of migraine: a double-blind study versus placebo. Cephalalgia 1992;12(2):81–4.
91. Jensen R, Brinck T, Olesen J. Sodium valproate has a prophylactic effect in migraine without aura: a triple-blind, placebo-controlled crossover study. Neurology 1994;44(4):647–51.
92. Mathew NT, Saper JR, Silberstein SD, et al. Migraine prophylaxis with divalproex. Arch Neurol 1995;52(3):281–6.
93. Silberstein SD, Collins SD. Safety of divalproex sodium in migraine prophylaxis: an open-label, long-term study. Long-term safety of Depakote in Headache Prophylaxis Study Group. Headache 1999;39(9):633–43.
94. Linde M, Mulleners WM, Chronicle EP, et al. Valproate (valproic acid or sodium valproate or a combination of the two) for the prophylaxis of episodic migraine in adults. Cochrane Database Syst Rev 2013;(6):CD010611.
95. Hesami O, Shams MR, Ayazkhoo L, et al. Comparison of pregabalin and sodium valproate in migraine prophylaxis: a randomized double-blinded study. Iran J Pharm Res 2018;17(2):783–9.
96. Sadeghian H, Motiei-Langroudi R. Comparison of levetiracetam and sodium valproate in migraine prophylaxis: a randomized placebo-controlled study. Ann Indian Acad Neurol 2015;18(1):45–8.

97. Silberstein SD. Divalproex sodium in headache: literature review and clinical guidelines. Headache 1996;36(9):547–55.
98. Pellock JM, Willmore LJ. A rational guide to routine blood monitoring in patients receiving antiepileptic drugs. Neurology 1991;41(7):961–4.
99. Vainionpää LK, Rättyä J, Knip M, et al. Valproate-induced hyperandrogenism during pubertal maturation in girls with epilepsy. Ann Neurol 1999;45(4):444–50.
100. Mohammadianinejad SE, Abbasi V, Sajedi SA, et al. Zonisamide versus topiramate in migraine prophylaxis: a double-blind randomized clinical trial. Clin Neuropharmacol 2011;34(4):174–7.
101. Bermejo PE, Dorado R. Zonisamide for migraine prophylaxis in patients refractory to topiramate. Clin Neuropharmacol 2009;32(2):103–6.
102. Drake ME, Greathouse NI, Renner JB, et al. Open-label zonisamide for refractory migraine. Clin Neuropharmacol 2004;27(6):278–80.
103. Villani V, Ciuffoli A, Prosperini L, et al. Zonisamide for migraine prophylaxis in topiramate-intolerant patients: an observational study. Headache 2011;51(2): 287–91.
104. Ashkenazi A, Benlifer A, Korenblit J, et al. Zonisamide for migraine prophylaxis in refractory patients. Cephalalgia 2006;26(10):1199–202.
105. Schrader H, Stovner LJ, Helde G, et al. Prophylactic treatment of migraine with angiotensin converting enzyme inhibitor (lisinopril): randomised, placebo controlled, crossover study. BMJ 2001;322(7277):19–22.
106. Tronvik E, Stovner LJ, Helde G, et al. Prophylactic treatment of migraine with an angiotensin II receptor blocker: a randomized controlled trial. JAMA 2003; 289(1):65–9.
107. Stovner LJ, Linde M, Gravdahl GB, et al. A comparative study of candesartan versus propranolol for migraine prophylaxis: a randomised, triple-blind, placebo-controlled, double cross-over study. Cephalalgia 2014;34(7):523–32.

Inpatient Management of Migraine

Michael J. Marmura, MD*, Angela Hou, MD

KEYWORDS

- Chronic migraine • Inpatient management • Refractory headache
- Medication overuse

KEY POINTS

- Indications for inpatient admission include chronic headache refractory to aggressive outpatient management, intractable nausea or vomiting, severe disability, medication overuse requiring detoxification, and complex medical or psychiatric comorbidities.
- Multiple medications have been studied for inpatient headache treatment, including dihydroergotamine, nonsteroidal anti-inflammatory drugs, magnesium, intravenous anticonvulsants such as valproate sodium, corticosteroids, diphenhydramine, intravenous lidocaine, and antiemetics, including neuroleptics, propofol, and ketamine.
- A multidisciplinary approach, including psychological evaluation during the inpatient stay, is recommended.
- The treatment of migraine in children is largely based on protocols used in adults.
- Follow-up with a practitioner skilled in headache management is the key to continue progress initiated during the inpatient stay, including continuing preventive treatments.

INTRODUCTION

Outpatient treatment is the mainstay of migraine management. Clinicians choose appropriate acute and preventive medications, lifestyle and behavioral therapies, and interventional procedures, such as neurotoxins, trigger point injections or nerve blocks, and neuromodulation devices as necessary to improve outcomes and quality of life for migraine and headache diseases.[1,2] These modalities are all available in the outpatient setting.

Like other common diseases, migraine disease may affect day-to-day function with variable levels of severity: more than 11 million in the US population have moderate to severe disability.[3] In 2008, more than 50 thousand patients were admitted for migraine

The authors have nothing to disclose.
Thomas Jefferson University, Jefferson Headache Center, 900 Walnut Street #200, Philadelphia, PA 19107, USA
* Corresponding author.
E-mail address: Michael.Marmura@jefferson.edu
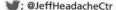; @JeffHeadacheCtr

Neurol Clin 37 (2019) 771–788
https://doi.org/10.1016/j.ncl.2019.07.007
0733-8619/19/© 2019 Elsevier Inc. All rights reserved.

in the United States, representing 63% of all admissions for headache.[4] Emergency department (ED) care for those with refractory migraine is often ineffective because of undertreatment,[5] which is reflected by high rates of dissatisfaction among patients and headache specialists.[6] Lucado and colleagues[7] determined there were more than 3 million ED visits for migraine in 2008 and that migraine was the most common diagnosis leading to admission. The average length of stay in this study for migraine was 2.7 days, significantly less than the 4.6-day average for overall admissions. Many factors may lead to the decision to admit persons with migraine. Inadequate treatment of migraine may lead to unnecessary testing, ED visit, and loss of functioning.[8] A small minority of those with migraine account for a large percentage of missed work days,[9] and missed or impaired function at work accounts for most of the cost of migraine disease.[10] In addition, overuse of acute medications, particularly opioids or barbiturates, are likely to worsen the disorder.[11] These medications often lead to dependence and severe withdrawal when discontinued, making outpatient management difficult.[12] Chronic pain and migraine are also linked to severe mood disorders, which can affect the likelihood of successful outpatient treatment.[13]

ADMISSION CRITERIA AND INITIAL EVALUATION

Given the emergence of outpatient infusion centers and comprehensive outpatient migraine programs, the costs of inpatient migraine care have come under increasing scrutiny.[14] For patients without significant comorbidities and disability, outpatient infusion with medication management may be successful.[15,16] Surveys and guidelines have attempted to identify indications for inpatient management of migraine. A survey distributed to American Headache Society members highlighted that nausea or vomiting (63.4%) and medication overuse with either opioids (61.3%) or barbiturates (58.1%) were the most popular factors favoring inpatient care.[17] Most thought other medication overuse, including overuse of triptans or simple analgesics, could typically be managed in the outpatient setting. Expert criteria and guidelines recommend considering inpatient treatment with intravenous (IV) medication for any of the following: (1) intractable nausea and/or vomiting or dehydration, (2) opioid or barbiturate dependence requiring detoxification, (3) failed outpatient treatment or frequent ED visits requiring inpatient management, including psychiatric care, (4) status migrainosus, and (5) medical disease or treatment requiring careful observation.[18,19]

Just as in the outpatient setting, a complete history and physical examination is the first step in the assessment of hospitalized patients with migraine.[20] Red flags include symptoms such as progressive or thunderclap headache, new-onset headache in elderly, gravid, or immunosuppressed, and signs such as papilledema, and all require further evaluation. In patients presenting to the ED with a new headache or change in pattern, secondary headache is not rare.[21] In patients with a long history of migraine, revisiting the diagnosis may provide reassurance. Diagnostic uncertainty contributes to anxiety and disability in chronic pain disorders, such as low back pain.[22] It may be helpful for clinicians to explain that refractory migraine is not rare and is a serious disease.[23] Although routine neuroimaging is not recommended for patients with migraine, at least 1 study has suggested it may alleviate short-term anxiety about secondary causes of headache.[24]

ED visits comprise most admissions for migraine, but in many cases an elective admission for intractable migraine is preferable. Planned, elective admissions allow for better planning and staffing, starting preventive treatment before the hospital, establishing a therapeutic relationship, and setting expectations and reviewing long-term goals,[25,26] not to mention obtaining insurance approval. Obtaining a complete history of acute medication use is important. Medication-overuse headache commonly worsens migraine and can trigger the need for inpatient hospitalization. Withdrawal of opioids, barbiturates, and even caffeine may cause worsening of migraine during a hospitalization.[27] It is essential to review the rationale for discontinuing medications and provide an alternative plan after discharge. **Table 1** lists the fundamental principles for inpatient migraine treatment.

PHARMACOLOGIC TREATMENTS

Inpatient protocols for migraine are based on infusion or ED studies, and inpatient case series that are largely uncontrolled and observational. The most commonly used IV medications in the inpatient settings include dihydroergotamine (DHE), neuroleptics, diphenhydramine, nonsteroidal anti-inflammatory drugs (NSAIDs), anticonvulsants, corticosteroids, and magnesium. In some cases, clinicians may introduce one or a series of medications in a stepwise fashion every day or so to assess for effectiveness and side effects. The other strategy is to start an aggressive plan from admission with multiple medications from different classes with a plan to titrate to effectiveness. For either approach, comprehensive headache care centers promote multidisciplinary treatment combining behavioral therapies, such as biofeedback, relaxation, or psychotherapy, together with medication treatment of migraine.[28,29] The use of nerve blocks or other procedures should be considered as a way to complement the pharmacologic approach and reduce length of stay.[30] A knowledgeable nursing staff that can recognize common and serious adverse events (AEs) can help by reassuring patients or alerting physicians when appropriate. Response to treatment may lead to the discovery of effective rescue medications to use in the future. At the time of discharge, patients should receive education and a written plan for treating migraine with medications using the principles of stratified care.[31] **Table 2** provides a proposed inpatient treatment strategy for migraine.

Dihydroergotamine

DHE is one of the best studied treatments for the inpatient treatment of migraine. Raskin[32] was the first to describe the use of IV DHE for intractable migraine in 1986. In his initial study, he treated 55 patients with continuous headache for more than 2 months with between 0.3 and 1 mg of IV DHE every 8 hours for 2 days. Most of the patients also had acute medication overuse. Of the 55 patients, 49 (89%) became headache-free in 2 days, with most reporting long-term relief.[32] Silberstein and

Table 1	
General principles for inpatient treatment of migraine	
Nonmedication Related	**Medication Related**
Review the diagnosis and decide if further tests are needed at admission	Review all medications carefully at admission, especially acute medication use
Establish a therapeutic relationship and set goals after discharge	Use long-acting medications to break cycle of daily headache, such as DHE
Review relevant other medical problems, such as depression, anxiety, obesity, or sleep disturbance	Ask about AEs during treatment. Monitor ECG and blood pressure and consider telemetry depending on drugs used
Use mental health providers to assist with pain-coping strategies	Withdraw opioids and barbiturates
Provide a clear discharge plan for acute migraine after discharge	Start or titrate preventive medication

Table 2	
Proposed protocol for the inpatient treatment of migraine	
Treatment/Medication and Dose	**Clinical Pearls**
Ensure adequate IV access	Consider a peripherally inserted central catheter, double lumen if using continuous IV treatment (lidocaine)
Start antiemetic 30 min before DHE 0.1–1 mg q8h unless contraindicated	Balance choice of antiemetic based on effectiveness and potential AEs. Consider delay × 1–2 d if triptan overuse
Start ketorolac 30 mg q8h unless contraindicated	Avoid prolonged use to reduce AEs
Start lidocaine 1 mg/min for 4 h, then 2 mg/min. Adjust dose based on levels q24h to effectiveness	Ensure telemetry monitoring, frequent monitoring of levels. Requires dedicated IV, may take days to work
Use diphenhydramine 25–50mg oral or IV before antiemetics or as a rescue for akathisia	Use with caution in elderly and in those with history of opioid addiction
Consider adjunctive medications on admission, such as magnesium 2 g IV, valproate 500–1000 mg q8-12h or levetiracetam 1 g q12h	Valproate may reduce metabolism medications, such as lidocaine, increasing AEs
Save corticosteroids, such as methylprednisolone 125 mg IV, or other drugs, such as ketamine, for nonresponders	Avoid using NSAIDs and corticosteroids together

colleagues[33] retrospectively reviewed results of 50 patients with chronic daily headache treated with DHE, including 37 with chronic migraine. All subjects had acute medication overuse. Overall, 91% of patients became headache-free, usually within 3 days, with a mean duration of hospitalization of 7.4 days. Most patients had an excellent or good result at 6 months and 24 months of follow-up.[34] Nagy and colleagues[35] described results from treatment of 114 chronic migraine patients with cumulative doses of between 8.25 and 11.25 mg IV DHE, with 84 (74%) reporting improvement, including 76 (67%) with headache freedom. Relja and colleagues[36] reported the results of DHE and metoclopramide in 111 patients with chronic daily headache, mostly migraine, with coexisting acute medication overuse. Treatment was effective as reflected by the fact that no patient relapsed to medication overuse. Patients overusing triptans had a faster response, with a mean length of stay of 10 days. In almost all cases, patients are treated with antiemetics, some of which may also treat migraine, about 30 minutes before getting DHE.[37]

DHE AEs are not infrequent and may lead to dose adjustments or occasionally discontinuation. Nausea is the most common side effect, but chest tightness, leg cramps, and hypertension are also common.[33] Headache may temporarily worsen immediately after DHE administration, but worsening does not necessarily predict poor response as long as nausea can be controlled.[38] Although DHE is typically given intermittently, continuous DHE infusion is also reportedly effective with fewer AEs.[39] Although DHE is contraindicated in those with significant coronary or peripheral artery disease, serious or permanent AEs, such as vasospasm, ischemia, or uncontrolled hypertension, are rare.[40]

Nonsteroidal Anti-Inflammatory Drugs

Aspirin and other NSAIDs are among the most proven[41] and commonly used drugs for migraine. Unlike with triptans, there is no evidence that frequent NSAID use triggers migraine progression.[42] Weatherall and colleagues[43] reviewed outcomes using IV lysine acetylsalicylate (aspirin) 1000 mg for the inpatient treatment of 91 subjects with migraine, most of whom also had acute medication overuse. They reported moderate improvement in 62% of subjects and good response in 27%. Aspirin was well tolerated with no major AEs: only 1 of the 14 patients with asthma had an exacerbation and 3 (14%) reported nausea or abdominal pain. In another study, ketorolac 30 mg was as effective as 10 mg metoclopramide as an infusion in the ED with greater effectiveness than 1000 mg sodium valproate.[44] Another small ED study found dexketoprofen 50 mg IV to be superior to and faster acting than ibuprofen IV 800 mg and metoclopramide IV 10 mg.[45]

Magnesium

Several studies have produced conflicting data regarding the use of IV magnesium for the treatment of acute migraine as an infusion. In 1 study, Bigal and colleagues[46] found that IV magnesium sulfate 1 g improved migraine in those with aura versus placebo and improved associated symptoms in those without aura as an adjuvant therapy, but was not effective for migraine headache in those without aura. Demirkaya and colleagues[47] performed a randomized, single-blind, placebo-controlled trial comparing 1 g IV magnesium sulfate with placebo with 2 groups of 15 subjects. Magnesium sulfate was superior to placebo with a pain-free rate of 87% for magnesium sulfate compared with 0% for placebo. On the other hand, Frank and colleagues[48] found no differences in a randomized double-blind placebo-controlled trial between 2 g of IV magnesium versus placebo for the treatment of 42 patients (21 in each treatment group) with acute benign headache in the ED. In comparative studies, IV magnesium was inferior to IV metoclopramide for acute migraine in 1 study[49] and had statistically similar efficacy to IV prochlorperazine in another.[50]

Intravenous Anticonvulsants: Valproate and Levetiracetam

Valproic acid and its derivatives are effective in migraine prophylaxis and may have a role as an IV treatment of migraine. Schwartz and colleagues[51] administered IV valproate sodium to 10 patients with chronic migraine and reported improvement in 8 (80%) of the 10 patients. Each received a loading dose of 15 mg/kg followed by 5 mg/kg every 8 hours. Four of the subjects reported marked improvement or pain freedom. Stillman and colleagues[52] reported effectiveness of IV valproate as an outpatient infusion in a study of 106 patients, 45 of whom had a diagnosis of chronic or "transformed" migraine. Although valproate doses ranged between 300 and 1200 mg, 61 patients (57.5%) responded to the initial treatment. Levetiracetam as an IV infusion may have a role in acute migraine treatment, but has little evidence to support its use.[53]

Corticosteroids

Corticosteroids, such as dexamethasone and methylprednisolone, may have a role in migraine management. The primary benefit of corticosteroids in headache management appears to be reducing headache recurrence. A meta-analysis of 25 studies (n = 3989) spanning from 1950 to 2014 showed that treatment with corticosteroids reduced headache recurrence in 78.6% of studies and reduced acute pain in 61.2% of studies with a median absolute risk reduction of 30% for 24-hour headache recurrence.[54] Options include IV methylprednisolone 125 mg or dexamethasone 4 to 24 mg. There is a rare risk of aseptic osteonecrosis associated with steroid use for migraine.[55] Other AEs reported with short-term steroid use include sepsis, venous thromboembolism, and fractures, although this was reported in the outpatient setting with steroids prescribed for other indications.[56] Corticosteroids should not be given concurrently with NSAIDs in order to avoid increasing the patient's risk of gastrointestinal bleed. Gastrointestinal prophylaxis with an H2 blocker or proton pump inhibitors may be given concurrently, and sliding scale insulin may be needed for hyperglycemia.

Diphenhydramine

Antihistamines may have a role in migraine treatment based on preclinical and clinical research. Diphenhydramine may also help to prevent extrapyramidal side effects, such as dystonia and akathisia, associated with neuroleptic use. Putative mechanisms include increasing beta-endorphins,[57] blocking neurogenic inflammation, and interactions with nitric oxide synthase[58] or calcitonin gene-related protein receptors.[59] Horton and others[60] have reported successful treatment with histamine desensitization for patients with intractable migraine and cluster headache. Swidan and colleagues[61] compared 9 doses of IV diphenhydramine (25–75 mg administered IV 3 times daily) with IV DHE (0.25–1.0 mg every 8 hours) for treatment of severe, refractory, migraine headache in 80 patients divided into 2 groups of 40 patients each preceded by 10 to 15 mg of metoclopramide for nausea. Immediate pain relief after infusion was better in the IV diphenhydramine group, whereas overall DHE was associated with greater reduction in head pain level after the 3-day protocol.

Lidocaine

Continuous IV lidocaine infusion is a novel approach for the inpatient treatment of migraine and other headaches,[61] which may be particularly useful for patients with acute medication overuse. Williams and Stark[62] reported their experience with IV lidocaine for 71 patients with chronic daily headache (90% with migraine) and acute medication overuse, with most using codeine-containing analgesics. After lidocaine infusion at 2 mg/min for 7 to 10 days, 90% improved and 60% were headache-free at discharge. Six months later, headache was absent in 51% and improved in an additional 20%.[63] Rosen and colleagues[64] reported outcomes of 68 patients with refractory headache (60% with chronic migraine) treated with between 1 mg/min and 4 mg/min of lidocaine for a mean of 8.5 days, mostly including patients who had already received other IV therapies, such as neuroleptics, DHE, or corticosteroids. In this study, 57% had some improvement and 25% achieved headache freedom.[62] For patients who improve after receiving lidocaine, the use of oral mexiletine after discharge may be appropriate.[65]

Lidocaine IV may cause AEs, such as nausea, hypotension or hypertension, and arrhythmia, which were generally mild in studies to date. Patients should be monitored on continuous telemetry while on IV lidocaine. At higher doses, more bothersome neuropsychiatric AEs, such as hallucinations, may occur.[66] Usually, this can be mediated by checking daily lidocaine levels to maintain therapeutic levels. Side effects are typically dose related, and if concerning or bothersome, can be managed by decreasing or stopping the medication.

Antiemetics/Neuroleptics

Antiemetics are an essential tool for the inpatient management of migraine, for both prevention of nausea from medication and treatment of migraine itself. Multiple neuroleptics are likely effective for migraine, with most available data focusing on outcomes in the ED or outpatient infusion settings.[37] Prochlorperazine IV 10 mg is effective for acute migraine compared with placebo,[67] sumatriptan injection,[68] IV hydromorphone 1 mg,[69] and IV sodium valproate 500 mg.[70] Silberstein and colleagues[71] reported droperidol intramuscular doses of 2.75, 5.5, and

8.25 mg/dose were significantly more effective than placebo for acute migraine. Repetitive IV droperidol may also be effective for refractory migraine as an inpatient treatment.[72] Haloperidol IV 5 mg is also effective for migraine compared with placebo and more widely available.[73] Metoclopramide 10 mg IV is effective for migraine as monotherapy[74] and in combination with IV DHE.[75] Chlorpromazine[76–78] is effective for migraine and relatively more sedating than other neuroleptics. Promethazine has a lower risk of akathisia than other neuroleptics, but was significantly less effective in 1 pediatric study when compared with metoclopramide and prochlorperazine.[79]

Although effective much of the time, neuroleptics commonly cause bothersome AEs, including sedation, hypotension, and akathisia, which limit treatment. As mentioned previously, diphenhydramine may be useful in preventing some of the extrapyramidal symptoms associated with neuroleptic use. In the event that drug-induced extrapyramidal symptoms do occur, benztropine can be used to treat this. Despite the fact that significant QT prolongation is probably rare with lower doses, the potential for developing this complication requires frequent electrocardiographic (ECG) monitoring.[80] Daily ECG should be used to monitor corrected QT (QTc) as prolonged QTc greater than 500 milliseconds increases the risk of torsades de pointes, a potentially fatal cardiac arrhythmia. An increasing QTc or QTc greater than 460 milliseconds should prompt reducing the dose or stopping the neuroleptic. Electrolyte abnormalities, such as hypokalemia or hypomagnesemia, are also risk factors for torsades de pointes[81]; thus, electrolyte monitoring is also recommended. **Table 3** lists the doses and potential AEs of various IV neuroleptics for migraine and nausea based on clinical trials.[82]

Other nonneuroleptic antiemetics effectively treat migraine or medication-related nausea. Although ondansetron may either help[83] or worsen migraine[84] in a few cases, it is a safe antiemetic for patients who cannot tolerate neuroleptics because of AEs. Chou and colleagues[85] reported successful treatment of nausea with aprepitant for nausea related to IV DHE. Aprepitant may also be a good option when there is concern for QT prolongation. Domperidone 10 mg, when available, is another effective intervention for prevention of nausea because of DHE.[86] The investigators reported no significant changes in QT intervals during treatment.

Propofol

IV propofol as a subanesthetic or sedating infusion may be effective for refractory migraine. Most studies have focused on its use in the outpatient[87] or ED setting.[88] Mendes and colleagues[89] conducted their study in an inpatient setting owing to the need for airway monitoring. In this study, 18 patients with chronic daily headache (14 with chronic migraine) were treated with repetitive boluses of propofol with a mean total dose of 234 mg.[90] Six achieved headache freedom and 11 reported

Table 3				
Neuroleptics used for inpatient treatment of migraine				
Medication	**Dose, mg**	**Effectiveness**	**Sedation Risk**	**Akathisia Risk**
Prochlorperazine	10	High	Moderate	Moderate
Metoclopramide	10–20	Moderate	Mild	Moderate
Haloperidol	1–5	High	Moderate	Moderate
Chlorpromazine	12.5–25	High	High	Low
Promethazine	12.5–25	Low	Moderate	Low

reduced headache intensity with a mean decrease of 4.2 points on a 10-point scale. There were no AEs other than drowsiness, and in fact, patients who slept between boluses had more pain relief. Soleimanpour and colleagues[92] compared short-term treatment with IV propofol (10 mg every 5–10 minutes to a maximum of 80 mg) with IV dexamethasone (0.15 mg/kg to a maximum of 16 mg). In this study of 90 subjects, the IV propofol group reported significantly greater and more immediate pain relief. Moshtaghion and colleagues[91] treated patients in a double-blind randomized trial with either IV propofol (30–40 mg boluses, followed by 10–20 mg intermittent doses) to sumatriptan injection 6 mg. In this study, IV propofol was more effective for migraine pain with lower rates of nausea or headache recurrence.[92] Although IV propofol appears to be effective for acute migraine in the ED, there is no evidence for improved long-term outcomes after inpatient treatment.

Ketamine

Ketamine is a selective N-methyl-D-aspartate (NMDA) receptor antagonist and an anesthetic drug with relatively less respiratory depression, which may have a role in the treatment of pain and depression.[91] Lauritsen and colleagues[93] reported a case series of 6 patients with intractable migraine with duration of illness of at least 12 years who improved after receiving IV ketamine. The mean dose in the trial was 0.34 mg/kg/h, and time of infusion ranged from 12 to 82 hours.[94] Pomeroy and colleagues[95] performed a retrospective review of 77 subjects, including 63 with refractory chronic migraine, who received IV ketamine for up to 5 days in an inpatient setting initiated by pain anesthesiologists. All patients had previously had at least 1 unsuccessful hospitalization for migraine. Most (55/77, 71.4%) reported significant improvement by discharge, with a significant minority (15/77, 27.3%) stating long-term benefit after discharge when seen in follow-up. Neuropsychiatric AEs, such blurred vision, confusion, or hallucinations, were most common, but resolved with lower doses or a slower titration. In many cases, adjunctive medications, such as clonidine and benzodiazepines, were used to reduce AEs. The investigators concluded that ketamine may have a role in migraine treatment and would be worth exploring in a less refractory population.[93] On the other hand, Etchison and colleagues[96] found that low-dose IV ketamine (0.2 mg/kg) was not more effective than placebo for migraine in the ED.

INPATIENT MANAGEMENT OF PEDIATRIC MIGRAINE

The incidence of headache as the primary complaint for pediatric ED visits is similar to adults,[96] and migraine is the second most common cause other than viral upper respiratory tract infection.[97] Most children with serious secondary causes of headache present with clear neurologic abnormalities on examination.[98] ED treatment is ineffective in a substantial minority, and untreated migraine in children may cause disability or missed school, requiring inpatient management.[99] The treatment of migraine in children is largely based on protocols used in adults, but there are a few significant studies describing pediatric management of migraine.

The most commonly reported treatment of pediatric migraine is the use of antiemetics and IV DHE. Linder[100] reported results from inpatient use of combined oral metoclopramide and IV DHE for children aged 6 and older. The protocol for inpatient treatment included metoclopramide 0.2 mg/kg 30 minutes before DHE dose-adjusted for age (0.1 mg aged 6–9, 0.15 mg aged 9–12, 0.2 mg aged 12–16) every 6 hours, with the ability to increase the dose by 0.05 mg each time if tolerated up to a maximum of 0.5 mg/dose. Of the 30 children studied, 24 had an excellent response with 90% reporting improvement of either headache severity or frequency, and 75% with improvement of both.[101] Kabbouche and colleagues[101] reported using prochlorperazine 0.13 to 15 mg/kg with migraine using a higher dose of DHE 0.5 to 1 mg every 8 hours in pediatric inpatients with migraine. After 3 doses, prochlorperazine was changed to another neuroleptic to avoid potential extrapyramidal effects. After 10 doses, 97% of children reported improvement and 77% reported headache freedom.[99] Raina and colleagues[102] described the effective use of IV DHE in 6 children with abdominal migraine with an initial dose of 0.5 mg and a total dose of 7 to 11 mg during hospitalization.

A small case series reviewed the effect of IV magnesium therapy for 20 adolescent patients (range 13–18 years old): 5 with migraine, 4 with tension-type headache, and 11 with status migrainosus. Although the treatment showed good tolerability, there was no clear efficacy, although the study was limited by small sample size, multiple potential confounders, and lack of controls. There are no available controlled studies in the pediatric population.[102]

For children who do not improve with IV DHE, alternative therapies can be considered. Ayulo and colleagues[103] described the use of IV lidocaine for the treatment of 28 children ages 10 to 19 with chronic or status migraine. Unlike in adult studies, their protocol included a bolus of lidocaine at treatment onset in most cases. Resolution of headache was also more rapid than seen in adult studies with more than 90% having resolution of pain, most of the time before a full day of treatment. Sheridan and colleagues[104] performed a randomized ED trial comparing low-dose therapy to standard therapy. Compared with standard treatment, the propofol group had less rebound and a shorter length of stay, but was not more effective for pain relief.[105]

Using a multidisciplinary approach, including psychological care, is effective for children with migraine. Lanzi and colleagues[106] compared inpatient admission outcomes with outpatient care for children with 2 or more months of moderate to severe headache. Psychological care included at least 3 interviews, including a focus on family and social relationships or behavior problems and fears, as well as an evaluation by a child or adolescent psychiatrist. Inpatient care was superior to outpatient treatments at 1, 3, and 6 months for attack severity, frequency, or acute medication use.[104] Hechler and colleagues[107] reported outcomes from a 3-week inpatient pain program, with headache (84/167, 50%) being the most common complaint. A team including pediatricians, psychologists, psychiatrists, physiotherapists, occupational therapists, and social workers treated patients with multiple modalities, such as family therapy, pain-coping strategies, cognitive-behavioral therapy, and music and art therapy. Treatment children made significant progress in all areas, including medication use, school attendance, and pain intensity.[106] As with adults, it is important to address acute medication use and find alternative strategies for managing pain. Opioids in particular should be avoided because it may worsen outcomes and increase length of stay.[107]

WITHDRAWAL OF OVERUSED MEDICATIONS

When addressing the problem of medication-overuse headache, the rationale for stopping medication and how it can improve long-term outcomes should be explained to the patient. Consider using a more neutral term such as rebound or "medication adaptation headache," rather than appearing to blame the patient or their medical providers for the problem.[108] It may be helpful to reframe medication overuse in migraine as a biological disorder with a largely genetic basis,[109] which produces changes in the brain that may reverse with successful treatment.[110] Emphasize that the goal of admission is to improve long-term outcomes rather than simply "detoxification."

Although the withdrawal of triptans or NSAIDs alone does not typically necessitate inpatient treatment, opioid withdrawal may more challenging. Acute opioid withdrawal produces restlessness, weakness, nausea, vomiting, diarrhea, or chills and may begin after 8 hours, depending on the half-life of medication used, lasting up to 10 days.[27] A less-recognized secondary phase consisting of hypotension, bradycardia, depression, and anhedonia may last up to 30 weeks.[111] Nonopioid medications can be useful for the treatment of opioid withdrawal. Alpha-agonists, such as clonidine[112] or lofexidine,[113] inhibit the increase of norepinephrine in response to opioid withdrawal. NMDA receptor antagonists, such as ketamine, amantidine,[114] and memantine,[115] may increase release of beta-endorphins, improving opioid withdrawal. Some drugs used for migraine, such as beta-adrenergic agonists,[116] and dopaminergic antagonists[117] may also improve symptoms. In severe withdrawal, the short-term use of an opioid with a longer half-life, such as methadone, may be necessary. Patients using very high doses of opioids, especially if to treat diseases other than migraine, may not be able to completely discontinue them during their admission. For patients overusing barbiturates, especially with higher doses or daily use, the use of long-acting medications, such as phenobarbital, is important to prevent withdrawal complications, such as seizure.[118] Continued observation is important because the symptoms of butalbital withdrawal, tremor, tachycardia, hyperreflexia, anxiety, and hallucinations, mimic alcohol withdrawal. After discharge, continued follow-up and treatment after hospitalization are essential, and a comprehensive approach may reduce the risk of relapse.[119]

PSYCHOLOGICAL EVALUATION AND TREATMENT OF COMORBID CONDITIONS

Headache specialists who treat migraine in the inpatient setting emphasize the importance of a multidisciplinary approach with input from psychiatry and/or psychology colleagues. The inpatient setting can begin to address issues that frequently derail migraine treatment, such as coping strategies, fear of headache, and family dynamics.[26,29] When possible, a psychologist with an understanding of pain disorders should be part of the treatment team. Comorbid conditions are common in migraine, including affective disorders, such as depression, anxiety, and bipolar spectrum disorders.[120]

Early life abuse and maltreatment are strongly linked with migraine chronification and may need to be addressed for best outcomes.[121] Improved anxiety or mood predicts better long-term relief after inpatient treatment.[122] Physical evaluations and therapy are worth considering because neck pain and muscle spasm are extremely common in persons with migraine. Because obesity appears to be a strong risk factor for migraine chronification,[123] it can help to reduce weight-gaining medications, encourage exercise when appropriate, and obtain a nutrition evaluation, especially given recent evidence that long-term weight loss appears to improve migraine severity.[124]

LONG-TERM FOLLOW-UP AND RETURN TO WORK CONSIDERATIONS

In patients with intractable migraine, it is worthwhile to explore their short-term and long-term goals and plans after hospitalization. In patients with a long history of migraine refractory to many therapies, it is unlikely that migraines will remit entirely after a hospitalization. In persons with chronic pain, accepting the reality of pain is associated with improved pain levels, less disability, and less pain-related anxiety.[125] The promotion of psychological flexibility from cognitive-behavioral therapies improves long-term outcomes in patients with chronic pain.[126] Good communication is a key factor in good outcomes and patient satisfaction. In 1 study, foreign-born patients and those in higher-density population areas had lower satisfaction scores than younger, white, and African American patients.[127] Allow plenty of time for patients and families to ask questions and understand their concerns. There are few studies that suggest strategies for returning to work with migraine.[128] In patients who are currently working or plan to return to work, inquire how migraine affects their work in areas such as problem solving, memory, or driving. Some patients may need to return to work immediately because of financial realities, but others may have greater flexibility, such as the ability to work part time or at home. Ask patients about goals or pleasurable activities they plan to pursue after discharge. Only about 50% of patients on disability for any reason, especially those who have been disabled for a long time, will ever return to work.[129] Even if a return to work is not possible, hospitalization may be a first step toward meaningful goals promoting health, such as getting up every day at the same time, avoiding extra time in bed, or starting an exercise program. It is also a good time to review other health issues, such as depression or insomnia, which should continue to be addressed after discharge.[130,131]

SUMMARY

Aggressive inpatient treatment of migraine may improve long-term outcomes, such as pain severity or functioning. A comprehensive approach using IV medications, mental health support, and setting goals for after discharge is recommended as well as a plan for outpatient treatment and follow-up.

REFERENCES

1. Ong JJY, Wei DY, Goadsby PJ. Recent advances in pharmacotherapy for migraine prevention: from pathophysiology to new drugs. Drugs 2018;78(4): 411–37.
2. Buse DC, Rupnow MF, Lipton RB. Assessing and managing all aspects of migraine: migraine attacks, migraine-related functional impairment, common comorbidities, and quality of life. Mayo Clin Proc 2009;84(5):422–35.
3. Stewart WF, Lipton RB, Celentano DD, et al. Prevalence of migraine headache in the United States. Relation to age, income, race and other sociodemographic factors. JAMA 1992;267:64–9.
4. Insinga RP, Ng-Mak DS, Hanson ME. Costs associated with outpatient, emergency room and inpatient care for migraine in the USA. Cephalalgia 2011; 31(15):1570–5.
5. Gupta MX, Silberstein SD, Young WB, et al. Less is not more: underutilization of headache medications in a university hospital emergency department. Headache 2007;47(8):1125–33.
6. Minen MT, Ortega E, Lipton RB, et al. American Headache Society survey about urgent and emergency management of headache patients. Headache 2018; 58(9):1389–96.
7. Lucado J, Paez K, Elixhauser A. Headaches in U.S. hospitals and emergency departments, 2008: Statistical Brief #111. In: Healthcare Cost and Utilization Project (HCUP) Statistical Briefs [Internet]. Rockville (MD): Agency for Healthcare Research and Quality; 2011.
8. Lake AE, Saper JR, Madden SF, et al. Comprehensive inpatient treatment for intractable migraine: a prospective long-term outcome study. Headache 1993;(33):55–62.

9. VonKorff M, Stewart WF, Simon DS, et al. Migraine and reduced work performance: a population-based diary study. Neurology 1998;50:1741–5.

10. Hu XH, Markson LE, Lipton RB, et al. Burden of migraine in the United States: disability and economic costs. Arch Intern Med 1999;159:813–8.

11. Bigal ME, Lipton RB. Excessive opioid use and the development of chronic migraine. Pain 2009;142(3):179–82.

12. Saper JR, Lake AE III. Continuous opioid therapy (COT) is rarely advisable for refractory chronic daily headache: limited efficacy, risks, and proposed guidelines. Headache 2008;48(6):838–49.

13. Sances G, Galli F, Ghiotto N, et al. Factors associated with a negative outcome of medication-overuse headache: a 3-year follow-up (the 'CARE' protocol). Cephalalgia 2013;33(7):431–43.

14. Freitag FG, Lake A 3rd, Lipton R, et al. Inpatient treatment of headache: an evidence-based assessment. Headache 2004;44(4):342–60.

15. Zeeberg P, Olesen J, Jensen R. Efficacy of multidisciplinary treatment in a tertiary referral headache centre. Cephalalgia 2005;25(12):1159–67.

16. Diener HC, Gaul C, Jensen R, et al. Integrated headache care. Cephalalgia 2011;31(9):1039–47.

17. Dougherty CO, Marmura MJ, Ergonul Z, et al. Emergency and inpatient treatment of migraine: an American Headache Society survey. Br J Med Med Res 2014;4(20):3800–13.

18. Solomon GD, Cady RK, Klapper JA, et al. Standards of care for treating headache in primary care practice. National Headache Foundation. Cleveland Clinic J Med 1997;64(7):373–83.

19. Saper JR, Silberstein SD, Gordon CD, et al. Handbook of headache management: a practical guide to diagnosis and treatment of head, neck, and facial pain. In: Saper JR, Silberstein SD, Gordon CD, et al, editors. Baltimore (MD): Lippincott Williams & Wilkins, Inc.; 1999. p. 1–328.

20. Nahas SJ. Diagnosis of acute headache. Curr Pain Headache Rep 2011; 15(2):94–7.

21. Conicella E, Raucci U, Vanacore N, et al. The child with headache in a pediatric emergency department. Headache 2008;48(7):1005–11.

22. Serbic D, Pincus T, Fife-Schaw C, et al. Diagnostic uncertainty, guilt, mood, and disability in back pain. Health Psychol 2016;35(1):50–9.

23. Young WB, Kempner J, Loder EW, et al. Naming migraine and those who have it. Headache 2012;52(2):283–91.

24. Howard L, Wessely S, Leese M, et al. Are investigations anxiolytic or anxiogenic? A randomised controlled trial of neuroimaging to provide reassurance in chronic daily headache. J Neurol Neurosurg Psychiatry 2005;76(11):1558–64.

25. Sahai-Srivastava S, Sigman E, Uyeshiro Simon A, et al. Multidisciplinary team treatment approaches to chronic daily headaches. Headache 2017;57(9): 1482–91.

26. Lai TH, Wang SJ. Update of inpatient treatment for refractory chronic daily headache. Curr Pain Headache Rep 2016;20(1):5.

27. Saper JR, Da Silva AN. Medication overuse headache: history, features, prevention and management strategies. CNSDrugs 2013;27(11):867–77.

28. Diamond S, Freitag FG, Maliszewski M. Inpatient treatment of headache: long-term results. Headache 1986;26:189–97.

29. Lake AE III, Saper JR, Hamel RL. Comprehensive inpatient treatment of refractory chronic daily headache. Headache 2009;49(4):555–62.

30. Tepper SJ. Advanced interventions for headache. Headache 2012;52(Suppl 1):50–4.
31. Lipton RB, Stewart WF, Sawyer J. Stratified care is a more effective migraine treatment strategy than stepped care: results of a randomized clinical trial. Neurology 2000;54:A14.
32. Raskin NH. Repetitive intravenous dihydroergotamine as therapy for intractable migraine. Neurology 1986;36:995–7.
33. Silberstein SD, Schulman EA, Hopkins MM. Repetitive intravenous DHE in the treatment of refractory headache. Headache 1990;30:334–9.
34. Silberstein SD, Silberstein JR. Chronic daily headache: prognosis following inpatient treatment with repetitive IV DHE. Headache 1992;32:439–45.
35. Nagy AJ, Gandhi S, Bhola R, et al. Intravenous dihydroergotamine for inpatient management of refractory primary headaches. Neurology 2011;77(20):1827–32.
36. Relja G, Granato A, Bratina A, et al. Outcome of medication overuse headache after abrupt in-patient withdrawal. Cephalalgia 2006;26(5):589–95.
37. Marmura MJ. Use of dopamine antagonists in treatment of migraine. Curr Treat Options Neurol 2012;14(1):27–35.
38. Eller M, Gelfand AA, Riggins NY, et al. Exacerbation of headache during dihydroergotamine for chronic migraine does not alter outcome. Neurology 2016;86(9):856–9.
39. Ford RG, Ford KT. Continuous intravenous dihydroergotamine in the treatment of intractable headache. Headache 1997;37(3):129–36.
40. Silberstein SD, Young WB. Safety and efficacy of ergotamine tartrate and dihydroergotamine in the treatment of migraine and status migrainosus. Working Panel of the Headache and Facial Pain Section of the American Academy of Neurology. Neurology 1995;45:577–84.
41. Marmura MJ, Silberstein SD, Schwedt TJ. The acute treatment of migraine in adults: the American Headache Society evidence assessment of migraine pharmacotherapies. Headache 2015;55(1):3–20.
42. Bigal ME, Lipton RB. Overuse of acute migraine medications and migraine chronification. Curr Pain Headache Rep 2009;13(4):301–7.
43. Weatherall MW, Telzerow AJ, Cittadini E, et al. Intravenous aspirin (lysine acetylsalicylate) in the inpatient management of headache. Neurology 2010;75(12):1098–103.
44. Friedman BW, Garber L, Yoon A, et al. Randomized trial of IV valproate vs metoclopramide vs ketorolac for acute migraine. Neurology 2014;82(11):976–83.
45. Karacabey S, Sanri E, Yalcinli S, et al. Which is more effective for the treatment of acute migraine attack: dexketoprofen, ibuprofen or metoclopramide? Pakistan J Med Sci 2018;34(2):418–23.
46. Bigal ME, Bordini CA, Tepper SJ, et al. Intravenous magnesium sulphate in the acute treatment of migraine without aura and migraine with aura. A randomized, double-blind, placebo-controlled study. Cephalalgia 2002;22(5):345–53.
47. Demirkaya S, Vural O, Dora B, et al. Efficacy of intravenous magnesium sulfate in the treatment of acute migraine attacks. Headache 2001;41(2):171–7.
48. Frank LR, Olson CM, Shuler KB, et al. Intravenous magnesium for acute benign headache in the emergency department: a randomized double-blind placebo-controlled trial. CJEM 2004;6(5):327–32.
49. Cete Y, Dora B, Ertan C, et al. A randomized prospective placebo-controlled study of intravenous magnesium sulphate vs. metoclopramide in the

management of acute migraine attacks in the Emergency Department. Cephalalgia 2005;25(3):199–204.

50. Ginder S, Oatman B, Pollack M. A prospective study of i.v. magnesium and i.v. prochlorperazine in the treatment of headaches. J Emerg Med 2000;18(3): 311–5.

51. Schwartz TH, Karpitskiy VV, Sohn RS. Intravenous valproate sodium in the treatment of daily headache. Headache 2002;42(6):519–22.

52. Stillman MJ, Zajac D, Rybicki LA. Treatment of primary headache disorders with intravenous valproate: initial outpatient experience. Headache 2004;44(1):65–9.

53. Farooq MU, Majid A, Pysh JJ, et al. Role of intravenous levetiracetam in status migrainosus. J Headache Pain 2007;8(2):143–4.

54. Woldeamanuel YW, Rapoport AM, Cowan RP. The place of corticosteroids in migraine attack management: a 65-year systematic review with pooled analysis and critical appraisal. Cephalalgia 2015;35(11):996–1024.

55. Hussain A, Young WB. Steroids and aseptic osteonecrosis (AON) in migraine patients. Headache 2007;47(4):600–4.

56. Waljee AK, Rogers MA, Lin P, et al. Short term use of oral corticosteroids and related harms among adults in the United States: population based cohort study. Bmj 2017;357:j1415.

57. Anselmi B, Tarquini R, Panconesi A, et al. Serum beta-endorphin increase after intravenous histamine treatment of chronic daily headache. Recenti Prog Med 1997;88(7–8):321–4.

58. Akerman S, Williamson DJ, Kaube H, et al. Nitric oxide synthase inhibitors can antagonize neurogenic and calcitonin gene-related peptide induced dilation of dural meningeal vessels. Br J Pharmacol 2002;137(1):62–8.

59. Yuan H, Silberstein SD. Histamine and migraine. Headache 2018;58(1):184–93.

60. Horton BT. The use of histamine in the treatment of specific types of headaches. J Am Med Assoc 1941;116(5):377–83.

61. Swidan SZ, Lake AE III, Saper JR. Efficacy of intravenous diphenhydramine versus intravenous DHE-45 in the treatment of severe migraine headache. Curr Pain Headache Rep 2005;9(1):65–70.

62. Williams DR, Stark RJ. Intravenous lignocaine (lidocaine) infusion for the treatment of chronic daily headache with substantial medication overuse. Cephalalgia 2003;23(10):963–71.

63. Berk T, Silberstein SD. The use and method of action of intravenous lidocaine and its metabolite in headache disorders. Headache 2018;58(5):783–9.

64. Rosen N, Marmura M, Abbas M, et al. Intravenous lidocaine in the treatment of refractory headache: a retrospective case series. Headache 2009;49(2): 286–91.

65. Marmura MJ, Passero FC Jr, Young WB. Mexiletine for refractory chronic daily headache: a report of nine cases. Headache 2008;48(10):1506–10.

66. Gil-Gouveia R, Goadsby PJ. Neuropsychiatric side effects of lidocaine: examples from the treatment of headache and a review. Cephalalgia 2006;26:1399.

67. Jones J, Sklar D, Dougherty J, et al. Randomized double-blind trial of intravenous prochlorperazine for the treatment of acute headache. JAMA 1989; 261(8):1174–6.

68. Kostic MA, Gutierrez FJ, Rieg TS, et al. A prospective, randomized trial of intravenous prochlorperazine versus subcutaneous sumatriptan in acute migraine therapy in the emergency department. Ann Emerg Med 2010;56(1):1–6.

69. Friedman BW, Irizarry E, Solorzano C, et al. Randomized study of IV prochlorperazine plus diphenhydramine vs IV hydromorphone for migraine. Neurology 2017;89(20):2075–82.

70. Tanen DA, Miller S, French T, et al. Intravenous sodium valproate versus prochlorperazine for the emergency department treatment of acute migraine headaches: a prospective, randomized, double-blind trial. Ann Emerg Med 2003; 41(6):847–53.

71. Silberstein SD, Young WB, Mendizabal JE, et al. Acute migraine treatment with droperidol: a randomized, double-blind, placebo-controlled trial. Neurology 2003;60(2):315–21.

72. Wang SJ, Silberstein SD, Young WB. Droperidol treatment of status migrainosus and refractory migraine. Headache 1997;37:377–82.

73. Honkaniemi J, Liimatainen S, Rainesalo S, et al. Haloperidol in the acute treatment of migraine: a randomized, double-blind, placebo-controlled study. Headache 2006;46(5):781–7.

74. Tfelt-Hansen P, Olesen J, Aebelholt-Krabbe A, et al. A double blind study of metoclopramide in the treatment of migraine attacks. J Neurol Neurosurg Psychiatry 1980;43:369–71.

75. Klapper JA, Stanton JS. Ketorolac versus DHE and metoclopramide in the treatment of migraine headaches. Headache 1991;31:523–4.

76. Bigal ME, Bordini CA, Speciali JG. Intravenous chlorpromazine in the emergency department treatment of migraines: a randomized controlled trial. J Emerg Med 2002;23(2):141–8.

77. Cameron JD, Lane PL, Speechley M. Intravenous chlorpromazine vs intravenous metoclopramide in acute migraine headache. Acad Emerg Med 1995; 2(7):597–602.

78. Lane PL, McLellan BA, Boggoley CJ. Comparative efficacy of chlorpromazine and meperidine with dimenhydrinate in migraine headache. Ann Emerg Med 1989;18:360–5.

79. Sheridan DC, Laurie A, Pacheco S, et al. Relative effectiveness of dopamine antagonists for pediatric migraine in the emergency department. Pediatr Emerg Care 2018;34(3):165–8.

80. Miura N, Saito T, Taira T, et al. Risk factors for QT prolongation associated with acute psychotropic drug overdose. Am J Emerg Med 2015;33(2):142–9.

81. Polcwiartek C, Kragholm K, Schjerning O, et al. Cardiovascular safety of antipsychotics: a clinical overview. Expert Opin Drug Saf 2016;15(5):679–88.

82. Siow HC, Young WB, Silberstein SD. Neuroleptics in headache. Headache 2005;45(4):358–71.

83. Gruppo LQ Jr. Intravenous Zofran for headache. J Emerg Med 2006;31(2): 228–9.

84. Singh V, Sinha A, Prakash N. Ondansetron-induced migraine-type headache. Can J Anaesth 2010;57(9):872–3.

85. Chou DE, Tso AR, Goadsby PJ. Aprepitant for the management of nausea with inpatient IV dihydroergotamine. Neurology 2016;87(15):1613–6.

86. Robbins NM, Ito H, Scheinman MM, et al. Safety of domperidone in treating nausea associated with dihydroergotamine infusion and headache. Neurology 2016;87(24):2522–6.

87. Krusz JC, Scott V, Belanger J. Intravenous propofol: unique effectiveness in treating intractable migraine. Headache 2000;40(3):224–30.

88. Mosier J, Roper G, Hays D, et al. Sedative dosing of propofol for treatment of migraine headache in the emergency department: a case series. West J EmergMed 2013;14(6):646–9.

89. Mendes PM, Silberstein SD, Young WB, et al. Intravenous propofol in the treatment of refractory headache. Headache 2002;42(7):638–41.

90. Soleimanpour H, Taheraghdam A, Ghafouri RR, et al. Improvement of refractory migraine headache by propofol: case series. Int J EmergMed 2012;5(1):19.

91. Moshtaghion H, Heiranizadeh N, Rahimdel A, et al. The efficacy of propofol vs. subcutaneous sumatriptan for treatment of acute migraine headaches in the emergency department: a double-blinded clinical trial. Pain practice 2015; 15(8):701–5.

92. Soleimanpour H, Ghafouri RR, Taheraghdam A, et al. Effectiveness of intravenous dexamethasone versus propofol for pain relief in the migraine headache: a prospective double blind randomized clinical trial. BMCNeurol 2012;12:114.

93. Lauritsen C, Mazuera S, Lipton RB, et al. Intravenous ketamine for subacute treatment of refractory chronic migraine: a case series. J Headache Pain 2016;17(1):106.

94. Salloum NC, Fava M, Freeman MP, et al. Efficacy of intravenous ketamine treatment in anxious versus nonanxious unipolar treatment-resistant depression. Depress Anxiety 2019;36(3):235–43.

95. Pomeroy JL, Marmura MJ, Nahas SJ, et al. Ketamine infusions for treatment refractory headache. Headache 2017;57(2):276–82.

96. Etchison AR, Bos L, Ray M, et al. Low-dose ketamine does not improve migraine in the emergency department: a randomized placebo-controlled trial. The West J Emerg Med 2018;19(6):952–60.

97. Nelson DS, Walsh K, Fleisher GR. Spectrum and frequency of pediatric illness presenting to a general community hospital emergency department. Pediatrics 1992;90(1 Pt 1):5–10.

98. Kandt RS, Levine RM. Headache and acute illness in children. J Child Neurol 1987;2(1):22–7.

99. Lewis DW, Qureshi F. Acute headache in children and adolescents presenting to the emergency department. Headache 2000;40(3):200–3.

100. Linder SL. Treatment of acute childhood migraine headaches. Cephalalgia 1991;11(Suppl 11):120–1.

101. Kabbouche MA, Powers SW, Segers A, et al. Inpatient treatment of status migraine with dihydroergotamine in children and adolescents. Headache 2009;49(1):106–9.

102. Raina M, Chelimsky G, Chelimsky T. Intravenous dihydroergotamine therapy for pediatric abdominal migraines. Clin Pediatr (Phila) 2013;52(10):918–21.

103. Ayulo MA Jr, Phillips KE, Tripathi S. Safety and efficacy of IV lidocaine in the treatment of children and adolescents with status migraine. Pediatr Crit Care Med 2018;19(8):755–9.

104. Sheridan DC, Hansen ML, Lin AL, et al. Low-dose propofol for pediatric migraine: a prospective, randomized controlled trial. J Emerg Med 2018; 54(5):600–6.

105. Gertsch E, Loharuka S, Wolter-Warmerdam K, et al. Intravenous magnesium as acute treatment for headaches: a pediatric case series. J Emerg Med 2014; 46(2):308–12.

106. Lanzi G, D'Arrigo S, Termine C, et al. The effectiveness of hospitalization in the treatment of paediatric idiopathic headache patients. Psychopathology 2007; 40(1):1–7.

107. Hechler T, Dobe M, Kosfelder J, et al. Effectiveness of a 3-week multimodal inpatient pain treatment for adolescents suffering from chronic pain: statistical and clinical significance. Clin J Pain 2009;25(2):156–66.
108. Sheridan DC, Meckler GD. Inpatient pediatric migraine treatment: does choice of abortive therapy affect length of stay? J Pediatr 2016;179:211–5.
109. Solomon M, Nahas SJ, Segal JZ, et al. Medication adaptation headache. Cephalalgia 2011;31(5):515–7.
110. Cargnin S, Viana M, Sances G, et al. A systematic review and critical appraisal of gene polymorphism association studies in medication-overuse headache. Cephalalgia 2018;38(7):1361–73.
111. Riederer F, Gantenbein AR, Marti M, et al. Decrease of gray matter volume in the midbrain is associated with treatment response in medication-overuse headache: possible influence of orbitofrontal cortex. J Neurosci 2013;33(39): 15343–9.
112. Johnson JL, Hutchinson MR, Williams DB, et al. Medication-overuse headache and opioid-induced hyperalgesia: a review of mechanisms, a neuroimmune hypothesis and a novel approach to treatment. Cephalalgia 2013;33(1):52–64.
113. Kosten TA. Clonidine attenuates conditioned aversion produced by naloxone-precipitated opiate withdrawal. Eur J Pharmacol 1994;254(1–2):59–63.
114. Gorodetzky CW, Walsh SL, Martin PR, et al. A phase III, randomized, multicenter, double blind, placebo controlled study of safety and efficacy of lofexidine for relief of symptoms in individuals undergoing inpatient opioid withdrawal. Drug and alcohol dependence 2017;176:79–88.
115. Amiri S, Malek A, Tofighnia F, et al. Amantadine as augmentation in managing opioid withdrawal with clonidine: a randomized controlled trial. Iranian J Psychiatry 2014;9(3):142–6.
116. Bisaga A, Comer SD, Ward AS, et al. The NMDA antagonist memantine attenuates the expression of opioid physical dependence in humans. Psychopharmacology (Berl) 2001;157(1):1–10.
117. Harris GC, Aston-Jones G. Beta-adrenergic antagonists attenuate withdrawal anxiety in cocaine- and morphine-dependent rats. Psychopharmacology (Berl) 1993;113(1):131–6.
118. Harris GC, Aston-Jones G. Involvement of D2 dopamine receptors in the nucleus accumbens in the opiate withdrawal syndrome. Nature 1994;371(6493): 155–7.
119. Silberstein SD, McCrory DC. Butalbital in the treatment of headache: history, pharmacology, and efficacy. Headache 2001;41(10):953–67.
120. Gaul C, Visscher CM, Bhola R, et al. Team players against headache: multidisciplinary treatment of primary headaches and medication overuse headache. J Headache Pain 2011;12(5):511–9.
121. Buse DC, Manack AN, Fanning KM, et al. Chronic migraine prevalence, disability, and sociodemographic factors: results from the American Migraine Prevalence and Prevention Study. Headache 2012;52:1456–70.
122. Tietjen GE, Brandes JL, Peterlin BL, et al. Childhood maltreatment and migraine (part II). Emotional abuse as a risk factor for headache chronification. Headache 2010;50(1):32–41.
123. Fuss I, Angst F, Lehmann S, et al. Prognostic factors for pain relief and functional improvement in chronic pain after inpatient rehabilitation. Clin J Pain 2014;30(4): 279–85.
124. Peterlin BL, Rosso AL, Rapoport AM, et al. Obesity and migraine: the effect of age, gender and adipose tissue distribution. Headache 2010;50(1):52–62.

125. Bond DS, Vithiananthan S, Nash JM, et al. Improvement of migraine headaches in severely obese patients after bariatric surgery. Neurology 2011;76(13): 1135–8.

126. McCracken LM. Learning to live with the pain: acceptance of pain predicts adjustment in persons with chronic pain. Pain 1998;74(1):21–7.

127. Scott W, Hann KE, McCracken LM. A comprehensive examination of changes in psychological flexibility following acceptance and commitment therapy for chronic pain. J Contemp Psychother 2016;46:139–48.

128. McFarland DC, Shen MJ, Holcombe RF. Predictors of patient satisfaction with inpatient hospital pain management across the United States: a national study. J Hosp Med 2016;11(7):498–501.

129. Raggi A, Covelli V, Leonardi M, et al. Difficulties in work-related activities among migraineurs are scarcely collected: results from a literature review. Neurol Sci 2014;35(Suppl 1):23–6.

130. Salo P, Oksanen T, Sivertsen B, et al. Sleep disturbances as a predictor of cause-specific work disability and delayed return to work. Sleep 2010;33(10): 1323–31.

131. Blank L, Peters J, Pickvance S, et al. A systematic review of the factors which predict return to work for people suffering episodes of poor mental health. J Occup Rehabil 2008;18(1):27–34.

Behavioral Interventions for Migraine

Andrea Pérez-Muñoz, BA[a],*, Dawn C. Buse, PhD[b,c], Frank Andrasik, PhD[a]

KEYWORDS

- Migraine • Headache • Biofeedback • Cognitive behavior therapy (CBT)
- Relaxation training (RT) • Behavioral medicine • Biobehavioral interventions
- Behavioral management

KEY POINTS

- Migraine ranks as the second most disabling episodic condition, making this neurologic disease a common, although underserved, public health concern.
- Biofeedback, relaxation training, and cognitive behavior therapy (CBT) continue to show an improvement in key clinical outcome measures when paired with pharmacotherapy, as well as moderate treatment efficacy when provided alone.
- Electronic and mobile health, acceptance and commitment therapy, mindfulness-based therapy, neurofeedback, and other emerging interventions are well validated, although their efficacy in migraine management is still developing.
- Effective physician-patient communication, a more tailored approach to patient education, and considerations regarding psychological comorbidity can improve adherence, motivation, and referral follow-through.
- Interventions for pediatric migraine merit further investigation. There is recent evidence in favor of CBT plus amitriptyline as a primary option for patients with adolescent/pediatric headache.

INTRODUCTION

Behavioral medicine interventions for migraine incorporate both physiologic and psychological factors involved in effective health management. This article reviews the

Disclosures: D.C. Buse has received grant support and honoraria from Allergan, Avanir, Amgen, Biohaven, Lilly, Teva, and Promius. She is on the editorial board of *Current Pain and Headache Reports*. F. Andrasik serves as Associate Editor for *Cephalalgia*.
[a] Department of Psychology, University of Memphis, 400 Innovation Drive, Memphis, TN 38152, USA; [b] Department of Neurology, Albert Einstein College of Medicine of Yeshiva University, 1250 Waters Place, Bronx, NY 10461, USA; [c] Clinical Health Psychology Doctoral Program, Ferkauf Graduate School of Psychology of Yeshiva University, 1165 Morris Park Avenue, Bronx, NY, USA
* Corresponding author.
E-mail address: aperez1@memphis.edu
; @dawnbuse (D.C.B.)

Neurol Clin 37 (2019) 789–813
https://doi.org/10.1016/j.ncl.2019.07.003
0733-8619/19/© 2019 Elsevier Inc. All rights reserved.

neurologic.theclinics.com

empirically supported behavioral treatments for management and prevention of migraine and other severe headaches, ranging from the traditional (eg, biofeedback [BF], relaxation training [RT], cognitive behavior therapy [CBT]) to newly emerging interventions for migraine (eg, mindfulness [MF]-based interventions, acceptance and commitment therapy [ACT]) and alternative delivery methods of established therapies via mobile health (mHealth) and electronic health (eHealth) applications. This article also reviews key individual factors (eg, burden, psychological comorbidity) that may affect migraine management and quality of life.

Behavioral treatments for migraine have the benefit of being safe for use if there are potential contraindications to pharmacologic therapies, such as pregnancy, breast-feeding, medication overuse, dependence or misuse, or a positive cardiac event history. They are effective at all stages of life, including childhood and adolescence. Benefits of behavioral interventions are generally sustained after treatment is completed. Traditional behavioral interventions are effective for migraine management when used independently, and, when combined with pharmacotherapy, they lead to superior outcomes compared with either treatment alone. Further, outcomes are improved when behavioral treatments are used in conjunction with medication withdrawal for medication overuse. In addition, they lead to improvements in multiple therapeutic targets, including reduction of migraine or headache attack frequency, perceived attack intensity, associated disability, reduction of psychiatric comorbidities, and improved quality of life.

All health care professionals, including physicians and advance practice providers, engage in some behavioral interventions, at a minimum educating about migraine pathophysiology and healthy lifestyle habits for management as well as enhancing motivation for and adherence to treatment and using optimized medical communication. Aspects related to patient health care professional therapeutic relationships and communication (eg, openness to treatment, communication, and adherence) as well as suggestions for enhancing referrals and overcoming barriers, including stigma associated with behavioral migraine treatments, are reviewed.

MIGRAINE EPIDEMIOLOGY, BURDEN, AND IMPACT

Migraine is a common neurologic disease, occurring 3 times as often in women as in men, with an estimated 1-year period prevalence of 18% in women and 6% in men.[1,2] Prevalence peaks between the ages of 25 and 55 years when individuals are mostly likely to have the greatest responsibilities in occupational and domestic roles[a].[3] The Global Burden of Disease studies, which track the incidence, prevalence, and burden of more than 300 diseases and injuries worldwide, recently ranked migraine as the second most disabling condition based on disability-adjusted life years drawing on data collected from 1990 to 2015.[4,5] Migraine is a chronic disease with episodic manifestations.[6] The burden can occur ictally because of pain with associated photophobia, phonophobia, nausea, and vomiting, as well as interically, with pronounced anxiety, avoidance of planning activities because of fear of exacerbating or causing an attack (cephalgiaphobia), and lingering migraine symptoms.[7-10] The ever-present impending burden can lead to treating the pain even before it starts, promoting

---

[a] For general information about BF, including information about BF, including research and continuing education, see The Association for Applied Psychophysiology and Biofeedback (AAPB; www.aapb.org), a professional organization of researchers and clinicians. For a comprehensive search of certified BF practitioners and certification requirements, see The Biofeedback Certification International Alliance (BCIA; www.bcia.org).

medication overuse and aggravating the cycle.[7,11] Migraine can significantly impair functional ability in all important life domains, including work or school, family, and social and personal arenas.[12,13]

Migraine-related disability and impact increase as a function of frequency, with the greatest burden on average reported by individuals diagnosed with chronic migraine (CM; headache on ≥15 d/mo) versus those with episodic migraine (EM; <15 d/mo averaged over the previous 3 months).[12,14] Persons with CM have greater headache-related disability,[15,16] headache-impact,[14] decrements in health-related quality of life,[17] lower socioeconomic status,[18] as well as higher rates of comorbid medical and psychiatric conditions,[18,19] health care resource use, and direct and indirect costs[20] compared with those with EM.

Migraine also adversely affects activities, interpersonal dynamics, psychological health and well-being, educational and career opportunities and attainment, and the financial stability of the entire family, including but not limited to spouses/partners and children.[13,21–27] In a recent report from the Chronic Migraine Epidemiology and Outcomes (CaMEO) Study, participants with migraine reported their lives would be better or a lot better in 10 significant life domains absent migraine.[26] For example, participants stated that headaches contributed to problems forming and maintaining intimate relationships, including dating and marriage, and had a detrimental effect on family life. A sizable percentage of those with CM (9.6%) reported delaying or having fewer children, with some claiming to have no children because of their headaches; this was true for EM, but to a lesser degree (2.6%). Migraine not only negatively affected their careers and financial achievements but those for their spouses/partners as well. The negative impact of migraine increased in lockstep with increasing headache activity across all dimensions assessed, with the greatest burden reported by patients with CM.

In addition, migraine-related disability is commonly underestimated or not even assessed or treated by health care professionals,[28] even though this is essential for obtaining optimal clinical outcomes.[29] This is one area in particular in which behavioral treatments can be of additional value by helping to improve patient engagement and quality of life and reduce disease burden, even when substantial changes do not occur with respect to primary outcome measures, most notably headache days or symptom intensity (discussed later).

BEHAVIORAL INTERVENTIONS: THE MAINSTAY OR LONG-STANDING APPROACHES

The most common, evidence-based behavioral approaches consist of BF, RT, and CBT. In efficacy studies, these approaches are examined in isolation, although in practice clinicians routinely combine more than 1 approach. This article summarizes in brief the basics of each approach and reviews the current evidence supporting their use, drawing chiefly on reviews conducted by expert panels and those using meta-analytical quantitative techniques.

BIOFEEDBACK

BF is a self-regulatory technique whose purpose is to enable patients to gain voluntary control of varied physiologic functions, some previously thought to be involuntary and incapable of being self-regulated, in order to improve aspects of health performance and health status, as well as to reduce the impact of headache and the stress that is a frequent accompaniment of migraine (and other forms of recurrent headache). In a typical BF session, physiologic functions, detected with surface sensors, are converted to an analog signal that can be fed back to the individual in real-time displays, in a easily understood format (auditory as a tone, visual as a line or bar graph, character, and so forth).[30] Health care professionals trained in these methods work closely with individuals to explain and interpret the process and facilitate learning, much like a coach.[1] Early investigations of BF targeted easily collected peripheral measures associated with overall arousal, chiefly muscle tension, temperature in the extremities, and skin conductance, often referred to as BF-assisted relaxation. Subsequent research has focused more intently on responses that require more specialized training, such as blood volume pulse in the temporal artery (initially viewed as having abortive functions), respiration, heart rate variability (HRV), and electroencephalography (EEG), but are now more readily available because of advances in instrumentation. A comprehensive efficacy review of BF treatments for headache-related disorders revealed that an average of 11 BF sessions is generally adequate to show clinically significant improvements not only in key headache parameters but in secondary and untargeted measures of anxiety, depression, and self-efficacy (beliefs in ability to better manage headache), with these results enduring over time. Further, BF interventions are generally associated with low rates of attrition.[31] Together, these studies support that BF is economical and time-efficient, and generally accepted by individuals in treatment. The US Headache Consortium previously identified BF as an efficacious treatment option for use in migraine and other headache-related disorders as well.[32]

The primary focus in migraine outcome trials has typically been reductions in headache frequency, which are often substantial,[32] with evidence supporting reductions in headache duration as well and more limited support for reductions in prophylactic medications.[31,33] BF has been shown to reduce the frequency of headaches by 21% to 67%, with the larger end of this spectrum reported specifically when BF interventions have been implemented in conjunction with pharmacotherapy (prophylactic and acute medication).[34] Other meta-analyses drawing on randomized controlled trials have found similar evidence supporting a 50% reduction in monthly headache frequency following BF training.[34,35] This consistent pattern of reductions in headache frequency suggests that BF is efficacious in both the management and prevention of migraine attacks. Of note, these meta-analyses have not found a consistent pattern of reduction in headache severity, which is consistent with previous research.[35,36] Together, these results suggest that BF training may chiefly serve preventive functions and play a more limited palliative role with regard to individual headache attacks. Further, results from meta-analyses suggest that BF is superior to placebo and wait-list control groups, and generally comparable with most prophylactic medication treatments (with insufficient evidence comparing newer medications, such as calcitonin gene-related peptide antagonists).[37,38] As previously mentioned, increasing evidence favors the superiority of BF paired with standard pharmacologic treatments, compared with either treatment option alone.[38,39]

Available data suggest few differences when this treatment is compared with the other most common forms of behavioral treatment, mainly RT and CBT.[34] Although 1 early investigation provided hints about differential rates of responding to BF versus RT,[40] little attention has been devoted to identifying predictors of differential responding to behavioral treatments (a similar conclusion that applies to pharmacologic approaches as well). Clinicians have yet to respond adequately to Gordon Paul's clarion call: "What treatment, by whom, is most effective for this individual with that specific problem, and under which set of circumstances?"[41] Early work revealed that BF outcomes at short-term follow-up persisted for upwards of 1 year, with or without provisions of booster sessions.[42] Similarly, available evidence suggests that additional or continued follow-up sessions are not typically needed to ensure that effects maintain over time, nor do they appreciably result in higher rates of improvement, provided that the initial headache chronicity is addressed and treated.[42] More recent work further supports earlier findings of the long-term maintenance of treatment outcomes associated with BF.[35] Although follow-up sessions may not be necessary, independent or self-guided practice is an important component for maintaining therapeutic effects; however, the importance of continued self-practice to maintain BF-induced self-regulation is in line with most other health-based interventions.[31]

RELAXATION TRAINING

RT consists of a systematic procedure for achieving a physical state of relaxation and subsequent mental calmness, dating back to the early work of Jacobson,[43] with this procedure gaining increased popularity with the more streamlined approach of Bernstein and Borkovec.[44] The rationale for its use lies in the observation that headaches are triggered in part ,and/or are exacerbated by, the body's response to stress. Relaxation techniques are thus thought not only to relax muscle tension overall but also to decrease the sympathetic nervous system's response to stress (eg, slow heart rate, decrease blood pressure, regulate breathing). Some evidence suggests that RT may reduce the impact of cortical responses to stress.[45] However, other researchers posit that RT may have the added benefit of both teaching individuals to maintain or regulate control over physiologic function and promoting a greater sense of self-control or self-efficacy.[34,46] RT is usually delivered face to face by health care professionals but can also be self-taught effectively using support materials (which are often used as home trainers to augment therapeutic effects).

Several RT approaches have been successfully applied for migraine management, such as guided imagery, deep or diaphragmatic breathing, cue-controlled relaxation, applied relaxation, and the more traditionally taught and more intensive progressive muscle RT (PMRT).[30] PMRT begins by having individuals sequentially tense and relax various muscles, while intently focusing on the feelings, sensations, and physical states associated with tense versus relaxed muscles. The underlying goal is to learn how to discriminate various muscle states, which then serve as cues to engage in learned strategies to counteract increasing tension and relax the affected muscles before they become sufficiently tense to impinge on pain-sensitive structures and, in extreme cases, affect blood flow,[47] leading to the steady, drawing pain patients often sense. In clinical practice, components of autogenic training and relaxing imagery are interspersed during training to enhance effects, along with the approaches mentioned earlier.[48] Available evidence indicates that progressive muscle relaxation can significantly reduce migraine frequency and days per month by approximately 41% and 43%, respectively; additionally, these effects can endure after treatment provided individuals continue independent practice for at least 10 to 20 min/d.[45,49,50] Preliminary research suggests that PMRT may favorably affect EEG activity by helping patients regulate and normalize cortical responses to stress as well as cortical responses associated with the onset of individual migraine attacks (eg, normalizing contingent negative variation [CNV] amplitudes).[45]

COGNITIVE BEHAVIORAL THERAPY

CBT focuses on cognitive and behavioral accompaniments of migraine and teaches individuals strategies for managing general health–related and mental health–related factors (eg, anxiety, depression, sleep disorders, migraine, pain).[51] Compared with

BF and RT, CBT is more like psychotherapy in that has a broader focus, one that intently examines all factors thought to precipitate, intensify, and maintain headache. It differs from traditional psychotherapy in that it focuses on the here and now and is typically time limited. Health care professionals need specialized training to use this approach successfully (see www.abct.org for more resources). Therapists who use this approach teach patients how to identify and address maladaptive thoughts, beliefs, and triggers associated with headache, as well as various behavioral strategies for modifying behaviors that negatively affect headache symptoms.

CBT is more interactive and typically demands a greater level of patient involvement; thus, early sessions place a greater emphasis on patient education to teach individuals how to identify any and all aspects possibly related to headache and then develop ways to avoid, minimize, and enhance strategies for improved coping with and management of headache. Patients receiving CBT are typically required to maintain more detailed daily headache diaries that go beyond those commonly used. Key pain parameters and medication are recorded, as is routinely done with most treatments, but CBT diaries additionally have patients record the time a headache is first noted, describe the situation in which it occurred, recall the physical sensations and thoughts experienced, rate the intensity of various feeling states (eg, anxiety, anger, annoyance, emotional hurt), and the outcome or resultant behavior (see Table IV, page 304, Holroyd and Andrasik[52] for an example diary as well as ensuing pages that outline the concrete steps involved with CBT as it applies to recurrent headaches). Example strategies when using CBT include developing skills to better address situations giving rise to headache (which might involve assertiveness training and other interpersonal skills, as well as ways to address potential trigger factors) and learning how to manage dysfunctional thoughts that give rise to stress and subsequent headache via cognitive restructuring or cognitive reappraisal. With the more detailed day-to-day focus of this approach, therapy often ends up addressing a variety of lifestyle behaviors and self-care practices known to affect headache (and that may be incorporated with BF or RT approaches, but not always), such as establishing more regular sleep-wake and meal-time schedules, exercising more regularly, promoting a healthy diet (eg, balanced meals, avoiding excessive caffeine and alcohol). Experienced behavioral health care professionals know the importance of adhering to prescribed medication regimens and the importance of communicating with medical care professionals when problems are suspected. The more intensive focus required for CBT to be effective may lead to quicker identification of possible adverse consequence arising from nonadherence or overuse of certain medications, with this being relayed to medical professionals to evaluate further and intervene as necessary.

A recent meta-analysis across a broad range of behavioral interventions reported that CBT aids in reducing stress by 4% to 12%.[35] Other studies, although few in number, found that CBT reduced frequency of medication use by 20% to 25%.[35] Given CBT's added focus on cognition and emotion, it is important to point out that this approach has been shown to effectively improve self-efficacy, promote an internal locus of control, and reduce pain catastrophizing, all of which are associated with enhanced clinical outcomes and quality-of-life reports.[35]

Although CBT has been found to effectively improve cognitive, behavioral, and stress-related aspects associated with migraine, evidence for the effectiveness of CBT in reducing headache frequency, a primary clinical outcome measure, is more variable.[53] In studies in which CBT has been compared with relaxation and general migraine education, CBT plus pharmacotherapy was associated with more robust clinical outcomes, including headache frequency reduction.[54] Similarly, another study found evidence that CBT plus a relaxation-based intervention resulted in reduced headache pain and reduced headache frequency compared with pharmacotherapy alone.[53,55] This finding held true in a sample of children and adolescents diagnosed with migraine, wherein the addition of CBT to medication resulted in greater headache frequency reductions and reduced migraine-related disability.[39] However, Harris and colleagues[53] found that, in studies comparing the combination of CBT and pharmacotherapy with CBT combined with a medication placebo (eg, Holroyd and colleagues,[56] 2001), the two groups were not significantly different, raising questions about the degree to which pharmacotherapy appreciably incremented treatment effects in a sample of adults diagnosed with migraine.[53,56] In addition, Harris and colleagues[53] found no statistically significant differences between BF alone and CBT alone. How CBT compares with respect to more basic forms of relaxation and general education is unknown and awaits further study.

In summary, available evidence suggests that CBT is another efficacious treatment option for use in migraine populations, although additional research is needed in this area, particularly to examine migraine-specific outcome measures. However, CBT may be appropriately used as a method for reducing the overall impact, or burden, of migraine for promoting lifestyle changes and managing migraine symptoms. In addition, available evidence suggests that CBT-based approaches can be effectively adapted for independent at-home use (eg, CBT conducted by a health care professional compared with self-managed CBT was not found to differ significantly).[53,57]

PATIENT EDUCATION

As with any effective treatment, patient education is foundational. Education has several interrelated goals designed to (1) provide information about aspects underlying and contributing to headache onset and maintenance; (2) address and help begin to counteract symptoms of depression, demoralization, and resignation, which are frequently a result of enduring repeated bouts of headache with minimal change; (3) stress the importance of patients becoming actively involved in treatment; and (4) overview what treatment entails.[52] Our approach views headaches as arising from a complex interplay of biological, psychological (cognitions and emotions), social, and environmental factors,[58] or the increasingly well-accepted biopsychosocial model. Evidence is accruing to support the therapeutic value of education alone.[59]

BEHAVIORAL INTERVENTIONS WITH CHILDREN AND ADOLESCENTS WITH MIGRAINE

Important evidence has recently been gathered on the efficacy of behavioral treatments for the management of migraine in children and adolescents. In the first major trial of note, youth with CM (but absent mediation overuse headache [MOH]), ranging in age from 10 to 17 years, were all provided a standard course of amitriptyline, supplemented by 10 sessions of either headache education or a more specific, tailored program of CBT that incorporated aspects of BF, with assignments determined randomly.[39] Multiple outcomes were assessed at various intervals, with the longest occurring 12 months after treatment. At this time point, 86% of the youth receiving CBT along with medication had 50% or greater reductions in headache days, with a similar percentage, 88%, reporting marked reductions in disability (obtained scores <20 on the Pediatric Migraine Disability Assessment [PedMIDAS]). Youth receiving headache education combined with amitriptyline improved as well, but to a lesser degree (69% reduction in headache days, with 76% scoring <20 on the PedMIDAS). A subsequent, more fine-grained analysis that tracked change trajectories over the initial 20 weeks of youth in this clinical trial consistently revealed more rapid and sizable reductions in headache days over time.[60] Although these encouraging findings support the investigators' claims that CBT plus amitriptyline merits consideration as a first-line treatment of youth with CM, CBT remains underused. Readers interested in learning more about the provider/system/patient-related barriers limiting access and ways to confront them in order to optimize comprehensive care are referred to Ernst and colleagues'[61] work.

Marcon and Labbé[62] long ago discussed important differences between youth and adults when assessing and treating headaches, regardless of the approach. Nonetheless, many researchers continue to hold onto the myth that children with headaches are merely tiny adults with headache. Recent publications provide more compelling evidence of key differences that merit serious consideration, to which interested readers are referred.[63,64]

ALTERNATIVE DELIVERY MODALITIES

The aforementioned behaviorally based migraine interventions, although efficacious, are viewed by many as expensive in terms of time and cost (with typical regimens involving 8–16 individual, face-to-face office visits) and are not widely available.[65] These considerations led researchers early on to explore the utility of alternative methods for delivering interventions, ones that not only address cost-related and time-related factors but are capable of reaching patients residing at a distance from a treatment center. To meet these challenges, researchers have explored the viability of a host of alternatives. The first wave of alternative delivery models followed what has become best known as the PLOT(Prudent Limited Office Treatment) model, wherein intensive in-office delivery formats markedly trimmed the number of face-to-face appointments.[66] To accomplish this, office contacts were reduced to 3 to 5 total (vs the more typical 8–16) and scheduled at critical time points to keep patients engaged and minimize attrition (which had surfaced as a major problem in studies absent any personal contact). Patients were provided with manuals and relaxation or home BF devices to augment effects. Time devoted to treatment was not appreciably decreased; instead, it was scheduled to occur at times convenient to the patients and in locations of their choice. These early approaches were influenced in part by studies finding higher levels of engagement and outcomes when patients become more involved in treatment.[67] An early meta-analysis showed similar levels of improvement and attrition when comparing PLOT with the more intensive clinic-based treatments.[68]

More recently behavioral interventions have expanded to incorporate applications and programs for mHealth using digital technology such as mobile phones, Internet, smart phone apps, and, most recently, virtual reality–based applications, with Internet use being the most common delivery modality.[65,69] With the exception of online and mobile headache diaries, few studies have investigated the efficacy of mHealth programs for migraine interventions; however, the limited existing studies suggest that mHealth applications (apps) for migraine management are generally useful and time-efficient for users. These apps have generally been judged to be effective for managing symptoms, recognizing potential triggers, and improving medication adherence among adolescents and young adults with migraine from the perspective of individuals diagnosed with a primary headache disorder as well as treating health care professionals.[70,71] An early study that incorporated the PLOT approach eliminated in-person contact, relying instead on mail, telephone, and Web-based communication.[72,73] This hybrid approach resulted in at least a 50% reduction in in-person therapist time as well more reported headache reduction per in-person hour, compared with more traditional forms of in-office intervention sessions.[72,73] Similarly,

Internet-delivered CBT was also found to be effective at reducing headache frequency by approximately 50% compared with control conditions.[74] A recent quantitative review of individualized health care and mHealth interventions examined 23 studies that incorporated usability outcome measures, such as satisfaction, tolerability, adherence, and engagement with the online or mobile program.[74] This meta-analysis revealed that electronic headache diaries, as opposed to the more standard pencil-and-paper headache diaries, were associated with less burden and greater participation on the part of the individuals using the program.[74]

Entirely self-administered mHealth applications have met with low adherence and high dropout rates.[74] Contact with a therapist did not significantly improve adherence to an Internet-based self-help program.[75] Research suggests that the high rates of attrition observed for Internet delivery may be caused more by limited experience with technology or perceived lack of competence when using technology versus the nature of the behavioral intervention.[65,72] These reported high rates of attrition may also suggest a need for occasional booster sessions and scheduled check-ins to help maintain individuals' motivation and engagement with the program. This need is not unique to mHealth, but it seems especially true for mHealth-based interventions in which contact with therapists and health care professionals is limited.

A study evaluating a headache management app (Curelator Headache)[76] merits more in-depth mention. This study is unique in that it directly compared rates of adherence across 3 groups: individuals who downloaded the app using a health care professional coupon code, those who downloaded the app for free, and others who downloaded the app entirely with their own funds (out-of-pocket costs). Although adherence rates were low overall, rates were highest for both groups of participants that paid some form of out-of-pocket cost to use the app.[76] This finding departs from previous research suggesting a linear relationship between the amount of financial investment and the rate of adherence, but it does comport with research suggesting motivation as a significant factor of adherence[76,77]; individuals willing to pay for a service, no matter the cost, may be more motivated to be active in their health care and, therefore, more willing to complete and comply with a program.

In summary, research on mHealth and Internet-based intervention methods to date suggests home delivery modalities generally require greater attention to methods to enhance motivation and involvement, as well as more extensive supplemental materials, particularly given that these interventions are self-administered and self-paced.[72] Although the efficacy of behaviorally and psychologically based interventions for migraine management has already been established in previous research, these findings further show that these interventions can be effective using other treatment delivery modalities.[34,53,78] Together, these studies suggest that these behavioral interventions can be adapted for both self-administration and mHealth applications, although further research into commercially available and empirically validated programs is clearly needed. In addition, patients have already begun to use social media and Web-based platforms as both formal and informal sources of information, support, and communication with regard to their headaches.[79–81]

EMERGING APPROACHES: MINDFULNESS AND ACCEPTANCE AND COMMITMENT THERAPY–BASED INTERVENTIONS

Some of the therapies briefly reviewed here are well validated for other psychological and medical conditions, but only now are being adapted and tested for migraine. This article reviews in brief the progress made to date with respect to approaches deriving from MF and ACT perspectives, the most rapidly growing new approaches.

MF, which has its roots in Hinduism, Daoism, and Buddhism, has been practiced for centuries but only recently has become a focus of intense study in the United States. Langer and colleagues[82] were among the first US researchers to show the value of MF for addressing stress and well-being in medical patients. MF grew in popularity following the ground-breaking work of Kabat-Zinn[83] with varied pain disorders, in an approach termed MF-based stress reduction (MBSR). MBSR draws heavily on RT, commonly used within pain management,[84,85] but adds specific components of MF designed to promote nonjudgmental acceptance and awareness of oneself, one's present situation, and pain; to increase self-efficacy when faced with difficult day-to-day situations[84]; as well as improve symptom management (ie, reduce the frequency of prophylactic and acute medication use). The major distinguishing feature of all MF-based approaches is the focus on accepting one's present state and not attempting to directly alter or confront aspects related to headache. The newest member of the family of MF-based interventions is ACT. Because this originated from clinical trials in which pain was not the chief focus, it may be informative to provide further background on what it entails.

ACT is based on the theoretic model of psychological flexibility (PF), commonly defined as being fully in the present by way of addressing obstacles and other life circumstances as they occur.[86] In line with the concept of PF, ACT focuses on the therapeutic process of developing and concretely conceptualizing the self. ACT further incorporates aspects of MF, particularly the concept of acceptance, in order to facilitate behavioral change and the development of PF; ACT has also often been thought of as a third-wave CBT-based intervention because of its different approach for addressing cognitive patterns of thought and emotion. ACT is typically divided into 6 core processes: acceptance, cognitive defusion, contact with the present, self, values, and committed action.[87] These processes are typically viewed as mediators in ACT that promote the process of changing the function of individual thoughts and, at times, reducing the overall impact of thoughts in order to motivate behavior change.[87]

To facilitate the discussion, this article summarizes key aspects of the various MF-based approaches for migraine to date, grouping them by the specific approach used and listing them within their categories in the order of their publication (**Table 1**). Several trends and findings have emerged to date.[88] First, the approaches investigated to date have varied considerably, including spiritual meditation; comprehensive MBSR; MF-based therapy combined with elements of cognitive therapy (MBCT); MBSR combined with MBCT, termed MF-based therapy (MBT); ACT, arising from a different area of application and subsequently extended to migraine; and "stripped down" versions of MF (incorporating only a few components). Second, the primary designs have examined the benefits of adding some form of MF to routine care/treatment as usual (TAU; which is often not well specified) to TAU alone, with exceedingly brief follow-up evaluations (immediately after treatment to 8 weeks most typically). Third, and surprisingly, certain studies have incorporated components that have derived from other theoretic models, which greatly complicates examination of mechanisms or mediators of treatment. Fourth, delivery formats, number of sessions, and total time in therapy show similar variability. Fifth, given the goals of MF, chiefly to learn to accept the present condition, it is surprising that the primary measures of outcome continue to focus on pain frequency and intensity. Researchers have long known that pain is multidimensional, with at least 2 main aspects: the sensory or intensity dimension versus the affective or reactive dimension.[89] Given the stated intent of MF, measures designed to assess the affective/reactive dimension might be more appropriate.[90]

Table 1
Studies of mindfulness-based treatments for migraine

Study	Design	Intervention	Conditions	Participants, Attrition (%)	Inclusion Criteria	Follow-up	Outcome Measures
Wachholtz & Pargament,[120] 2008	RCT	Spiritual meditation	E$_1$: spiritual meditation C$_2$: internal secular meditation C$_3$: external secular meditation C$_4$: relaxation	E$_1$: 22 (14) C$_2$: 21 (5) C$_3$: 20 (15) C$_4$: 20 (10)	Individuals (≥18 y old) with a diagnosis of migraine or mixed migraine. Experienced at least 2 migraine attacks in prior month	1 mo	Headache frequency* Headache severity Pain tolerance* Affect* Anxiety Depression Quality of life Self-efficacy* Spirituality*
Tonelli & Wachholtz,[121] 2014	RT	Spiritual meditation	E: brief meditation based on loving kindness meditation	E: 27	Meditation-naive individuals (≥18 y old) that reported 2–10 migraine attacks per month. Current migraine diagnosis	Baseline, posttest	Pain perception* Emotional tension*
Feuille & Pargament,[122] 2015	RCT	Spiritual meditation	E: standard MF C$_1$: spiritualized MF C$_2$: relaxation	E: 35 (37) C$_1$: 37 (27) C$_2$: 35 (29)	Individuals (≥18 y old) reporting at least 2 migraine attacks in the past month. Current migraine diagnosis	2–3 wk	Pain perception* MF*
Wachholtz et al,[123] 2017	ET	Spiritual meditation	E: spiritual meditation C$_1$: internally focused secular meditation C$_2$: externally focused secular meditation C$_3$: progressive muscle relaxation	E: 25 C$_1$: 23 C$_2$: 22 C$_3$: 22	Meditation-naive individuals (≥18 y old) meeting criteria for vascular headache (including migraine)	1 mo	Headache frequency* Headache severity Pain medication use* Spirituality

(continued on next page)

Table 1
(continued)

Study	Design	Intervention	Conditions	Participants, Attrition (%)	Inclusion Criteria	Follow-up	Outcome Measures
Rosenzweig et al,[124] 2010	CCT	MBSR	E: MBSR	E: 34	Individuals (≥18 y old) diagnosed with a chronic pain condition	8 wk	Health-related quality of life*
Wells et al,[125] 2014	RCT	MBSR	E: MBSR C: TAU	E: 10 C: 9	Individuals (≥18 y old) with a diagnosis of migraine (with/without aura). No other medical or psychological condition that may affect ability to participate	8 wk	Migraine frequency Adherence Headache impact Migraine disability Quality of life Depression Self-efficacy Anxiety MF ability*
Bakhshani et al,[126] 2016	RCT	MBSR	E: MBSR + pharma C: wait-list + pharma	E: 20 C: 20	Individuals (≥18 y old) diagnosed with CM	8 wk	Headache intensity* Quality of life
Cathcart et al,[127] 2014	RCT	MBT	E: MBT C: wait-list	E: 29 (20.7) C: 29 (34.5)	Individuals (≥18 y old) meeting criteria for chronic tension-type headache. Could not have been receiving an intervention at the time of the study. No other psychiatric diagnosis or comorbid pain/headache diagnosis	3 wk	Headache frequency* Headache duration Headache intensity Depression Anxiety* Stress
Day et al,[94] 2014	RCT	MBCT	E: MBCT C: delayed treatment	E: 19 C: 17	Individuals (≥19 y old) with headache pain	8 wk	Headache frequency Headache duration Headache intensity MF Pain acceptance* Pain catastrophizing* Self-efficacy*

Study	Design		Groups	E/C (n)	Population	Duration	Outcomes
Day et al,[128] 2014	ET	MBCT	E: treatment responders C: treatment nonresponders	E: 14 C: 7	Follow-up study to Day et al[128] (2014). Individuals (≥19 y old) with headache. Responders included individuals with >50% improvement; nonresponders included individuals with <50% improvement	8 wk	Pain acceptance* Pain catastrophizing*
Day & Thorn,[129] 2016	RCT	MBCT	E: MBCT C: TAU	E: 19 C: 17	Individuals (≥19 y old) with a primary headache diagnosis	8 wk	Pain acceptance* Pain catastrophizing Self-efficacy
Seng et al,[95] in press	RCT	MBCT	E: MBCT for migraine C: wait-list/TAU	E: 31 (19) C: 29 (3)	Individuals (18–65 y old) diagnosed with migraine. >6 headache days per month. Individuals with continuous headache, severe psychiatric illness, or that began a preventive migraine medication regimen 4 wk before study were excluded	Baseline, 1, 2, and 4 mo	Headache-related disability (HDI)* Headache-related disability (MIDAS) Migraine disability (MIDI)* Headache days per month Pain intensity
Dindo et al,[130] 2012	RCT	ACT	E: 1-d ACT + migraine education workshop C: wait-list/TAU (pharma)	E: 31 C: 14	Individuals (≥18 y old) with a history of migraine that also endorsed depression	2, 6, and 12 wk	Depression* General functioning* Medication change

(continued on next page)

Table 1
(continued)

Study	Design	Intervention	Conditions	Participants, Attrition (%)	Inclusion Criteria	Follow-up	Outcome Measures
Mo'tamedi et al,[131] 2012	RCT	ACT	E: ACT C: TAU (pharma)	E: 15 C: 15 (25)	Individuals (≥18 y old) with a primary headache diagnosis	<1 wk	Pain perception Migraine disability* Distress*
Dindo et al,[132] 2014	RCT	ACT	E: 1-d ACT + migraine education workshop C: TAU (pharma)	E: 38 C: 22	Adults (≥18 y old) with a self-reported and/or clinician-reported diagnosis of migraine	3 mo	Headache frequency* Headache severity* Medication use* Headache disability*
Azam et al,[133] 2016	RCT	MF meditation	E: audio-guided MF meditation C: MF meditation description	E: 39 (0) C: 41 (0)	E: individuals self-reporting recurrent migraine or headache C: individuals not reporting migraine of recurrent headache	Baseline, posttest	HRV* Respiration Self-reported stress*
Grazzi et al,[91] 2017	CCT	Abbreviated MF	E: MF C: TAU (pharma)	E: 22 (5) C: 22 (14)	Individuals (18–65 y old) diagnosed with CM and medication overuse	3, 6, 12 wk	Headache impact* Headache disability Depression Anxiety

The table reflects randomized clinical trials, controlled clinical trials, and effectiveness trials that examine the effectiveness of ACT, spiritual meditation, and other forms of MF-based interventions (MF meditation, MF-based therapy combined with cognitive therapy, MBSR, and so forth) in a migraine population. Asterisks denote that differences are significant.

Abbreviations: C, control; CCT, controlled clinical trial; E, experimental; ET, effectiveness trial; HDI, headache disability inventory; MIDAS, migraine disability assessment questionnaire; MIDI, migraine disability index; pharma, pharmacotherapy; RCT, randomized controlled trial; TAU, treatment as usual.

One of the more recent investigations attempted to assess the independent effects of MF by comparing prophylactic pharmacotherapy alone in a sample of individuals diagnosed with MOH with those receiving a modified version of MF alone.[91] Although the design was more consistent with an effectiveness trial, it is the first to our knowledge to compare MF with pharmacology in a head-to-head approach.[92] MF was administered in a briefer format in an attempt to equate time demands across conditions. This trial consisted of 6 small group sessions in which participants were instructed to practice meditation by focusing on their breathing and body awareness while maintaining a relaxed position.[35,91] This study found comparable results for headache reductions. Fifty percent (50%) of individuals receiving MF alone experienced at least a 50% reduction in headache frequency, with a similar level of improvement for standard pharmacotherapy (53%).[91] However, MF had the added benefit of reducing acute medication use frequency from an average of 17.7 to 10.3 intakes per month. MF has also been shown to produce both functional and structural changes in brain regions associated with pain and emotion regulation (eg, amygdala, prefrontal cortex). In a follow-up study, MF was shown to influence the expression of interleukin-6, a biomarker of inflammation that is thought to signal pain sensory information during migraine attacks.[91] In addition, a more recent follow-up to this study found a marked increase in catecholamine levels and improved regulation of tyrosine metabolism, which is typically associated with migraine chronification; these physiologic changes were similar in both pharmacotherapy groups and groups engaging in MF alone.[93]

Two studies merit specific mention because of their inclusion of novel treatment components and measures. Day and colleagues[94] added key components of CBT to their MF-based study techniques known to affect co-occurring psychological symptoms (chiefly depression and anxiety) and reduce maladaptive thoughts that can exacerbate headache and pain, such as catastrophizing. Patients with various forms of primary headaches were randomized to receive MBCT at the start of treatment or following a delay, with all receiving concurrent routine medical care (unspecified). Immediate posttreatment assessments revealed significant gains in self-efficacy and pain acceptance, but no appreciable changes in headache outcomes or medication intake. Similar findings occurred when the patients initially assigned to the delayed condition were provided MBCT. Because dropout rates were high (around 25%), subsequent analyses were conducted to compare completers with noncompleters, with similar findings reported. A final analysis, comparing treatment responders (50% or greater improvement) with nonresponders revealed that patients reporting the greatest improvement were those able to most reduce catastrophizing and come to accept the presence of pain, a concept underlying all MF-based approaches and something mentioned earlier as being perhaps most salient to include. Similarly, Seng and colleagues[95] further adapted a migraine-specific form of MBCT (MBCT for migraine). Results of this clinical trial found significant reductions in headache-related disability, but not a reduction in headache days or pain intensity.

Together, these studies provide evidence to suggest that MF-based interventions can significantly improve primary treatment outcomes in headache populations. Both MBSR and MBCT have been found to reduce headache frequency, the primary clinical outcome measure in headache research. In addition, there is some evidence in support of reductions in headache duration, reductions in acute medication use, as well as changes in neurologic processes associated with migraine chronification (ie, changes in stress-response hormones). Although more research in this area is needed, these studies support the view that MF-based intervention reduces the impact of symptoms associated with chronic pain, and that MF-based interventions may work to change how individuals experience and approach pain management by way of increasing mindful and nonjudgmental awareness of their physical and cognitive selves.[35]

A NOD TO THE FUTURE: HEART RATE VARIABILITY AND NEUROFEEDBACK

Controlled trials may soon rigorously evaluate 2 new forms of BF that are growing in popularity, one of which is based on HRV. HRV is typically defined as the variation between heart rate beats, with greater ranges of increased and decreased heart rate associated with greater abilities in heart rate self-regulation.[96] Therefore, in most otherwise healthy individuals, heart rate and respiration vary throughout the day; however, individuals with health problems, including migraine, tend to experience a narrower range of HRV (ie, steady heart rate throughout the day).[96] Given this information, the primary goal of HRV BF is to teach individuals to regulate heart rate and maintain respiratory control more efficiently.[96] The role of HRV in migraine and other primary headache disorders has been investigated, although much of this research has examined HRV as an outcome measure in relaxation-based BF studies. More research is needed to determine whether respiratory and cardiac regulation are efficacious in treating migraine and whether these methods produce clinically significant outcomes, particularly with regard to reducing migraine frequency.

With the development of more recent technological advancements, BF has expanded to include methods for monitoring endogenous brain-wave activity using modern brain imaging techniques, such as EEG. This type of BF is more commonly referred to as neurofeedback.[97,98] Although research investigating the clinical utility of neurofeedback modalities in migraine is limited, this approach has been found to be of value with regard to other health topics, such as various psychopathologic disorders (eg, anxiety, attention-deficit/hyperactivity disorder) as well as pain management.[98] Neurofeedback methods may allow further investigations into migraine-related brain activity, such as the CNV[99,100] and cortical spreading depression,[101,102] two common "biomarkers" of migraine. However, neurofeedback equipment can be expensive, equipment setup is lengthier, and the help of a technician may be necessary for attaching electrodes and acquiring, processing, and interpreting data, and so forth. To date, options for home use are limited.

TREATMENT ADHERENCE, MOTIVATION, AND REFERRALS

Enhancing motivation for adherence to all types of migraine treatments is an important element in achieving good outcomes.[103,104] Some unique challenges exist in making successful referrals and continuing engagement in behavioral therapies. Biobehavioral interventions have shown efficacy and positive clinical outcomes in treating migraine and other primary headache disorders; however, access and openness to treatment may be complicated by a myriad of factors. Factors related to patient openness can be broken down into 2 broad categories: (1) factors related to broader health care systems, and (2) factors related to the patient.[61] With regard to factors related to broader health care systems, health care professional knowledge of biobehavioral interventions, previous patient exposure to biobehavioral interventions, and health care professional–patient communication are key factors related to promoting patient openness. Ernst and colleagues[61] (2015) suggest that knowledgeable health care professionals may be more likely to effectively refer patients to biobehavioral interventions. Persuasive communication, combined with an empathic understanding of the patient's concerns, perspective, and general autonomy, may prove beneficial in promoting treatment openness. Related to this, assessing readiness to change (from the motivational interviewing model[105]) can aid in assessing a patient's motivation to change, openness to treatment, and likelihood of referral follow-through.[106] For example, a patient in the precontemplation stage of the readiness to change model may not be ready for a referral but may be ready to hear about other, nonpharmacologic treatment options.

Considering the prevalence of psychiatric comorbidity in individuals diagnosed with a primary headache disorder,[107,108] it is likely that individuals being referred for biobehavioral interventions have some experience with these forms of treatment.[109,110] Similarly, individuals with previous experience seeing a psychologist or other health care professional for migraine are more likely to initiate behavioral interventions than individuals who have not had this experience.[111] Although previous exposure may increase openness to these interventions, a referral to a pain-focused intervention may be more beneficial with individuals diagnosed with migraine.[61] In the case of individuals that have not had previous exposure to psychology-based interventions or that are less open to these interventions, the social stigma related to receiving treatment from a psychologist may increase patient hesitancy and, as a result, decrease patient openness to biobehavioral interventions.[61] In either case, discussing associated risks and benefits of biobehavioral interventions in a similar manner to that in which medical interventions are discussed may be beneficial. Other patient-related barriers that may affect openness are distance, time, stress related to the nature of intervention, and financial burden, time constraints being the most cited reason for not pursuing behavioral interventions.[111]

Building rapport with patients and establishing therapeutic relationships based on a collaborative approach to health care and migraine management is important to the referral process, because patients may be more open to suggestions and more likely to follow through with appointments and referrals if they have a greater sense of trust in their health care professionals or medical teams.[28,112] As such, it is equally important to promote ongoing discussions about treatment in order to monitor patient concerns over the course of treatment. Open, 2-way communication is also helpful in establishing and maintaining rapport. Adherence to all treatments and medical advice is greater when the treatments and goals are mutually agreed on, taking into account the patient's goals, values, and preferences. Because the diagnosis and management of migraine is symptom driven and relies entirely on patient report, as does the assessment of disability, optimized medical communication is essential for both the diagnosis and the ongoing effective management of migraine. Simple strategies, such as asking open-ended questions and using the ask-tell-ask technique to confirm understanding, can facilitate improved patient outcomes.[28,112,113]

PSYCHOLOGICAL COMORBIDITIES

Migraine is comorbid with many neurologic, medical, and psychiatric conditions. For example, when people with migraine are compared with those without migraine, the former have 2 to 4 times greater odds of having depression, anxiety disorders, posttraumatic stress disorder, bipolar disorder, personality disorders, and suicide attempts.[114-116] Rates of psychiatric comorbidities are highest among patients with CM and those seen at specialty headache clinics.[18,114] In an analysis of data from the American Migraine Prevalence and Prevention (AMPP) study, respondents with CM were approximately twice as likely to have depression and anxiety as those with EM.[18] This pattern has also been found in international studies, such as those conducted in Taiwan, where rates of depression and anxiety were almost 4-fold higher among people with CM.[14,19] Anxiety and depression have both been identified as risk factors for chronification from EM to CM.[117]

Given the high rates of psychiatric comorbidity with migraine, patients should routinely be screened minimally for depression and anxiety,[118] along with any other suspected associated disorders. The following screeners have been well validated among medical patients and are free for use: the Patient Health Questionnaire Depression Module (PHQ-9) for depression and the Generalized Anxiety Disorder 7-item scale (GAD-7) for anxiety.[119] Positive screens should be followed by a more thorough diagnostic evaluation and, when confirmed, should be concurrently addressed when possible; lacking resources to do so, a referral for adjunctive treatment by a qualified provider is indicated. It is well established that biobehavioral treatments for migraine have the added advantage of positively affecting depression and anxiety, as well as other important variables affecting treatment outcomes, such as self-efficacy and medication overuse,[31] even when these aspects are not targeted directly. The authors suspect that the more wide-ranging approach embodied by CBT is more likely to affect psychological accompaniments of headache than the single use of BF or RL.[52] More direct, intensive therapeutic interventions may be needed when these symptoms are more severe.

SUMMARY

All health care professionals use various behavioral techniques to enhance treatment outcomes. Traditional empirically supported behavioral treatments for migraine, including CBT, BF, and relaxation therapies, are well established in their ability to positively affect migraine attack frequency and intensity, associated disability, quality of life, and treatment adherence when practiced in combination with pharmacotherapy or, under some conditions, when practiced alone. They are most effective when used prophylactically and practiced regularly. Given its emphasis on both psychological and behavioral modification, CBT has continued to show efficacy in treating cases of psychiatric comorbidity; similarly, evidence is emerging in favor of CBT combined with amitriptyline as a first-line treatment option for children and adolescents diagnosed with migraine or other primary headache conditions. Early data on developing treatments, including MF and acceptance-based therapies, point to treatment efficacy in reducing perceived impact and disability and improving quality of life in people with migraine. Despite the proven efficacy of traditional behavioral treatments for migraine, challenges exist in successful referral and participation in these therapies because of factors including cost, access, and stigma. Information and encouragement given by the physician or health care professional making the referral are very helpful in facilitating successful referrals and outcomes.

REFERENCES

1. Lipton RB, Bigal ME, Diamond M, et al. Migraine prevalence, disease burden, and the need for preventive therapy. Neurology 2007;68(5):343–9.

2. Buse DC, Loder EW, Gorman JA, et al. Sex differences in prevalence, symptoms, and other features of migraine, probable migraine and other severe headache: Results of the American Migraine Prevalence and Prevention study. Headache 2013;53(8):1278–99.

3. Burch R, Rizzoli P, Loder E. The prevalence and impact of migraine and severe headache in the United States: figures and trends from government health studies. Headache 2018;58:496–505.

4. World Health Organization. Global Health Estimates 2015: disease burden by cause, age, sex, by country and by region, 2000-2015 2016. Geneva (Switzerland). Available at: http://www.who.int/healthinfo/global_burden_disease/estimates/en/index2.html. Accessed December 17, 2018.

5. GBD 2015 Neurological Disorders Collaborator Group. Global, regional, and national burden of neurological disorders during 1990-2015: a systematic analysis for the Global Burden of Disease Study 2015. Lancet Neurol 2017;16(11): 877–97.

6. Haut SR, Bigal ME, Lipton RB. Chronic disorders with episodic manifestations: focus on epilepsy and migraine. Lancet Neurol 2006;5(2):148–57.

7. Dahlöf CGH, Dimenäs E. Migraine patients experience poorer subjective well-being/quality of life even between attacks. Cephalalgia 1995;15(1):31–6.

8. Buse DC, Rupnow MFT, Lipton RB. Assessing and managing all aspects of migraine: migraine attacks, migraine-related functional impairment, common comorbidities, and quality of life. Mayo Clin Proc 2009;84(5):422–35.

9. Peres MFP, Mercante JPP, Guendler VZ, et al. Cephalalgiaphobia: a possible specific phobia of illness. J Headache Pain 2007;8(1):56–9.

10. Brandes JL. The migraine cycle: patient burden of migraine during and between migraine attacks. Headache 2008;48(3):430–41.

11. Buse DC, Manack AN, Fanning K, et al. Chronic migraine prevalence, disability, and sociodemographic factors: results from the American Migraine Prevalence and Prevention Study. Headache 2012;52:1456–70.

12. Buse D, Manack A, Serrano D, et al. Headache impact of chronic and episodic migraine: results from the American Migraine Prevalence and Prevention study. Headache 2012;52(1):3–17.

13. Buse DC, Scher AI, Dodick DW, et al. Impact of migraine on the family: perspectives of people with migraine and their spouse/domestic partner in the CaMEO study. Mayo Clin Proc 2016 [pii:S0025-6196(16)00126-9].

14. Blumenfeld AM, Varon SF, Wilcox TK, et al. Disability, HRQoL and resource use among chronic and episodic people with migraine: results from the International Burden of Migraine Study (IBMS). Cephalalgia 2011;31(3):301–15.

15. Bigal ME, Rapoport AM, Lipton RB, et al. Assessment of migraine disability using the Migraine Disability Assessment (MIDAS) questionnaire: a comparison of chronic migraine with episodic migraine. Headache 2003;3:336–42.

16. Bigal ME, Serrano D, Reed M, et al. Chronic migraine in the population: burden, diagnosis, and satisfaction with treatment. Neurology 2008;71:559–66.

17. Meletiche DM, Lofland JH, Young WB. Quality of life differences between patients with episodic and transformed migraine. Headache 2001;41:573–8.

18. Buse DC, Manack A, Serrano D, et al. Sociodemographic and comorbidity profiles of chronic migraine and episodic migraine sufferers. J Neurol Neurosurg Psychiatry 2010;81:428–32.

19. Chen YC, Tang CH, Ng K, et al. Comorbidity profiles of chronic migraine sufferers in a national database in Taiwan. J Headache Pain 2012;13:311–9.

20. Stewart WF, Wood GC, Manack A, et al. Employment and work impact of chronic migraine and episodic migraine. J Occup Environ Med 2010;52:8–14.

21. Seng EK, Mauser ED, Marzouk M, et al. When mom has migraine: an observational study of the impact of parental migraine on adolescent children. Headache 2018. https://doi.org/10.1111/head.13433.

22. Smith R. Impact of migraine on the family. Headache 1998;38:423–6.

23. MacGregor EA, Brandes J, Eikermann A, et al. Impact of migraine on patients and their families: the migraine and zolmitriptan evaluation (MAZE) survey–Phase III. Curr Med Res Opin 2004;20:1143–50.

24. Lipton RB, Bigal ME, Kolodner K, et al. The family impact of migraine: population-based studies in the USA and UK. Cephalalgia 2003;23:429–40.

25. Buse DC, Powers SW, Gelfand AA, et al. Adolescent perspectives on the burden of a parent's migraine: results from the CaMEO Study. Headache 2018;58:512–24.

26. Buse DC, Fanning KM, Reed ML, et al. Life with migraine: results of the chronic migraine epidemiology and outcomes (CaMEO) study. Headache, in press.

27. Dueland AN, Leira R, Burke TA, et al. The impact of migraine on work, family, and leisure among young women – a multinational study. Curr Med Res Opin 2004;20:1595–604.

28. Lipton RB, Hahn SR, Cady RK, et al. In-office discussions of migraine: results from the American Migraine Communication Study. J Gen Intern Med 2008;23:1145–51.

29. Holmes WF, MacGregor EA, Sawyer JP, et al. Information about migraine disability influences healthcare professionals' perceptions of illness severity and treatment needs. Headache 2001;41(4):343–50.

30. Buse DC, Andrasik A. Behavioral medicine for migraine. Neurol Clin 2009;27(2):445–65.

31. Nestoriuc Y, Martin A, Rief W, et al. Biofeedback treatment for headache disorders: a comprehensive efficacy review. Appl Psychophysiol Biofeedback 2008;33:125–40.

32. Campbell JK, Penzien DB, Wall EM. Evidence-based guidelines for migraine headache: behavioral and physical treatments. US Headache Consortium; 2000. Available at: http://www.aan.com.

33. Nestoriuc Y, Martin A. Efficacy for biofeedback for migraine: a meta-analysis. Pain 2007;128:111–27.

34. Sullivan A, Cousins S, Ridsdale L. Psychological interventions for migraine: a systematic review. J Neurol 2016;256:2369–77.

35. Raggi A, Grignani E, Leonardi M, et al. Behavioral approaches for primary headaches: recent advances. Headache 2018;56(6):913–25.

36. Stokes DA, Lappin MS. Neurofeedback and biofeedback with 37 people with migraine: a clinical outcome study. Behav Brain Funct 2010;6:9.

37. Andrasik F, Grazzi L. Biofeedback and behavioral treatments: filling some gaps. Neurol Sem 2014;34:S121–7.

38. Holroyd KA, Penzien DB. Pharmacological versus non-pharmacological prophylaxis of recurrent migraine headache: a meta-analytic review of clinical trials. Pain 1990;42:1–13.

39. Powers SW, Kashikar-Zuck SM, Allen JR, et al. Cognitive behavioral therapy plus amitriptyline for chronic migraine in children and adolescents. JAMA 2013;310(24):2622–30.

40. Blanchard EB, Andrasik F, Neff DF, et al. Sequential comparisons of relaxation training and biofeedback in the treatment of three kinds of chronic headache or, the machines may be necessary some of the time. Behav Res Ther 1982;20:469–81.

41. Paul GL. Strategy outcome research in psychotherapy. J Consult Psychol 1967;31(2):109–18.

42. Andrasik F, Blanchard EB, Neff DF, et al. Biofeedback and relaxation training for chronic headache: a controlled comparison of booster treatments and regular contacts for long-term maintenance. J Consult Clin Psychol 1984;52(4):604–15.
43. Jacobson E. The technique of progressive relaxation. J Nerv Ment Dis 1924; 60(6):568–78.
44. Bernstein DA, Borkovec TD. Progressive relaxation training: a manual for the helping professions. Champaign (IL): Research Press; 1973.
45. Meyer B, Keller A, Wöhlbier H-G, et al. Progressive muscle relaxation reduces migraine frequency and normalizes amplitudes of contingent negative variation (CNV). J Headache Pain 2016;17:37.
46. Bandura A, Adams NE. Analysis of self-efficacy theory of behavioral change. Cognit Ther Res 1977;1(4):287–310.
47. Mauskop A. Nonmedication, alternative, and complimentary treatments for migraine. Continuum (Minneap Minn) 2012;18(4):796–806.
48. Luthe W, Schultz JH. Autogenic therapy. New York: Grune & Stratton; 1969.
49. Minen M, Boubour A, Powers S, et al. Introduction to progressive muscle relaxation for migraine in the emergency department: a pilot feasibility study. Neurology 2017;88(16 Suppl):P2.168.
50. Varkey E, Cider A, Carlsson J, et al. Exercise as migraine prophylaxis: a randomized study using relaxation and topiramate as controls. Cephalalgia 2011; 31(14):1428–38.
51. Holroyd KA, Andrasik F, Westbrook T. Cognitive control of tension headache. Cognit Ther Res 1977;1:121–33.
52. Holroyd KA, Andrasik F. A cognitive-behavioral approach to recurrent tension and migraine headache. In: Kendall PC, editor. Advances in cognitive-behavioral research and therapy. New York: Academic; 1982. p. 275–320.
53. Harris P, Loveman E, Clegg A, et al. Systematic review of cognitive behavioural therapy for the management of headaches and migraine attacks in adults. Br J Pain 2015;9(4):213–24.
54. Kroner JW, Peugh J, Kashikar-Zuck SM, et al. Trajectory of improvement in children and adolescents with chronic migraine: results from the cognitive-behavioral therapy and amitriptyline trial. J Pain 2017;18(6):637–44.
55. Holroyd KA, Nash JM, Pingel JD, et al. A comparison of pharmacological (amitriptyline HCL) and nonpharmacological (cognitive-behavioral) therapies for chronic tension headaches. J Consult Clin Psychol 1991;59(3):387–93.
56. Holroyd KA, O'Donnell FJ, Stensland M, et al. Management of chronic tension-type headache with tricyclic antidepressant medication, stress management therapy, and their combination: a randomized controlled trial. JAMA 2001; 285(17):2208–15.
57. Martin PR, Nathan PR, Milech D, et al. Cognitive therapy vs. self-management training in the treatment of chronic headaches. Br J Clin Psychol 1989;28: 347–61.
58. Andrasik F, Flor H, Turk DC. An expanded view of psychological aspects in head pain: the biopsychosocial model. Neurol Sci 2005;26:S87–91.
59. McClean A, Becker WJ, Vujadinovic Z. Making a new-patient headache education session more patient-centered: what participants want to know. Disabil Rehabil 2019;1–12 [Epub ahead of print].
60. Powers SW, Coffey CS, Chamberlin LA, et al. Trial of amitriptyline, topiramate, and placebo for pediatric migraine. N Engl J Med 2017;376:115–24.
61. Ernst MM, O'Brien H, Powers SW. Cognitive-behavioral therapy: how medical providers can increase patient and family openness and access to

evidence-based multimodal therapy for pediatric migraine. Headache 2015; 55(10):1382–96.

62. Marcon R, Labbé E. Assessment and treatment of children's headaches from a developmental perspective. Headache 1991;30:586–92.

63. Powers SW, Andrasik F. Biobehavioral treatment, disability, and psychological effects of pediatric headache. Pediatr Ann 2005;34:461–5.

64. Kroon Van Diest AM, Ernst MM, Vaughn L, et al. CBT for pediatric migraine: a qualitative study of patient and parent experience. Headache 2018;58:661–75.

65. Stubberud A, Linde M. Digital technology and mobile health in behavioral migraine therapy: a narrative review. Curr Pain Headache Rep 2018;22:66.

66. Andrasik F, Schwartz MS. Headache. In: Schwartz MS, Andrasik F, editors. Biofeedback: a practitioner's guide. 4th edition. New York: Guilford Press; 2016. p. 305–55.

67. Andrasik F. Behavioral management of migraine. Biomed Pharmacother 1996; 50:52–7.

68. Haddock CK, Rowan AB, Andrasik F, et al. Home-based behavioral treatment for chronic benign headache: a meta-analysis of controlled trials. Cephalalgia 1997;17(2):113–8.

69. Pourmand A, Davis S, Marchak A, et al. Virtual reality as a clinical tool for pain management. Curr Pain Headache Rep 2018;22:53.

70. Mosadeghi-Nik M, Askari MS, Fatehi F. Mobile health (mHealth) for headache disorders: a review of the evidence base. J Telemed Telecare 2016;22(8):4727.

71. Ramsey RR, Holbein CE, Powers SW, et al. A pilot investigation of a mobile phone application and progressive reminder system to improve adherence to daily prevention treatment in adolescents and young adults with migraine. Cephalalgia 2018;38(14):2035–44.

72. Andrasik F. Behavioral treatment of headaches: extending the reach. Neurol Sci 2012;33(Suppl 1):S127–30.

73. Folen RA, James LC, Earles JE, et al. Biofeedback via telehealth: a new frontier of applied psychophysiology. Appl Psychophysiol Biofeedback 2001;26(3): 195–204.

74. Minen M, Torous J, Raynowska J, et al. Electronic behavioral interventions for headache: a systematic review. J Headache Pain 2016;17:51.

75. Anderson G, Lundström P, Ström L. Internet-based treatment of headache: does telephone contact add anything. Headache 2003;43:353–61.

76. Seng EK, Prieto P, Boucher G, et al. Anxiety, incentives, and adherence to self-monitoring on a mobile health platform: a naturalistic longitudinal cohort study in people with headache. Headache 2018;58(10):1541–55.

77. Aziz H, Hatah E, Bakry MM, et al. How payment scheme affects patients' adherence to medications? A systematic review. Patient Prefer Adherence 2016;10: 837–50.

78. Richardson GM, McGrath PJ. Cognitive-behavioral therapy for migraine headaches: a minimal-therapist-contact approach versus a clinic-based approach. Headache 1989;29(6):352–7.

79. Nascimento TD, DosSantos MF, Danciu T, et al. Real-time sharing and expression of migraine headache suffering on Twitter: a cross-sectional infodemiology study. J Med Internet Res 2014;16(4):e96.

80. Hoedebecke K, Beaman L, Mugambi J, et al. Health care and social media: what patients really understand. F1000Res 2017;6:118.

81. Loder EW, Rayhill M, Burch RC. Safety problems with a transdermal patch for migraine: lessons from the development, approval, and marketing process. Headache 2018;58(10):1639–57.

82. Langer E, Blank E, Chanowitz B. The mindlessness of ostensibly thoughtful action: the role of placebic information in interpersonal interaction. J Pers Soc Psychol 1978;36:635–63.

83. Kabat-Zinn J. An outpatient program in behavioral medicine for chronic pain patients based on the practice of mindfulness meditation: theoretical considerations and preliminary results. Gen Hosp Psychiatry 1982;4:33–47.

84. Marchand WR. Mindfulness-based stress reduction, mindfulness-based cognitive therapy, and Zen meditation for depression, anxiety, pain, and psychological distress. J Psychiatr Pract 2012;18(4):233–52.

85. Kabat-Zinn J, Lipworth L, Burney R. The clinical use of mindfulness meditation for the self-regulation of chronic pain. J Behav Med 1985;8(2):163–90.

86. Yu L, McCracken LM. Model and processes of acceptance and commitment therapy (ACT) for chronic pain including a closer look at the self. Curr Pain Headache Rep 2016;20(2):12.

87. Hayes SC, Luoma JB, Bond FW, et al. Acceptance and commitment therapy: model, processes, and outcomes. Behav Res Ther 2006;44(1):1–25.

88. Andrasik F, Grazzi L, D'Amico D, et al. Mindfulness and headache: a "new" old treatment with new findings. Cephalalgia 2016;36(12):1192–205.

89. Beecher HK. Control of suffering in severe trauma: usefulness of a quantitative approach. JAMA 1960;173:534–6.

90. Andrasik F, Blanchard EB, Ahles T, et al. Assessing the reactive as well as the sensory component of headache pain. Headache 1981;21:218–21.

91. Grazzi L, Sansone E, Raggi A, et al. Mindfulness and pharmacological prophylaxis after withdrawal from medication overuse in patients with chronic migraine: an effectiveness trial with one-year follow-up. J Headache Pain 2017;18:15.

92. Nash JM, McCrory DC, Nicholson RA, et al. Efficacy and effectiveness approaches in behavioral treatment trials. Headache 2005;45:507–12.

93. Grazzi L, Raggi A, D'Amico D, et al. A prospective pilot study of the effect on catecholamines of mindfulness training vs pharmacological prophylaxis in patients with chronic migraine and medication overuse headache. Cephalalgia 2019;39(5):655–64.

94. Day MA, Thorn BE, Ward LC, et al. Mindfulness-based cognitive therapy for the treatment of headache pain: a pilot study. Clin J Pain 2014;30:152–61.

95. Seng EK, Singer AB, Metts C, et al. Does mindfulness-based cognitive therapy for migraine reduce migraine-related disability in people with episodic and chronic migraine? A phase 2b pilot randomized clinical trial. Headache, in press.

96. Lehrer PM, Gevirtz R. Heart rate variability biofeedback: how and why does it work. Front Psychol 2014;5:756–64.

97. Hammond DC. What is neurofeedback: an update. J Neurother 2011;15: 305–36.

98. Marzbani H, Marateb HR, Mansourian M. Neurofeedback: a comprehensive review on system design, methodology and clinical applications. Basic Clin Neurosci 2016;7(2):143–58.

99. Kropp P, Geber W-D. Is increased amplitude of contingent negative variation in migraine due to cortical hyperactivity or to reduced habituation. Cephalalgia 1993;13:37–41.

100. Kropp P, Siniatchkin M, Geber W-D. On the pathophysiology of migraine: links for the empirically based treatment with neurofeedback. Appl Psychophysiol Biofeedback 2002;27(3):203–13.
101. Ayata C, Jin H, Kudo C, et al. Suppression of cortical spreading depression in migraine prophylaxis. Ann Neurol 2006;59(4):652–61.
102. Noseda R, Burnstein R. Migraine pathophysiology: anatomy of the trigeminovascular pathway and associated neurological systems, cortical spreading depression, sensitization, and modulation of pain. Pain 2013;154(Suppl 1):S44–53.
103. Seng EK, Robbins MS, Nicholson RA. Acute migraine medication adherence, migraine disability and patient satisfaction: a naturalistic daily diary study. Cephalalgia 2017;37(10):955–64.
104. Seng EK, Rains JA, Nicholson RA, et al. Improving medication adherence in migraine treatment. Curr Pain Headache Rep 2015;19(6):24.
105. Rollnick S, Miller WR. What is motivational interviewing? Behav Cogn Psychother 1995;23:325–34.
106. Shinitzky HE, Kub J. The art of motivating behavior change: the use of motivational interviewing to promote health. Public Health Nurs 2001;18(3):178–85.
107. Antonaci F, Nappi G, Galli F, et al. Migraine and psychiatric comorbidity: a review of clinical findings. J Headache Pain 2011;12(2):115–25.
108. Hamelsky SW, Lipton RB. Psychiatric comorbidity of migraine. Headache 2006; 46(9):1327–33.
109. Seng EK, Holroyd KA. Optimal use of acute headache medication: a qualitative examination of behaviors and barriers to their performance. Headache 2013;53: 1438–50.
110. Minen MT, Seng EK, Holroyd KA. Influence of family psychiatric and headache history on migraine-related health care utilization. Headache 2014;54(3): 485–92.
111. Minen MT, Azarchi S, Sobolev R, et al. Factors related to migraine patients' decisions to initiate behavioral migraine treatment following a headache specialist's recommendation: a prospective study. Pain Med 2018;19:2274–82.
112. Hahn SR, Lipton RB, Sheftell FD, et al. Healthcare provider-patient communication and migraine assessment: results of the American migraine communication study, phase II. Curr Med Res Opin 2008;24(6):1711–8.
113. Buse DC, Lipton RB. Facilitating communication with patients for improved migraine outcomes. Curr Pain Headache Rep 2008;12:230–6.
114. Buse DC, Silberstein SD, Manack AN, et al. Psychiatric comorbidity of episodic and chronic migraine. J Neurol 2012;260(8):1960–9.
115. Jette N, Patten S, Williams J, et al. Comorbidity of migraine and psychiatric disorders–a national population-based study. Headache 2008;48:501–16.
116. Zwart OJA, Dyb G, Hagen K, et al. Depression and anxiety disorders associated with headache frequency. The Nord-Trøndelag Health Study. Eur J Neurol 2003; 10:147–52.
117. Buse DC, Greisman JD, Biagi K, et al. Migraine progression: a systematic review. Headache 2019;59(3):306–38.
118. Smitherman TA, Maizels M, Penzien DB. Headache chronification: screening and behavioral management of comorbid depressive and anxiety disorders. Headache 2008;48:45–50.
119. Kroenke K, Spitzer RL, Williams JBW, et al. The patient health questionnaire somatic, anxiety, and depression symptom scales: a systematic review. Gen Hosp Psychiatry 2010;32:345–59.

120. Wachholtz AB, Pargament KI. Migraine attacks and meditation: does spirituality matter. J Behav Med 2008;31(4):351–66.
121. Tonelli ME, Wachholtz AB. Meditation-based treatment yielding immediate relief for meditation-naïve people with migraine. Pain Manag Nurs 2014;15(1):36–40.
122. Feuille M, Pargament K. Pain, mindfulness, and spirituality: a randomized controlled trial comparing effects of mindfulness and relaxation on pain-related outcomes in people with migraine. J Health Psychol 2015;20(8): 1090–106.
123. Wachholtz AB, Malone CD, Pargament KI. Effect of different meditation types on migraine headache medication use. Behav Med 2017;43(1):1–8.
124. Rosenzweig S, Greeson JM, Reibel DK, et al. Mindfulness-based stress reduction for chronic pain conditions: variation in treatment outcomes and role of home meditation practice. J Psychosom Res 2010;68(1):29–36.
125. Wells RE, Burch R, Paulsen RH, et al. Meditation for migraine attacks: a pilot randomized controlled trial. Headache 2014;54(9):1484–95.
126. Bakhshani N-M, Amirani A, Amirifard H, et al. The effectiveness of mindfulness-based stress reduction on perceived pain intensity and quality of life in patients with chronic headache. Glob J Health Sci 2016;8(4):142–51.
127. Cathcart S, Galatis N, Immink M, et al. Brief mindfulness-based therapy for chronic tension-type headache: a randomized controlled pilot study. Behav Cogn Psychother 2014;42(1):1–15.
128. Day MA, Thorn BE, Rubin NJ. Mindfulness-based cognitive therapy for the treatment of headache pain: a mixed-methods analysis comparing treatment responders and treatment non-responders. Complement Ther Med 2014;22(2): 278–85.
129. Day MA, Thorn BE. The mediating role of pain acceptance during mindfulness-based cognitive therapy for headache. Complement Ther Med 2016;25:51–4.
130. Dindo L, Recober A, Marchman JN, et al. One-day behavioral treatment for patients with comorbid depression and migraine: A pilot study. Behav Res Ther 2012;50(9):537–43.
131. Mo'tamedi H, Rezaiemaram P, Tavallaie A. The effectiveness of a group-based acceptance and commitment additive therapy on rehabilitation of female outpatients with chronic headache: preliminary findings reducing 3 dimensions of headache impact. Headache 2012;52(7):1106–19.
132. Dindo L, Recober A, Marchman J, et al. One-day behavioral intervention in depressed migraine patients: effects on headache. Headache 2014;54(3): 528–38.
133. Azam MA, Katz J, Mohabir V, et al. Individuals with tension and migraine headache exhibit increased heart rate variability during post-stress mindfulness meditation practice but a decrease during a post-stress control condition: a randomized, controlled experiment. Int J Psychophysiol 2016;110:66–74.

Pediatric Migraine
An Update

Kaitlin Greene, MD, Samantha L. Irwin, MD, MSc, MB BCh BAO, FRCPC,
Amy A. Gelfand, MD*

KEYWORDS

- Migraine • Headache • Pediatric • Children • Adolescents

KEY POINTS

- Recognition and treatment of migraine in pediatrics is important given the high prevalence and associated disability in this population.
- Migraine in children is more likely to be bilateral and of shorter duration; however, other features are shared with adult migraine, including premonitory and cranial autonomic symptoms.
- The episodic syndromes that can be associated with migraine often present in childhood, and benign paroxysmal torticollis is associated with genetic variants seen in hemiplegic migraine.
- Triptans have been shown to be effective for acute treatment of migraine in children and adolescents. Preventive migraine treatment in this age group may include medication, behavioral treatment, and/or lifestyle management.

BACKGROUND

Migraine is common in the pediatric population, with an overall estimated prevalence of 7.7%.[1] The prevalence of migraine increases over the course of childhood and adolescence, from 5% among children 5 to 10 years old to approximately 15% among teens.[2] Chronic migraine, wherein headache occurs at least 15 d/mo, has a prevalence of 0.8% to 1.8% among children 12 to 17 years old.[2,3] In childhood and early adolescence, boys and girls are equally likely to be affected by migraine, but by late adolescence the prevalence of migraine is higher in girls, with a ratio similar to that seen in adults.[1] Migraine can cause significant disability in children and adolescents, resulting in absence from school, impaired school performance, and missed

Disclosure: See last page of article.
Department of Neurology, UCSF Pediatric Headache Center, University of California, San Francisco, UCSF Benioff Children's Hospital, Mission Hall Box 0137, 550 16th Street, 4th Floor, San Francisco, CA 94158, USA
* Corresponding author.
E-mail address: amy.gelfand@ucsf.edu

extracurricular activities.[4] Recognition and diagnosis of migraine is of increasing importance as more migraine-specific therapeutic interventions become available to children.

APPROACH TO THE PEDIATRIC HEADACHE HISTORY

Children and adolescents are generally capable of providing detailed and personally accurate headache histories, and it is important to obtain a first-hand account of headaches from the child whenever possible. To facilitate this, it can be helpful to identify the child as the primary historian at the beginning of the visit. At the same time, parents' insights into the headache history can be invaluable, particularly with respect to birth, developmental history, and family history, and the child should be encouraged to ask for parental input when required.

In younger children, it can be helpful to allow them the opportunity to draw what they experience during headaches. In one study, interpretation of drawings predicted clinical diagnosis of migraine versus nonmigraine headache in 90% of cases.[5] Because it can sometimes be difficult for children to articulate the experience of associated features such as photophobia and phonophobia or nausea, description of children's behavior during attacks can shed light on additional symptoms. For example, preference to lie down in a quiet, dark room suggests photophobia and phonophobia, whereas decreased appetite during attacks may suggest nausea.

DIAGNOSIS OF PEDIATRIC MIGRAINE AND ASSOCIATED CONDITIONS

The first goal of the headache history in pediatric patients is to identify red flags that may be a clue to the presence of secondary headache. Concerning features include new or worsening headache type, headaches with positional features, headaches with cough or strain, recurrent thunderclap headaches, focal neurologic symptoms or abnormal neurologic examination (including an abnormal visual examination, papilledema, ataxia, or incoordination), and side-locked headache. In addition, it is important to evaluate for signs of systemic disease or known systemic disorders. Specifically, in children, this includes assessment for neurocutaneous stigmata and the presence of developmental delay, as well as consideration of potential neurovascular and neurogenetic conditions that can be associated with secondary headache.

In pediatric patients, the diagnosis of migraine follows the International Classification of Headache Disorders, Third Edition (ICHD-3) diagnostic criteria for migraine in adults with a few key differences related to duration and location of symptoms.[6] Although migraine in adults lasts 4 to 72 hours (untreated or unsuccessfully treated), duration in pediatric patients can be as short as 2 hours.[6,7] Although unilateral location is typical of migraine in adult patients, more than 80% of children and adolescents have bilateral symptoms.[7] Although not included in the diagnostic criteria, osmophobia can also provide a historical clue in support of a migraine diagnosis. Osmophobia is thought to reflect an overall increased sensitivity to sensory stimuli in migraine, and is reported in up to 34.6% of pediatric patients with migraine compared with 14.3% of pediatric patients with tension-type headache.[8]

Cranial autonomic features are common among pediatric patients with migraine.[9,10] These symptoms have been attributed to activation of the trigeminal autonomic reflex consisting of trigeminal nociceptive afferents and parasympathetic efferents. In one study of 162 children and adolescents with migraine, two-thirds of patients had at least 1 cranial autonomic symptom and most had more than 1.[10] The most commonly reported symptoms were aural fullness, facial flushing or sweating, lacrimation, and conjunctival injection.[10]

Children and adolescents may also experience the premonitory and postdromal phases of migraine. Premonitory symptoms are reported in up to two-thirds of adolescent patients and may include fatigue, irritability/mood change, yawning, micturition changes, light sensitivity, nausea, neck stiffness, and facial changes such as pallor or shadowing under the eyes.[11] Identification of premonitory features can facilitate early recognition and treatment of migraine attacks. Following the headache phase, children can also have postdromal symptoms. In one study, 82% of patients reported postdromal symptoms, including thirst, somnolence, visual disturbances, and food cravings.[12]

Migraine with Aura

Migraine aura is characterized by recurrent attacks of reversible neurologic symptoms lasting between 5 and 60 minutes, with gradual spread over at least 5 minutes and accompanied by or followed within 60 minutes by headache. As in adults, visual aura is the most common aura type in children. A retrospective cohort study of 164 children aged 5 to 17 years with migraine with aura found that visual symptoms were reported in 93% of attacks with aura, whereas only 5.5% of patients experienced primary somatosensory aura and 0.6% of patients experienced primary motor or language aura.[13] An additional 25% of patients also experienced a second type of aura, including somatosensory (64.3%), speech (23.8%), and motor disturbance (11.9%).[13]

Although uncommon, it is important to assess for the presence of motor aura (ie, hemiplegic migraine) in pediatric patients given the potential for autosomal dominant inheritance in association with mutations in CACNA1A, ATP1A2, and SCN1A genes. Notably, CACNA1A mutations have also been identified in patients with benign paroxysmal torticollis of infancy.[14,15]

Episodic Conditions that May Be Associated with Migraine

The ICHD-3 identifies a group of disorders that were historically noted to occur in childhood and may be associated with increased likelihood of developing migraine. This group includes benign paroxysmal torticollis, benign paroxysmal vertigo of childhood, and recurrent gastrointestinal disturbance, which encompasses cyclic vomiting syndrome and abdominal migraine. Two additional childhood-onset conditions have been listed in the appendix of ICHD-3 as episodic syndromes that may be associated with migraine. These conditions are infantile colic and alternating hemiplegia of childhood. The episodic syndromes are characterized by recurrent stereotyped episodes of neurologic symptoms, with periods of being well in between, and normal interval development and examination. Obtaining a detailed history about these syndromes can be helpful in providing support for a migraine diagnosis. Clinical features of these conditions are outlined in **Table 1** and diagnostic criteria can be found in ICHD-3.[6]

Importantly, diagnosis of the episodic syndromes depends on careful clinical evaluation and exclusion of alternative diagnoses. For example, certain metabolic disorders can present with episodic vomiting, whereas certain seizure disorders can cause episodes of vertigo. Treatment of the episodic syndromes depends on frequency and severity of symptoms. There has been 1 positive randomized placebo-controlled trial of pizotifen, a serotonin and histamine antagonist, for preventive treatment of abdominal migraine.[16] Beyond this, there have been few controlled data to

Table 1
Episodic conditions that may be associated with migraine

	Age	Features	Duration	Associated Symptoms
Cyclic vomiting syndrome[102-105]	School age (mean onset at 4–9 y)	Episodes of recurrent vomiting	Hours to days	Vomiting up to 4 times/h Attacks ≥1 h to 10 d and ≥1 wk apart
Abdominal migraine[102,106-108]	School age (mean onset at 4–7 y)	Episodes of moderate to severe midline dull pain	Hours to days	Anorexia, nausea, vomiting, pallor
Benign paroxysmal vertigo[109-111]	Early childhood (mean onset at 2–4 y)	Abrupt onset of vertigo often manifested as ataxia or dizziness	Minutes to hours	Nystagmus, ataxia, vomiting, pallor, fearfulness Normal audiometric and vestibular function between attacks Exclusion of posterior fossa disorder, seizure and vestibular disorders
Benign paroxysmal torticollis[112-114]	Early infancy (median onset at 2–5 mo)	Episodes of unilateral head tilt occurring at regular intervals	Minutes to days	Irritability, ataxia, pallor, malaise, vomiting Genetic link to CACNA1A[14,15]
Infantile colic[a,115]	Infancy (peak at 6 wk)	Excessive crying	>3 h/d on >3 d/wk	Infants of mothers with migraine 2.6 times as likely to have colic vs infants of mothers without migraine[116]
Alternating hemiplegia of childhood[a]	Infancy (before 18 mo)	Episodes of alternating hemiplegia	Minutes to days[117]	Encephalopathy, paroxysmal spells, dystonic posturing, or choreoathetoid movements, autonomic disturbance Genetic link to ATP1A3[118]

[a] ICHD-3 appendix only.
Data from Refs. [6,100,101]

guide treatment selection and thus treatment is generally based on case reports and retrospective studies.

TREATMENT OF MIGRAINE IN PEDIATRIC PATIENTS

Over the past decade, there have been several developments in the acute and preventive treatment of migraine, including the US Food and Drug Administration (FDA) approval of 4 triptan medications for use in pediatric and adolescent populations and the development of novel targeted preventive therapies for migraine. At the same time, data from the Childhood and Adolescent Migraine Prevention (CHAMP) trial, a large, double-blind, multicentered, controlled trial of topiramate versus amitriptyline versus placebo, has reshaped the approach to first-line migraine prevention treatment in children and adolescents and redirected focus toward alternative preventive strategies with minimal side effects.[17,18]

Acute Treatment

Children and adolescents should be allowed to rest in a dark, quiet setting and sleep should be encouraged if possible. Hydration should be optimized.

Acute medications should be given as early as possible at the onset of headache, or as soon as possible following worsening of headache in patients with continuous headache. In school-aged children, this often means having the medication readily available at school, and health care providers play an important role in providing documentation and guidance regarding the appropriate administration of medications in the school setting. Medication dosage should be optimized for weight and age. Given that it is unlikely that any acute medication works for 100% of attacks, patients should be encouraged to try a medication at least 3 times to determine efficacy.

Patients should also be counseled about the potential risk of medication overuse headache. There is some debate as to whether frequent acute medication drives headache frequency.[19] It is possible that sometimes patients simply experience an increase in their headache frequency and their use of acute medications increases accordingly; in this type of scenario, acute medication use may be an effect rather than a cause of increased headache frequency. This distinction is important in order to avoid stigmatizing patients who have a difficult migraine problem by suggesting that the patient's own actions are contributing to the problem. Ultimately, people's susceptibility to medication overuse headache probably depends to a certain extent on their individual characteristics and on the type of medications being frequently used. For example, use of nonsteroidal antiinflammatory drugs (NSAIDs) on up to 9 d/mo is associated with lower risk of progression to chronic migraine in adults,[20] and there are small studies suggesting that daily use of naproxen is effective as a migraine preventive.[21–26] Nonetheless, conservative guidance supports limiting the use of simple analgesics (NSAIDs and acetaminophen) to ~4 d/wk or 15 d/mo, and limiting prescription medication use (triptans, opioids, combination, ergotamines) to ~2 d/wk or less than 10 d/mo.

Considerations around acute medication formulation are also important in this age group. Prominent nausea and vomiting during attacks may make it difficult to administer and absorb oral medications. It may be necessary to use alternative modes of administration, such as intranasal, subcutaneous, rectal, and/or dissolving tablets. In addition, young children may not be able to swallow pills. It can be helpful to encourage typically developing children to learn to swallow pills beginning around age 8 years in order to broaden their medication options.

First-line treatment options in children include NSAIDs and acetaminophen. Both acetaminophen (15 mg/kg) and ibuprofen (7.5–10 mg/kg) have been studied and found to be effective in randomized placebo-controlled trials for acute treatment of migraine in children as young as 4 years old.[27,28] Although both medications were superior to placebo, ibuprofen was superior to acetaminophen in the primary end point of pain reduction at 2 hours.[27] In the United States, both of these medications are available in liquid and chewable tablet formulations for young children who are unable to swallow pills. Another option in the NSAID category is naproxen (5–10 mg/kg), which has the advantage of a longer dosing interval of 12 hours. The combination of naproxen with sumatriptan has been shown to be more effective than either medication alone in adults,[29] and this combination is safe and effective in adolescent patients.[30]

Triptans

In patients with inadequate response to acetaminophen or ibuprofen, triptans should be considered (**Table 2**). A Cochrane Review in 2016 found that triptans as a class were superior to placebo in the treatment of migraine in children and adolescents.[31] Notably, 4 triptans are now FDA approved for use in adolescents aged 12 to 17 years: almotriptan oral tablets, zolmitriptan nasal spray, rizatriptan oral melts, and combination sumatriptan/naproxen oral tablets. In addition, for younger children with migraine, rizatriptan oral melts have been approved for use in children aged 6 years and older. For children who are unable to tolerate oral medications because of nausea or inability to swallow pills, alternative formulations such as nasal spray (sumatriptan,

Table 2
Triptan dosing in children and adolescents

	Form	Available Dose (mg)	<40 kg Dose (mg)	>40 kg Dose (mg)	Notes
Shorter-acting Triptans					
Sumatriptan[119–122]	SQ	3, 6	0.1/kg	4–6	Combined sumatriptan/naproxen oral tablet (10 mg/60 mg to 85 mg/500 mg) FDA approved for ages 12–17 y[30]
	NS	5, 20	5	10–20	
	Tablet	25, 50, 100	12.5–25	50	
Rizatriptan[123,124]	Tablet	5, 10	5	10	Oral dissolving tablet FDA approved for ages 6–17 y
	MLT	5, 10			
Almotriptan[125]	Tablet	6.25	6.25	12.5	Oral tablet FDA approved for ages 12–17 y
		12.5			
Zolmitriptan[126–128]	Tablet	2.5, 5	2.5	5	Nasal spray FDA approved for ages 12–17 y
	ODT	2.5, 5			
	NS	2.5, 5			
Eletriptan[129]	Tablet	20, 40, 80	20	40–80	—
Longer-acting Triptans					
Frovatriptan[130]	Tablet	2.5	1.25	2.5	—
Naratriptan[131]	Tablet	1, 2.5	1	2.5	—

Abbreviations: MLT, dissolving tablet (melt); NS, nasal spray; ODT, oral dissolving tablet; SQ, subcutaneous injection.

zolmitriptan), melt (rizatriptan), or subcutaneous injection (sumatriptan) may be considered (see **Table 2**).

Contraindications to triptans are generally less common in the pediatric population than in adults, but should be excluded before use. These contraindications include uncontrolled hypertension, vascular disease, cerebral vascular abnormalities, and pregnancy. In addition, there is a labeled contraindication to triptans for patients with hemiplegic or basilar migraine subtypes, although studies have shown no adverse effect of triptan use in these populations.[32]

Antiemetics

In children with prominent migraine-related nausea and/or vomiting, the dopamine receptor antagonist prochlorperazine can be beneficial. Intravenous (IV) prochlorperazine has been studied in pediatric patients who present to the emergency room with migraine and has been shown to be more effective than IV ketorolac in this setting.[33] Prochlorperazine can also be administered as an oral tablet or as a suppository when oral formulations are not tolerated (0.25–0.5 mg/kg/dose). Coadministration of diphenhydramine with prochlorperazine can be effective in preventing or minimizing extrapyramidal side effects.[34]

Additional dopamine antagonists used in the acute treatment of migraine include chlorpromazine, promethazine, and metoclopramide. Retrospective studies have suggested that chlorpromazine and metoclopramide are less effective than prochlorperazine in children and/or adolescents presenting to the emergency room for acute treatment of migraine,[35–37] but further controlled studies are needed to determine efficacy in this population. Of note, the dopamine antagonists carry a risk of prolongation of the QT interval, and electrocardiogram is recommended before use. Additional options for management of nausea include the serotonin (5-hydroxytryptamine) antagonists ondansetron and granisetron; in one retrospective review of children treated for acute migraine in the emergency department, those treated with IV ondansetron had similar revisit rates to those treated with dopamine antagonists.[36]

Preventive Treatment

The aim of migraine preventive treatment is to decrease migraine frequency. The CHAMP trial has provided new insight into the preventive management of migraine in the pediatric population.[18] This large, multisite, randomized, double-blind trial compared placebo with amitriptyline (1 mg/kg/d) and topiramate (2 mg/kg/d) in children and adolescents aged 8 to 17 years with migraine. Approximately three-quarters of the participants had episodic migraine. Inclusion criteria required a PedMIDAS (Pediatric Migraine Disability Assessment) score (measure of headache-related disability) of at least 10, indicating mild or greater migraine-related disability. Children were excluded if they had continuous headache, medication overuse headache, PedMIDAS score greater than or equal to 140, psychiatric illness, or a previous adequate trial of either of the medications. The CHAMP study was discontinued early because of futility, with more than half of patients in each treatment arm meeting the primary end point of at least 50% reduction in headache frequency at the 24-week time point and more frequent adverse events in the topiramate and amitriptyline treatment arms.[18]

There has been much contemplation about how to interpret the results of the CHAMP trial.[38] It is worth noting that there were potentially active cointerventions that may have contributed to the high placebo response rate. First, there were monthly study visits with reinforcement of lifestyle management strategies at each visit. In addition, participants in the CHAMP trial received evidence-based acute migraine treatment, specifically NSAIDs and/or triptans. Data in adults suggest that effective acute treatments may also have a preventive effect.[39,40] In addition, children with refractory headache disorders, including those with high levels of migraine-related disability (PedMIDAS ≥ 140) and those with continuous headaches, were excluded from the study. This population may ultimately have the greatest benefit from use of preventive medications, and may be more willing to tolerate medication side effects in order to decrease migraine burden.

Ultimately, the findings from CHAMP have led to reevaluation of how migraine preventive medications are prescribed in the pediatric population. In particular, there has been increasing emphasis on optimization of preventive medications with the fewest side effects and the most supportive data, augmentation of lifestyle modifications, and use of behavioral approaches.

Lifestyle changes

Consistency and regularity of schedule are thought to be important in migraine management. However, achieving these goals can be challenging in light of the frequent changes children and adolescents experience related to school schedules, activities, and physical and emotional maturation. Patients should be counseled about sleep and hydration, regular meals, and consistent exercise. It can be helpful to identify whether dehydration, meal skipping, and/or inadequate sleep are perceived as triggers by the patient or family, and, if so, to use this as motivation for improvement in these areas.

A consensus statement published by the American Academy of Sleep Medicine outlines the optimal duration of sleep for children and adolescents based on age.[41] Adolescents need at least 8 hours of sleep nightly for optimal health; however, they often have difficulty obtaining this, in part because of their physiologically delayed sleep phase and because high schools often begin earlier than they would ideally wake up.[42] This situation can lead to substantial shifts in wake times and bedtimes between weekdays and weekends as teenagers attempt to catch up on sleep by sleeping in on Saturdays and Sundays. It can also be helpful to address screen time because this has been shown to have a negative impact on sleep quality and duration.[43] In particular, blue-light exposure from devices in the 2 hours before bedtime can suppress the body's melatonin release and disrupt sleep.[44,45] Screen time has also been associated with lower psychological well-being,[46] depression, and anxiety[47] in children and adolescents. Future research is warranted to investigate the impact of screen time on headache frequency in this population.

In addition, decreased levels of physical activity have been associated with higher prevalence of migraine in adults, and one study showed that 40 minutes of aerobic exercise 3 times weekly had equal benefit to topiramate in the preventive treatment of migraine in adults.[48,49]

In addition, it is important to address any potential stressors, including school stress, home stress, physical and/or emotional abuse, and bullying, because these have been shown to be risk factors for headache in children.[50] Both anxiety and mood disorders have been reported as common comorbidities in children with migraine, and it is important to address these given their potential impact on both headache and overall quality of life.[51]

Behavioral interventions

In addition to clinic-based counseling around routine and regularity, structured behavioral interventions have been shown to be beneficial for migraine prevention. In particular, cognitive behavior therapy (CBT) has been studied as an adjunctive therapy for adolescents with chronic migraine.[52] This type of therapy focuses on improved understanding of the connections between thoughts, emotions, body responses, and actions, and teaches adolescents to use positive realistic thinking strategies and specific skills to cope with migraine. In a study of children 10 to 17 years old with chronic migraine, those who received CBT plus amitriptyline had greater reduction in headache days and migraine-related disability compared with those who received CBT and headache education alone.[52] In addition, in adult patients with chronic migraine and insomnia, CBT therapy for insomnia has been shown to improve sleep and reduce headache frequency.[53,54]

Biofeedback has also been studied for migraine prevention in the pediatric population. This behavioral strategy teaches patients to mediate physical responses to stress through improved awareness and voluntary regulation of physiologic responses. A meta-analysis of 5 controlled studies of biofeedback for pediatric migraine prevention found that biofeedback reduced migraine frequency, attack duration, and headache intensity; however, the investigators acknowledge that the meta-analysis was limited by the risk of bias and variability in methods of randomization, techniques, and outcome measures used among the included studies.[55]

Pharmacologic preventives

In children who have at least 4 headache days per month, or in whom there is significant migraine-related disability, preventive medications may be considered in addition to the behavioral strategies outlined earlier. When using preventive medications in children, it is important to have open discussions with the family about the expectations for timing and extent of benefit. A medication trial of 6 to 8 weeks is recommended to determine efficacy, and a greater than or equal to 50% decrease in headache frequency is the most common measure of efficacy. Complete headache freedom is atypical. In light of findings from the CHAMP trial, the emphasis should be on identifying therapies with the most benefit and fewest side effects, and patients and their parents should be counseled about monitoring for side effects. To limit side effects, medications should be started at a low dose and titrated slowly to goal dose.

Supplements

Given their favorable side effect profile and overall tolerability, certain over-the-counter supplements can be used as first-line preventive therapies in children with migraine. Although they have been studied in children, note that these supplements are not subject to FDA regulation. It is helpful to provide families with recommendations for brands with validated dosages and minimal additives.

Riboflavin (vitamin B_2) Riboflavin plays a role in maintenance of cellular energy function through its role as an enzymatic cofactor in the electronic transport chain. In adults, mitochondrial DNA haplotype predicts migraine preventive benefit.[56] Controlled studies of efficacy in migraine prevention in children have been mixed. Although 2 prior trials in children have had high placebo response rates and failed to show superiority of riboflavin compared with placebo,[57,58] 1 placebo-controlled trial showed significantly greater reduction in headache frequency and duration in patients treated with 100 mg/d compared with those treated with 50 mg/d or placebo.[59] Riboflavin is generally well tolerated and the primary side effect is orange discoloration of the urine.

Magnesium Magnesium is important in neuronal function because it is a key metabolic cofactor in mitochondrial function, decreases membrane permeability, and may act as an antagonist at the N-methyl-D-aspartate (NMDA) glutamate receptor, thereby decreasing neuronal hyperexcitability.[60] A randomized, double-blind, placebo-controlled trial in children with migraine showed that magnesium but not placebo resulted in significant reduction in headache frequency over the study period, although ultimately there was no significant difference between the magnesium and placebo groups.[61] The most common side effect of magnesium is diarrhea. In addition, caution is warranted in the setting of renal impairment or neuromuscular junction disease.

Melatonin Melatonin is produced by the pineal gland and regulated by the suprachiasmatic nucleus of the hypothalamus; it plays an important role in maintenance of circadian rhythms and sleep-wake cycles. Although the mechanism of melatonin in treating headache is unknown, there is evidence for its use in several primary headache disorders, including trigeminal autonomic cephalalgias, primary stabbing headache, and migraine.[62] In pediatric patients, uncontrolled observational studies have suggested that melatonin therapy at doses of 3 to 6 mg nightly results in decreased headache frequency at 3 months.[63–65] A double-blind, randomized-controlled pilot study of melatonin versus placebo for migraine prevention in adolescents found that melatonin was safe and possibly effective in this population, although the study was not powered to detect significant benefit compared with placebo.[66] Further placebo-controlled trials are needed. Side effects are minimal and include daytime drowsiness in 7% to 12%.[63,65]

Coenzyme Q10 Like riboflavin, coenzyme Q10 is an essential enzyme in the mitochondrial electron transport chain and thereby plays a critical role in energy production in cells. Coenzyme Q10 has been studied for migraine prevention in the pediatric population. In one open-label study, children with migraine who were found to have low serum coenzyme Q10 levels were treated with enzyme supplementation at dosages of 1 to 3 mg/kg/d for 3 months, with subsequent increase in coenzyme Q10 levels and significant reduction in headache frequency.[67] A subsequent randomized, double-blind, placebo-controlled crossover trial showed a trend favoring coenzyme Q10 more than placebo in the first phase of the study (weeks 1–4), but there was a large participant dropout rate and the study did not meet its primary end point. Coenzyme Q10 is generally well tolerated in children and adolescents, although it should be used with caution in the setting of biliary obstruction or hepatic insufficiency.

Butterbur Butterbur is a plant extract with spasmolytic and analgesic effects. In children, butterbur was shown to reduce migraine frequency by 63% in one open-label study.[68] Later, a randomized, placebo-controlled trial of butterbur and music therapy in children found that only music therapy was superior to placebo at the specified posttreatment time point, although both were superior to placebo at 6-month follow-up.[69] However, if the pyrrolizidine alkaloids in the plant are not adequately removed they can cause significant hepatotoxicity, and therefore the use of butterbur is no longer recommended in pediatric populations.

Vitamin D Vitamin D is involved in bone metabolism and brain development. Children with migraine have been found to have significantly lower vitamin D levels than controls,[70] and one study found that vitamin D as an adjunct to amitriptyline resulted in lower headache frequency than amitriptyline alone in children with low, normal, and high vitamin D levels.[71] Further studies are needed to elucidate the role of vitamin D in migraine prevention.

Prescription medications
The medications included here are limited to those that have been studied in children and/or adolescents for migraine prevention.

Amitriptyline Before the CHAMP trial, amitriptyline (1 mg/kg/d) was shown to be effective in decreasing the frequency of migraine in a prospective observational study in pediatric patients with 3 or more headaches per month.[72] However, the larger placebo-controlled CHAMP trial found no benefit of amitriptyline compared with placebo, as noted earlier.[17] Side effects of tricyclic antidepressants include drowsiness, cardiac rhythm abnormalities, dry mouth, constipation, and urinary retention.

Propranolol Data for use of propranolol in pediatric migraine prevention are mixed. One prospective, double-blind, placebo-controlled study in children and adolescents with migraine showed greater decrease in headache frequency with propranolol compared with placebo,[73] but subsequent studies have not replicated this finding.[74,75] Side effects of propranolol include fatigue, sleep disturbance, and light-headedness.

Flunarizine The calcium channel blocker flunarizine has also been studied in children and was associated with significant reduction in headache frequency in 2 randomized, placebo-controlled studies.[76,77] Side effects of flunarizine include sedation and weight gain. The 2004 practice parameters from the American Academy of Neurology for migraine prevention in children concluded that this medication is probably effective for migraine in children[78]; however, flunarizine is not currently available in the United States.

Nimodipine Another calcium channel blocker, nimodipine, was studied in children in a placebo-controlled crossover trial; nimodipine was found to have no benefit compared with placebo during the primary treatment period, but was superior to placebo in the second treatment period.[79] The only side effect reported in this study was abdominal discomfort.[79]

Topiramate Topiramate was approved by the FDA for migraine prevention in children 12 to 17 years old while the CHAMP trial was ongoing, and it remains the only medication approved by the FDA for migraine prevention in adolescents. Three randomized, placebo-controlled trials previously showed superiority of topiramate compared with placebo in adolescents.[80–82] However, as discussed earlier, the CHAMP study did not replicate these findings.[18] In addition, side effects of topiramate are common and include cognitive slowing, paresthesias, and weight loss in addition to more serious potential side effects of glaucoma, renal stones, and teratogenicity.

Sodium valproate In children and adolescents, there have been multiple observational studies showing efficacy of valproic acid in reducing headache frequency,[83–85] with randomized trials showing similar efficacy to topiramate[86] and propranolol.[87] However, there have been no placebo-controlled trials of valproic acid for migraine prevention in the pediatric population. The side effect profile of valproic acid is extensive and includes alopecia, tremor, teratogenicity (pregnancy category X for migraine prevention), hepatotoxicity, pancreatitis, leukopenia, and thrombocytopenia.

New Directions

Antibodies against calcitonin gene–related peptide (CGRP) or its receptor have been developed as the first class of migraine-specific preventive therapy, and several of these are now FDA approved in the United States for use in adults. CGRP is expressed throughout the nervous system and is involved in the pathogenesis of migraine.[88] In a study of pediatric patients with migraine, CGRP levels were found to be increased during migraine attacks.[89] Anti-CGRP monoclonal antibodies have been found to be safe and effective for treatment of both episodic and chronic migraine in adults but have not yet been studied in children.[90–98] Based on review of safety data and potential long-term adverse effects, pediatric headache experts have recommended consideration of use of these medications in carefully selected patients with close clinical monitoring for adverse effects.[99]

SUMMARY

Migraine is common in children and adolescents and can be a source of significant disability. Important differences in migraine phenotype in children compared with adults are shorter attack duration and bilateral pain location. By taking a careful, child-directed history, important insight can be gained into associated features of headache as well as presence of childhood-onset syndromes that may be associated with migraine. Treatment of migraine in pediatric patients includes both acute and preventive strategies. With recent findings from the CHAMP trial showing that placebo had equal efficacy to amitriptyline and topiramate with fewer side effects, there is renewed emphasis on using treatments with the fewest side effects and best evidence for efficacy. This approach may include use of certain natural supplements as well as behavioral techniques such as CBT. Further research is needed to determine whether novel migraine-specific medications such as the anti-CGRP monoclonal antibodies are effective and well tolerated in the pediatric population.

DISCLOSURE

K. Greene, nothing to disclose. S.L. Irwin, CEO of HeadSoothe, a company that is working to develop a combination nutraceutical for headache. A.A. Gelfand has received consulting fees from Zosano, Eli Lilly, Impax, Theranica, Advanced Clinical, and Impel Neuropharma. She has received honoraria from UpToDate (for authorship) and *JAMA Neurology* (as an associate editor). She receives grant support from Amgen and research support from eNeura. She receives personal compensation for medical-legal consulting. Her spouse received consulting fees from Biogen (daclizumab) and Alexion (eculizumab), research support from Genentech (ocrevus), service contract support from MedDay, honoraria for editorial work from Dynamed Plus, and personal compensation for medical-legal consulting. This article discusses the unlabeled/investigational use of all listed medications for the treatment of headache in children and adolescents, with the exceptions of almotriptan oral tablets, sumatriptan/naproxen combination tablets, zolmitriptan nasal spray for adolescents 12 to 17 years of age, rizatriptan oral tablets or melts for acute migraine in children 6 years of age and older, as well as topiramate in adolescents 12 to 17 years of age for migraine prevention.

REFERENCES

1. Abu-Arafeh I, Razak S, Sivaraman B, et al. Prevalence of headache and migraine in children and adolescents: a systematic review of population-based studies. Dev Med Child Neurol 2010;52(12):1088–97.
2. Victor TW, Hu X, Campbell JC, et al. Migraine prevalence by age and sex in the United States: a life-span study. Cephalalgia 2010;30(9):1065–72.
3. Lipton RB, Manack A, Ricci JA, et al. Prevalence and burden of chronic migraine in adolescents: results of the chronic daily headache in adolescents study (C-dAS). Headache 2011;51(5):693–706.
4. Arruda MA, Bigal ME. Migraine and migraine subtypes in preadolescent children: association with school performance. Neurology 2012;79(18):1881–8.

5. Stafstrom CE, Goldenholz SR, Dulli DA. Serial headache drawings by children with migraine: correlation with clinical headache status. J Child Neurol 2005; 20(10):809–13.

6. Headache Classification Committee of the International Headache Society (IHS) The international classification of headache disorders, 3rd edition. Cephalalgia 2018;38(1):1–211.

7. Hershey AD, Winner P, Kabbouche MA, et al. Use of the ICHD-II criteria in the diagnosis of pediatric migraine. Headache 2005;45(10):1288–97.

8. De Carlo D, Dal Zotto L, Perissinotto E, et al. Osmophobia in migraine classification: a multicentre study in juvenile patients. Cephalalgia 2010;30(12): 1486–94.

9. Raieli V, Giordano G, Spitaleri C, et al. Migraine and cranial autonomic symptoms in children and adolescents: a clinical study. J Child Neurol 2015;30(2): 182–6.

10. Gelfand AA, Reider AC, Goadsby PJ. Cranial autonomic symptoms in pediatric migraine are the rule, not the exception. Neurology 2013;81(5):431–6.

11. Cuvellier JC, Mars A, Vallee L. The prevalence of premonitory symptoms in paediatric migraine: a questionnaire study in 103 children and adolescents. Cephalalgia 2009;29(11):1197–201.

12. Mamouri O, Cuvellier JC, Duhamel A, et al. Postdrome symptoms in pediatric migraine: a questionnaire retrospective study by phone in 100 patients. Cephalalgia 2018;38(5):943–8.

13. Balestri M, Papetti L, Maiorani D, et al. Features of aura in paediatric migraine diagnosed using the ICHD 3 beta criteria. Cephalalgia 2018;38(11):1742–7.

14. Giffin NJ, Benton S, Goadsby PJ. Benign paroxysmal torticollis of infancy: four new cases and linkage to CACNA1A mutation. Dev Med Child Neurol 2002; 44(7):490–3.

15. Roubertie A, Echenne B, Leydet J, et al. Benign paroxysmal tonic upgaze, benign paroxysmal torticollis, episodic ataxia and CACNA1A mutation in a family. J Neurol 2008;255(10):1600–2.

16. Symon DN, Russell G. Double blind placebo controlled trial of pizotifen syrup in the treatment of abdominal migraine. Arch Dis Child 1995;72(1):48–50.

17. Powers SW, Hershey AD, Coffey CS, et al. The childhood and adolescent migraine prevention (CHAMP) study: a report on Baseline characteristics of participants. Headache 2016;56(5):859–70.

18. Hershey AD, Powers SW, Coffey CS, et al. Childhood and Adolescent Migraine Prevention (CHAMP) study: a double-blinded, placebo-controlled, comparative effectiveness study of amitriptyline, topiramate, and placebo in the prevention of childhood and adolescent migraine. Headache 2013;53(5):799–816.

19. Scher AI, Rizzoli PB, Loder EW. Medication overuse headache: An entrenched idea in need of scrutiny. Neurology 2017;89(12):1296–304.

20. Bigal ME, Serrano D, Buse D, et al. Acute migraine medications and evolution from episodic to chronic migraine: a longitudinal population-based study. Headache 2008;48(8):1157–68.

21. Lewis D, Middlebrook M, Deline C. Naproxen sodium for chemoprophylaxis of adolescent migraine. Ann Neurol 1994;36:542.

22. Bellavance AJ, Meloche JP. A comparative study of naproxen sodium, pizotyline and placebo in migraine prophylaxis. Headache 1990;30(11):710–5.

23. Behan PO, Connelly K. Prophylaxis of migraine: a comparison between naproxen sodium and pizotifen. Headache 1986;26(5):237–9.

24. Ziegler DK, Ellis DJ. Naproxen in prophylaxis of migraine. Arch Neurol 1985; 42(6):582–4.
25. Welch KM, Ellis DJ, Keenan PA. Successful migraine prophylaxis with naproxen sodium. Neurology 1985;35(9):1304–10.
26. Sargent J, Solbach P, Damasio H, et al. A comparison of naproxen sodium to propranolol hydrochloride and a placebo control for the prophylaxis of migraine headache. Headache 1985;25(6):320–4.
27. Hamalainen ML, Hoppu K, Valkeila E, et al. Ibuprofen or acetaminophen for the acute treatment of migraine in children: a double-blind, randomized, placebo-controlled, crossover study. Neurology 1997;48(1):103–7.
28. Lewis DW, Kellstein D, Dahl G, et al. Children's ibuprofen suspension for the acute treatment of pediatric migraine. Headache 2002;42(8):780–6.
29. Brandes JL, Kudrow D, Stark SR, et al. Sumatriptan-naproxen for acute treatment of migraine: a randomized trial. JAMA 2007;297(13):1443–54.
30. McDonald SA, Hershey AD, Pearlman E, et al. Long-term evaluation of sumatriptan and naproxen sodium for the acute treatment of migraine in adolescents. Headache 2011;51(9):1374–87.
31. Richer L, Billinghurst L, Linsdell MA, et al. Drugs for the acute treatment of migraine in children and adolescents. Cochrane Database Syst Rev 2016;(4):CD005220.
32. Mathew PG, Krel R, Buddhdev B, et al. A retrospective analysis of triptan and dhe use for basilar and hemiplegic migraine. Headache 2016;56(5):841–8.
33. Brousseau DC, Duffy SJ, Anderson AC, et al. Treatment of pediatric migraine headaches: a randomized, double-blind trial of prochlorperazine versus ketorolac. Ann Emerg Med 2004;43(2):256–62.
34. Vinson DR, Drotts DL. Diphenhydramine for the prevention of akathisia induced by prochlorperazine: a randomized, controlled trial. Ann Emerg Med 2001;37(2): 125–31.
35. Kanis JM, Timm NL. Chlorpromazine for the treatment of migraine in a pediatric emergency department. Headache 2014;54(2):335–42.
36. Bachur RG, Monuteaux MC, Neuman MI. A comparison of acute treatment regimens for migraine in the emergency department. Pediatrics 2015;135(2):232–8.
37. Patniyot IR, Gelfand AA. Acute treatment therapies for pediatric migraine: a qualitative systematic review. Headache 2016;56(1):49–70.
38. Gelfand AA, Qubty W, Goadsby PJ. Pediatric migraine prevention-first, do no harm. JAMA Neurol 2017;74(8):893–4.
39. Lipton RB, Fanning KM, Serrano D, et al. Ineffective acute treatment of episodic migraine is associated with new-onset chronic migraine. Neurology 2015;84(7): 688–95.
40. Cady RK, Voirin J, Farmer K, et al. Two center, randomized pilot study of migraine prophylaxis comparing paradigms using pre-emptive frovatriptan or daily topiramate: research and clinical implications. Headache 2012;52(5): 749–64.
41. Paruthi S, Brooks LJ, D'Ambrosio C, et al. Recommended amount of sleep for pediatric populations: a consensus statement of the American Academy of Sleep Medicine. J Clin Sleep Med 2016;12(6):785–6.
42. Carskadon MA, Tarokh L. Developmental changes in sleep biology and potential effects on adolescent behavior and caffeine use. Nutr Rev 2014;72(Suppl 1):60–4.
43. Przybylski AK. Digital screen time and pediatric sleep: evidence from a preregistered cohort study. J Pediatr 2019;205:218–23.e1.

44. Figueiro MG, Bierman A, Rea MS. A train of blue light pulses delivered through closed eyelids suppresses melatonin and phase shifts the human circadian system. Nat Sci Sleep 2013;5:133–41.
45. Figueiro MG, Plitnick B, Rea MS. Pulsing blue light through closed eyelids: effects on acute melatonin suppression and phase shifting of dim light melatonin onset. Nat Sci Sleep 2014;6:149–56.
46. Twenge JM, Campbell WK. Associations between screen time and lower psychological well-being among children and adolescents: Evidence from a population-based study. Prev Med Rep 2018;12:271–83.
47. Maras D, Flament MF, Murray M, et al. Screen time is associated with depression and anxiety in Canadian youth. Prev Med 2015;73:133–8.
48. Varkey E, Cider A, Carlsson J, et al. Exercise as migraine prophylaxis: a randomized study using relaxation and topiramate as controls. Cephalalgia 2011;31(14):1428–38.
49. Varkey E, Cider A, Carlsson J, et al. A study to evaluate the feasibility of an aerobic exercise program in patients with migraine. Headache 2009;49(4):563–70.
50. Straube A, Heinen F, Ebinger F, et al. Headache in school children: prevalence and risk factors. Dtsch Arztebl Int 2013;110(48):811–8.
51. Orr SL, Potter BK, Ma J, et al. Migraine and mental health in a population-based sample of adolescents. Can J Neurol Sci 2017;44(1):44–50.
52. Powers SW, Kashikar-Zuck SM, Allen JR, et al. Cognitive behavioral therapy plus amitriptyline for chronic migraine in children and adolescents: a randomized clinical trial. JAMA 2013;310(24):2622–30.
53. Smitherman TA, Walters AB, Davis RE, et al. Randomized controlled pilot trial of behavioral insomnia treatment for chronic migraine with comorbid insomnia. Headache 2016;56(2):276–91.
54. Smitherman TA, Kuka AJ, Calhoun AH, et al. Cognitive-behavioral therapy for insomnia to reduce chronic migraine: a sequential bayesian analysis. Headache 2018;58(7):1052–9.
55. Stubberud A, Varkey E, McCrory DC, et al. Biofeedback as prophylaxis for pediatric migraine: a meta-analysis. Pediatrics 2016;138(2) [pii:e20160675].
56. Di Lorenzo C, Pierelli F, Coppola G, et al. Mitochondrial DNA haplogroups influence the therapeutic response to riboflavin in migraineurs. Neurology 2009;72(18):1588–94.
57. Bruijn J, Duivenvoorden H, Passchier J, et al. Medium-dose riboflavin as a prophylactic agent in children with migraine: a preliminary placebo-controlled, randomised, double-blind, cross-over trial. Cephalalgia 2010;30(12):1426–34.
58. MacLennan SC, Wade FM, Forrest KM, et al. High-dose riboflavin for migraine prophylaxis in children: a double-blind, randomized, placebo-controlled trial. J Child Neurol 2008;23(11):1300–4.
59. Talebian A, Soltani B, Banafshe HR, et al. Prophylactic effect of riboflavin on pediatric migraine: a randomized, double-blind, placebo-controlled trial. Electron Physician 2018;10(2):6279–85.
60. Kirkland AE, Sarlo GL, Holton KF. The role of magnesium in neurological disorders. Nutrients 2018;10(6) [pii:E730].
61. Wang F, Van Den Eeden SK, Ackerson LM, et al. Oral magnesium oxide prophylaxis of frequent migrainous headache in children: a randomized, double-blind, placebo-controlled trial. Headache 2003;43(6):601–10.
62. Gelfand AA, Goadsby PJ. The role of melatonin in the treatment of primary headache disorders. Headache 2016;56(8):1257–66.

63. Miano S, Parisi P, Pelliccia A, et al. Melatonin to prevent migraine or tension-type headache in children. Neurol Sci 2008;29(4):285–7.

64. Gelfand AA. Melatonin in the treatment of primary headache disorders. Headache 2017;57(6):848–9.

65. Fallah R, Shoroki FF, Ferdosian F. Safety and efficacy of melatonin in pediatric migraine prophylaxis. Curr Drug Saf 2015;10(2):132–5.

66. Gelfand AA, Qubty W, Patniyot I, et al. Home-based trials in adolescent migraine: a randomized clinical trial. JAMA Neurol 2017;74(6):744–5.

67. Hershey AD, Powers SW, Vockell AL, et al. Coenzyme Q10 deficiency and response to supplementation in pediatric and adolescent migraine. Headache 2007;47(1):73–80.

68. Pothmann R, Danesch U. Migraine prevention in children and adolescents: results of an open study with a special butterbur root extract. Headache 2005; 45(3):196–203.

69. Oelkers-Ax R, Leins A, Parzer P, et al. Butterbur root extract and music therapy in the prevention of childhood migraine: an explorative study. Eur J Pain 2008; 12(3):301–13.

70. Donmez A, Orun E, Sonmez FM. Vitamin D status in children with headache: a case-control study. Clin Nutr ESPEN 2018;23:222–7.

71. Cayir A, Turan MI, Tan H. Effect of vitamin D therapy in addition to amitriptyline on migraine attacks in pediatric patients. Braz J Med Biol Res 2014;47(4): 349–54.

72. Hershey AD, Powers SW, Bentti AL, et al. Effectiveness of amitriptyline in the prophylactic management of childhood headaches. Headache 2000;40(7): 539–49.

73. Ludvigsson J. Propranolol used in prophylaxis of migraine in children. Acta Neurol Scand 1974;50(1):109–15.

74. Forsythe WI, Gillies D, Sills MA. Propanolol ('Inderal') in the treatment of childhood migraine. Dev Med Child Neurol 1984;26(6):737–41.

75. Olness K, MacDonald JT, Uden DL. Comparison of self-hypnosis and propranolol in the treatment of juvenile classic migraine. Pediatrics 1987;79(4):593–7.

76. Sorge F, De Simone R, Marano E, et al. Flunarizine in prophylaxis of childhood migraine. A double-blind, placebo-controlled, crossover study. Cephalalgia 1988;8(1):1–6.

77. Sorge F, Marano E. Flunarizine v. placebo in childhood migraine. A double-blind study. Cephalalgia 1985;5(Suppl 2):145–8.

78. Lewis D, Ashwal S, Hershey A, et al. Practice parameter: pharmacological treatment of migraine headache in children and adolescents: report of the American Academy of Neurology Quality Standards Subcommittee and the Practice Committee of the Child Neurology Society. Neurology 2004;63(12):2215–24.

79. Battistella PA, Ruffilli R, Moro R, et al. A placebo-controlled crossover trial of nimodipine in pediatric migraine. Headache 1990;30(5):264–8.

80. Winner P, Pearlman EM, Linder SL, et al. Topiramate for migraine prevention in children: a randomized, double-blind, placebo-controlled trial. Headache 2005; 45(10):1304–12.

81. Lewis D, Winner P, Saper J, et al. Randomized, double-blind, placebo-controlled study to evaluate the efficacy and safety of topiramate for migraine prevention in pediatric subjects 12 to 17 years of age. Pediatrics 2009;123(3): 924–34.

82. Lakshmi CV, Singhi P, Malhi P, et al. Topiramate in the prophylaxis of pediatric migraine: a double-blind placebo-controlled trial. J Child Neurol 2007;22(7): 829–35.

83. Pakalnis A, Greenberg G, Drake ME Jr, et al. Pediatric migraine prophylaxis with divalproex. J Child Neurol 2001;16(10):731–4.

84. Serdaroglu G, Erhan E, Tekgul H, et al. Sodium valproate prophylaxis in childhood migraine. Headache 2002;42(8):819–22.

85. Caruso JM, Brown WD, Exil G, et al. The efficacy of divalproex sodium in the prophylactic treatment of children with migraine. Headache 2000;40(8):672–6.

86. Unalp A, Uran N, Ozturk A. Comparison of the effectiveness of topiramate and sodium valproate in pediatric migraine. J Child Neurol 2008;23(12):1377–81.

87. Bidabadi E, Mashouf M. A randomized trial of propranolol versus sodium valproate for the prophylaxis of migraine in pediatric patients. Paediatr Drugs 2010;12(4):269–75.

88. Goadsby PJ, Holland PR, Martins-Oliveira M, et al. Pathophysiology of migraine: a disorder of sensory processing. Physiol Rev 2017;97(2):553–622.

89. Fan PC, Kuo PH, Chang SH, et al. Plasma calcitonin gene-related peptide in diagnosing and predicting paediatric migraine. Cephalalgia 2009;29(8):883–90.

90. Goadsby PJ, Reuter U, Hallstrom Y, et al. A controlled trial of erenumab for episodic migraine. N Engl J Med 2017;377(22):2123–32.

91. Schwedt T, Reuter U, Tepper S, et al. Early onset of efficacy with erenumab in patients with episodic and chronic migraine. J Headache Pain 2018;19(1):92.

92. Tepper S, Ashina M, Reuter U, et al. Safety and efficacy of erenumab for preventive treatment of chronic migraine: a randomised, double-blind, placebo-controlled phase 2 trial. Lancet Neurol 2017;16(6):425–34.

93. Dodick DW, Ashina M, Brandes JL, et al. ARISE: a Phase 3 randomized trial of erenumab for episodic migraine. Cephalalgia 2018;38(6):1026–37.

94. Skljarevski V, Matharu M, Millen BA, et al. Efficacy and safety of galcanezumab for the prevention of episodic migraine: Results of the EVOLVE-2 Phase 3 randomized controlled clinical trial. Cephalalgia 2018;38(8):1442–54.

95. Aurora SK. Efficacy of Galcanezumab in patients who failed to Respond to preventives previously: results from EVOLVE-1, EVOLVE-2, and REGAIN studies. Paper presented at: American Academy of Neurology Annual Scientific Meeting 2018. Los Angeles, CA.

96. Stauffer VL, Dodick DW, Zhang Q, et al. Evaluation of galcanezumab for the prevention of episodic migraine: the EVOLVE-1 randomized clinical trial. JAMA Neurol 2018;75(9):1080–8.

97. Dodick DW, Silberstein SD, Bigal ME, et al. Effect of fremanezumab compared with placebo for prevention of episodic migraine: a randomized clinical trial. JAMA 2018;319(19):1999–2008.

98. Silberstein SD, Dodick DW, Bigal ME, et al. Fremanezumab for the preventive treatment of chronic migraine. N Engl J Med 2017;377(22):2113–22.

99. Szperka CL, VanderPluym J, Orr SL, et al. Recommendations on the use of anti-CGRP monoclonal antibodies in children and adolescents. Headache 2018; 58(10):1658–69.

100. Gelfand AA. Episodic syndromes that may be associated with migraine: A.K.A. "the Childhood Periodic Syndromes". Headache 2015;55(10):1358–64.

101. Gelfand AA. Episodic syndromes of childhood associated with migraine. Curr Opin Neurol 2018;31(3):281–5.

102. Irwin S, Barmherzig R, Gelfand A. Recurrent gastrointestinal disturbance: abdominal migraine and cyclic vomiting syndrome. Curr Neurol Neurosci Rep 2017;17(3):21.

103. Drumm BR, Bourke B, Drummond J, et al. Cyclical vomiting syndrome in children: a prospective study. Neurogastroenterol Motil 2012;24(10):922–7.

104. Lagman-Bartolome AM, Lay C. Pediatric migraine variants: a review of epidemiology, diagnosis, treatment, and outcome. Curr Neurol Neurosci Rep 2015; 15(6):34.

105. Catto-Smith AG, Ranuh R. Abdominal migraine and cyclical vomiting. Semin Pediatr Surg 2003;12(4):254–8.

106. Mortimer MJ, Kay J, Jaron A. Clinical epidemiology of childhood abdominal migraine in an urban general practice. Dev Med Child Neurol 1993;35(3):243–8.

107. Abu-Arafeh I, Russell G. Prevalence and clinical features of abdominal migraine compared with those of migraine headache. Arch Dis Child 1995;72(5):413–7.

108. Rasquin A, Di Lorenzo C, Forbes D, et al. Childhood functional gastrointestinal disorders: child/adolescent. Gastroenterology 2006;130(5):1527–37.

109. Batu ED, Anlar B, Topcu M, et al. Vertigo in childhood: a retrospective series of 100 children. Eur J Paediatr Neurol 2015;19(2):226–32.

110. Batuecas-Caletrio A, Martin-Sanchez V, Cordero-Civantos C, et al. Is benign paroxysmal vertigo of childhood a migraine precursor? Eur J Paediatr Neurol 2013;17(4):397–400.

111. Krams B, Echenne B, Leydet J, et al. Benign paroxysmal vertigo of childhood: long-term outcome. Cephalalgia 2011;31(4):439–43.

112. Rosman NP, Douglass LM, Sharif UM, et al. The neurology of benign paroxysmal torticollis of infancy: report of 10 new cases and review of the literature. J Child Neurol 2009;24(2):155–60.

113. Danielsson A, Anderlid BM, Stodberg T, et al. Benign paroxysmal torticollis of infancy does not lead to neurological sequelae. Dev Med Child Neurol 2018; 60(12):1251–5.

114. Humbertclaude V, Krams B, Nogue E, et al. Benign paroxysmal torticollis, benign paroxysmal vertigo, and benign tonic upward gaze are not benign disorders. Dev Med Child Neurol 2018;60(12):1256–63.

115. Johnson JD, Cocker K, Chang E. Infantile colic: recognition and treatment. Am Fam Physician 2015;92(7):577–82.

116. Gelfand AA, Thomas KC, Goadsby PJ. Before the headache: infant colic as an early life expression of migraine. Neurology 2012;79(13):1392–6.

117. Sweney MT, Silver K, Gerard-Blanluet M, et al. Alternating hemiplegia of childhood: early characteristics and evolution of a neurodevelopmental syndrome. Pediatrics 2009;123(3):e534–41.

118. Heinzen EL, Swoboda KJ, Hitomi Y, et al. De novo mutations in ATP1A3 cause alternating hemiplegia of childhood. Nat Genet 2012;44(9):1030–4.

119. Rothner AD, Winner P, Nett R, et al. One-year tolerability and efficacy of sumatriptan nasal spray in adolescents with migraine: results of a multicenter, open-label study. Clin Ther 2000;22(12):1533–46.

120. Winner P, Rothner AD, Saper J, et al. A randomized, double-blind, placebo-controlled study of sumatriptan nasal spray in the treatment of acute migraine in adolescents. Pediatrics 2000;106(5):989–97.

121. Ahonen K, Hamalainen ML, Rantala H, et al. Nasal sumatriptan is effective in treatment of migraine attacks in children: a randomized trial. Neurology 2004; 62(6):883–7.

122. Ueberall MA, Wenzel D. Intranasal sumatriptan for the acute treatment of migraine in children. Neurology 1999;52(7):1507–10.
123. Ho TW, Pearlman E, Lewis D, et al. Efficacy and tolerability of rizatriptan in pediatric migraineurs: results from a randomized, double-blind, placebo-controlled trial using a novel adaptive enrichment design. Cephalalgia 2012; 32(10):750–65.
124. Ahonen K, Hamalainen ML, Eerola M, et al. A randomized trial of rizatriptan in migraine attacks in children. Neurology 2006;67(7):1135–40.
125. Linder SL, Mathew NT, Cady RK, et al. Efficacy and tolerability of almotriptan in adolescents: a randomized, double-blind, placebo-controlled trial. Headache 2008;48(9):1326–36.
126. Evers S, Rahmann A, Kraemer C, et al. Treatment of childhood migraine attacks with oral zolmitriptan and ibuprofen. Neurology 2006;67(3):497–9.
127. Lewis DW, Winner P, Hershey AD, et al. Adolescent Migraine Steering C. Efficacy of zolmitriptan nasal spray in adolescent migraine. Pediatrics 2007; 120(2):390–6.
128. Rothner AD, Wasiewski W, Winner P, et al. Zolmitriptan oral tablet in migraine treatment: high placebo responses in adolescents. Headache 2006;46(1): 101–9.
129. Winner P, Linder SL, Lipton RB, et al. Eletriptan for the acute treatment of migraine in adolescents: results of a double-blind, placebo-controlled trial. Headache 2007;47(4):511–8.
130. Elkind AH, Wade A, Ishkanian G. Pharmacokinetics of frovatriptan in adolescent migraineurs. J Clin Pharmacol 2004;44(10):1158–65.
131. Christensen ML, Eades SK, Fuseau E, et al. Pharmacokinetics of naratriptan in adolescent subjects with a history of migraine. J Clin Pharmacol 2001;41(2): 170–5.

Migraine in Women

Ana Marissa Lagman-Bartolome, MD, FRCPC[a],*,
Christine Lay, MD, FRCPC[b]

KEYWORDS

- Migraine • Women • Hormones • Menarche • Menstrual migraine • Menopause
- Stroke • Hormonal treatment

KEY POINTS

- Migraine impacts women from early adolescence and puberty through the perimeno-pausal and postmenopausal years and is thus a lifelong disorder.
- Female hormones, in particular estrogen, fluctuate in a cyclical pattern every month, creating a monthly migraine in many women.
- Estrogen also fluctuates over a woman's lifetime and can impact migraine both posi-tively—in pregnancy—and negatively—in the perimenopause.
- Effective treatment, including hormonal therapies, may require individualized adjust-ments, but generally leads to effective migraine control.

Migraine disproportionately affects women 3 times more than men, with 18% of women and 6% of men being afflicted, which suggests that migraine is influenced by factors, including fluctuating hormones throughout the life of a female migraineur. These hormonal influences have an impact at menarche, menstruation, pregnancy, and menopause.[1,2] The onset of migraine typically occurs 1 to 2 years before or after menarche, with 1 study noting that those who underwent menarche by age 11 years have a 7% increased likelihood of developing migraine than those who reached menarche at 12 years of age or older.[3] This female predominance emerges after pu-berty with the prevalence of migraine reaching 24% in those aged 30 to 39 years.[4–6]

FACTORS IN THE GENDER DIFFERENCE

There remain knowledge gaps in understanding the detailed mechanism behind the sex and gender differences in migraine, but one of the most common theories is that fluctuations in female sex hormones play a key role.[5] The female hormones,

[a] Pediatric Neurology and Headache Medicine, Women's College Hospital, Hospital for Sick Children, University of Toronto, 76 Grenville Street, Toronto, Ontario M5S 1B2, Canada; [b] Neurology and Headache Medicine, Women's College Hospital, Hospital for Sick Children, University of Toronto, 76 Grenville Street, Toronto, Ontario M5S 1B2, Canada
* Corresponding author.
E-mail address: marissa.lagman@wchospital.ca

Neurol Clin 37 (2019) 835–845
https://doi.org/10.1016/j.ncl.2019.07.002
0733-8619/19/Crown Copyright © 2019 Published by Elsevier Inc. All rights reserved.

and in particular estrogen, fluctuate throughout a woman's life, in addition to the cyclical nature of the hormonal cycle, and it is these fluctuations that can provoke migraine attacks.

Compared with men, women also report more intense migraine attacks and migraine-related symptoms (ie, photophobia, phonophobia, nausea, visual aura, blurred vision) and more migraine-related disability.[1,6] One possible explanation for this, is that menstrually related migraine (MRM) has been shown to be more severe, longer lasting, more likely to be associated with cutaneous allodynia, more resistant to treatment, and carries higher associated disability.[7]

Several risk factors have been identified that increase migraine transformation from episodic to chronic migraine, including environmental, genetic, epigenetic, and social factors. Women are at higher risk of transforming to chronic migraine because they have higher reported rates of depression, anxiety as well as adverse childhood experiences.[8] Obese women are likely to have more than a 2-fold higher risk of episodic and chronic migraine, probably owing to the pathologic estrogen production in adipose tissue.[9] Estrogen withdrawal plays a role in triggering migraine and animal studies confirm that female gonadal hormones increase the susceptibility to migraine via an estrogen-dependent electrophysiological effect, as compared with testosterone, which suppresses migraine.[10,11] Although the role of testosterone in migraine pathophysiology remains unclear, it can potentially modulate cerebral blood flow, serotonergic tone, and susceptibility to cortical spreading depression.[12] Although men produce small quantities of estrogen via aromatization of androstenedione and testosterone, these estrogen quantities are much lower than in young women and they remain fairly stable with a much more gradual decline with age.[13]

Several neuroimaging studies have provided insights into the structural, chemical, and functional differences of women with migraine. Structural brain differences in areas involved in pain processing, sensation, affective processing, and autonomic function have been seen, including thicker left posterior insula and increased activation of the insula and precuneus.[2,8] A greater activation of areas of brain involved in emotional processing was also observed in women compared with men, suggesting a possible mechanism for higher subjective rating of headache unpleasantness experienced by female migraineurs.[8,14]

Serotonin, known to have a crucial role in migraine pathogenesis,[15] can be enhanced by estrogen, which increases the expression of tryptophan hydroxylase and decreases the expression of the serotonin reuptake transporter. Estrogen also can activate the endogenous opioid system, producing an analgesic effect.[8,16] Experimental studies suggest that progesterone plays a protective role by reducing nociception in the trigeminovascular system, by inhibiting neurogenic edema, and histamine secretion from mast cells as well as by decreasing prostaglandin production.[8]

MIGRAINE IN ADOLESCENCE

The lifetime prevalence of migraine is similar in girls and boys aged 7 to 9 years before puberty and it increases further over the course of adolescence.[17] By late adolescence, migraine affects more girls than boys, reaching the 3:1 ratio seen in adult women and men.[5,18,19]

Unlike adult migraine, pediatric migraine is most often nonthrobbing, bilateral, with a faster onset and shorter in duration (2–72 hours), with the photophobia and phonophobia often inferred by behavior.[20] During puberty, sex hormones affect neural circuits, which cause changes in the hypothalamus and insula.[21] At menarche, approximately 53% of adolescent girls reported headaches; hence, pubertal development and age seem to modulate the effect of ovarian hormones on migraine.[2] The incidence of migraine with aura peaks between 12 and 13 years of age, whereas migraine without aura presents a few years later. With respect to MRM, specific genomic patterns that have been identified suggest a probable genetic predisposition.[22]

The treatment of adolescent migraine is challenging owing to limited studies and high placebo rates. Currently no guidelines exist for the management of pediatric migraine. Some strategies that are beneficial in the pediatric population include avoiding medication overuse, drinking more fluids, regulating sleep rhythms, avoiding caffeine, eating regular meals, eating protein in the morning, regular exercise (30 minutes a day), decreasing stress with meditation, and the consideration of a trial of migraine supplements such as magnesium citrate or riboflavin.[22,23]

Pharmacologic abortive therapies should be used early in the pain phase when efficacy is highest. Low-quality evidence from 2 small trials shows that ibuprofen seems to improve pain freedom and triptans as a class are also safe and effective but are associated with higher rates of minor adverse events. Almotriptan (oral), rizatriptan (melt), zolmitriptan (nasal spray), and sumatriptan are approved by the US Food and Drug Administration (FDA) for acute migraine treatment in adolescents from 12 to 17 years of age. Sumatriptan plus naproxen sodium is also effective in treating adolescents with migraine.[19,22,24,25]

The decision to use preventative medication in adolescents is multifactorial, but it is rooted in how migraine impacts the teen's life. If deemed necessary, melatonin 3 mg nightly, riboflavin 400 mg/d, cognitive-behavioral therapy, or low-dose prescription medications could be considered. Topiramate is the only FDA-approved migraine prevention drug in adolescents 12 to 17 years of age; however, it and any other preventative should be used with caution in adolescent girls of reproductive age owing the drugs' potential teratogenicity.[19]

MENSTRUAL MIGRAINE

Menstrual migraine (MM), which encompasses both pure MM and MRM, is more typically without aura, and it most frequently occurs in the second decade of life around the onset of menarche. Studies show its prevalence varies from 4% to 70%,[26] but peaks around age 40 and as menopause approaches its prevalence declines. Pure MM attacks may occur before, during, or after menstruation (day −2 through day +3) and must occur in at least 2 out of 3 cycles with no migraine at any other time of the month.[20] It is estimated that only 7% to 35% of women experience pure MM and MRM is seen in 60% of women. MM attacks are often more severe, of longer duration, and less responsive to both acute and prophylactic treatment than nonmenstrual migraines. It is important to note that premenstrual headache is different because it typically resolves with the onset of menstruation. The diagnosis can be further verified by keeping a calendar or electronic diary.

The luteal phase with its abrupt decreases in estrogen and progesterone is believed to trigger migraine. This decrease in endogenous and exogenous estrogen concentrations precipitates MRM potentially by lowering the threshold for trigeminal activation.[27] The decrease in estrogen may also make blood vessels more permeable to proinflammatory mediators such as prostaglandins, which are increased by 3-fold in the luteal phase. As estrogen decreases, production of serotonin is reduced and elimination is accelerated. Furthermore, 5-hydroxytryptamine 1 receptors, which are the targets of triptans, decrease with low estrogen, which may explain why MM attacks are more resistant to acute therapy. As a result, the mainstay for MM treatment is preventive therapy to minimize or eliminate the premenstrual decrease in estrogen or to preemptively treat the attack. Effective measures include hormonal therapy such as estrogen implants, gonadotropin-releasing hormone agonists to suppress ovarian steroid production maintaining physiologic levels of estradiol by adding back estrogen,[28,29] or applying percutaneous estradiol gel for 1 week perimenstrually to minimize the magnitude of the decrease in estrogen.[30] Preventive regimens limiting the decrease in estrogen may be used. The low-dose oral contraceptive pills (containing 20 μg ethinylestradiol [EE] or less) can be given continuously for 12 weeks, followed by 7 days of 10 μg EE or alternatively, a 20-μg pill can be taken at bedtime on days 1 to 24 followed by 1.25 mg of conjugated equine estrogen at bedtime on days 25 to 27.[27] Another option is a commercially available pill pack that contains 21 days of 20 μg EE followed by 2 days of placebo and then 5 days of 10 μg EE. This pill can be used with the final week taken in reverse order to avoid the precipitous 20-μg EE decrease and instead provides two 10-μg EE doses (between days 21 and 22 and again between days 26 and 27).[27]

Several studies were done evaluating triptans for acute treatment of MM with some good evidence for sumatriptan and combination sumatriptan-naproxen (85–500 mg), zolmitriptan, rizatriptan, frovatriptan, or almotriptan with 1 to 4 hours of pain relief and a responder rate ranging from 30% to 81%.[31]

Guidelines on pharmacologic preventive therapy recommended several medications, which showed good evidence for MM prevention including frovatriptan (level A), naratriptan, and zolmitriptan (level B).[32] These medications are given 1 to 2 days before the onset of headaches for 3 to 5 days. Patients must monitor triptan use and limit it to less than 10 days a month to avoid medication overuse.[20] Several nonsteroidal anti-inflammatory drugs also have evidence in prevention including naproxen sodium 550 mg taken twice daily for 5 to 7 days (day −7 to day +6 was) significantly effective in decreasing headache frequency compared with placebo.[33] Neuromodulation therapy including noninvasive vagus nerve stimulation given at 2-minute stimulations to the cervical branch of the vagus nerve 3 times daily (performed from −3 days before estimated onset of menstruation through +3 days after the end of menstruation) was found to be effective treatment without safety or tolerability concerns.[34]

MIGRAINE, STROKE, AND HORMONAL TREATMENT

Peak estrogen levels are higher in women with migraine with aura compared with those without aura. It has also been noted that new onset of migraine aura or worsening of migraine with aura may occur with the initiation of oral contraceptive or hormone replacement therapy (HRT) as well as with pregnancy.[17,35]

The question of birth control will arise whether in the adolescent girl or in the young through older-aged premenopausal woman. The oral contraceptive pill might improve, worsen, or have no impact on migraine. Typically, the worsening occurs during the placebo week. Approximately 70% of combined hormonal contraceptive users experience headache on placebo days, with peak incidence on the third day of the placebo pill.[36] Oral contraceptive pills are considered safe in women with migraine without aura, migraine with simple aura, and in those women who are nonsmokers and have no cardiovascular risk factors.

Fluctuations in estrogen levels may impact migraine and thus contraceptive vaginal inserts, patches, and implants may decrease fluctuations and improve migraine. If prescribing an oral contraceptive, it is optimal to find a pill that is low dose and monophasic. The European Headache Federation and European Society of Contraception and Reproductive Health systematically reviewed the evidence of hormonal contraceptives and the risk of ischemic stroke in women with migraine. The group considered combined oral contraceptive pills (COC) containing more than 35 μg of EE as high-risk products for ischemic stroke; COCs containing 35 μg EE or less, combined patch, combined vaginal ring as medium risk; and progesterone-only contraceptives including the oral pill, subdermal implant, depot injection, and levonorgestrel-releasing intrauterine system as no risk products.[37]

For migraine with aura, the oral contraceptive pill, transdermal patch, and vaginal ring were cautioned against, preferring nonhormonal options such as condoms, the progestin-only pill, and the intrauterine device. A recent meta-analysis showed that a progesterone-only pill containing desogestrel 75 μg/d decreased the number of migraine attacks and number of days with migraine per month and decreased the intensity and duration of attacks, and analgesic and triptan use.[38] For migraine without aura, hormonal contraceptive methods can be considered provided there are no additional vascular risk factors. If aura develops, switching to a nonhormonal method is recommended.

It is believed that there is a 2- to 3-fold increased risk of ischemic stroke in women with migraine with aura who also take the COC.[37] Although multiple organizations including the World Health Organization, Centers for Disease Control and Prevention, European Headache Federation, and American College of Obstetricians and Gynecologists recommend that women with migraine with aura completely avoid combination contraceptive use because of an increased risk of stroke, the evidence supporting this recommendation remains controversial with mixed evidence and multiple confounding factors.[35,39] There is minimal direct evidence supporting the combined effects of migraine and hormonal contraceptives as they relate to an increased stroke risk, aside from a known theoretic concern based on the independent effects of migraine and estrogen on the cerebral vasculature.

A systematic review found that migraine with aura is associated with 2-fold increase risk of ischemic stroke in 9 population studies but not among patients with migraine without aura. The risk was further increased in women less than 45 years of age, smokers, and those on oral contraceptives.[40] A more recent review on the effects of migraine and hormonal contraceptive use on risk of stroke risk among females age 15 to 49 years showed a cumulative incidence of 11 strokes in 100,000 females. The combined effect of COC and migraine with aura was associated with a 6-fold increased risk of ischemic stroke, but the use of COC did not substantially further increase risk of stroke among female migraineurs without aura. It is therefore crucial to determine the type of migraine in the assessment of COC use among women with migraine.[41]

A meta-analysis that combined results from 4 studies showed that among oral contraceptive users, the odds ratio of stroke was 3.2 (95% confidence interval, 1.5–7.2) among women with migraine and 2.3 (95% confidence interval, 0.7–7.2) among women without migraine, both compared with nonusers without migraine.[42]

In these multiple studies, there is mixed evidence with multiple confounding factors, including the use of high estrogen containing pills, aura frequency, age, definitive confirmation of stroke diagnosis, and other stroke risk factors.[35] The use of COC in this population remains a complex issue and controversial, resulting in differences in clinical practice among experts in headache medicine. The results should be interpreted with caution, given that migraine may have been underestimated and oral contraceptive type may have included progesterone-only pills and the common comorbidities that are associated with stroke, such as hypertension and smoking, may not have been clearly determined.

Several hypotheses support the relationship between migraine with aura and ischemic stroke. The migraine may lead directly to stroke owing to cortical spreading depression related to the aura (migrainous infarction). Individuals with auras may have vascular risk factors, such as smoking and hypertension, which place them at higher risk of stroke.[42] Those individuals who suffer from migraine with aura are believed to have a high prevalence of other vasculopathies that include antiphospholipid syndrome and systemic lupus erythematosus. Migraine with aura has also been linked to patent foramen ovale, which can result in paradoxic microembolization. Evidence has demonstrated an increased risk of ischemic stroke among women who use COCs. The risk is greatest among women using high-dose COCs ($\geq$50 µg EE); however, the risk may still be increased among women using lower dose COCs. The increased risk of stroke in those who use oral contraceptive pills seems to be due to the estrogen component; however, some women find that migraine can often improve when using combine oral contraceptive medications and aura might possibly improve with stabilization of estrogen levels with low-dose COC.[39]

The longitudinal Women's Health Study analyzed data of women over age 45 years and found that migraine with aura conferred an increased risk of stroke that varied directly with aura frequency. Less frequent aura (less than once a month) showed a 2-fold increased risk of stroke compared with women without migraine, but the risk increased to more than 4-fold when aura frequency exceeded once a week.[43]

Although the risk of stroke may be increased among women with migraine who use COCs, the risk should be considered in the context of overall absolute risk among the population. The absolute risk of stroke among women of reproductive age is low, with an incidence of 4.3 to 8.9 per 100,000 per year. This risk increases with age, as well as the presence of cardiovascular risk factors such as smoking, hypertension, and diabetes. The attributable risk of stroke at the population level related to risk factors of migraine headaches or COC use is likely to be low overall.

MIGRAINE IN PREGNANCY AND THE PUERPERIUM

It is well-established that migraine typically occurs in women during their childbearing years. What poses a significant challenge in women with migraine during the childbearing years is the safe treatment of migraine before and after conception, because up to 50% of pregnancies are unplanned and it is up to care providers to take this into account in female migraineurs and consider choosing medications with a lesser risk of teratogenicity.[44]

In the evaluation of female migraineurs during pregnancy and within 6 weeks postpartum (puerperium), it is crucial to monitor for red flags to rule out secondary headache disorders that may present during pregnancy and the puerperium, including aneurysmal subarachnoid hemorrhage, acute stroke, cerebral venous thrombosis, cervical artery dissection, reversible cerebral vasoconstriction syndrome, a congenital or space-occupying lesion such as a pituitary tumor, preeclampsia, eclampsia, and posterior reversible encephalopathy syndrome, as well as high or low intracranial pressure.[45]

Migraine during pregnancy can be significantly impacted by hormonal changes, stress, disrupted sleep, nausea, and dehydration. A transient worsening may occur during the first trimester, but retrospective studies have shown a 60% to 70% improvement in headache symptoms, often by the second and third trimesters.[45] In patients with migraine with aura, hormonal effects related to pregnancy may increase attacks.

Studies suggest that severe maternal migraines may increase the occurrence of adverse delivery outcomes[46,47] with 1 retrospective study finding that pregnant migraineurs seeking acute migraine treatment had increased rates of preeclampsia, preterm birth, and low birthweight, but decreased cesarean delivery rates.[48] However, the management of headaches in pregnancy is both a therapeutic and diagnostic challenge. As noted, clinicians must first rule out any underlying pathology, then nonpharmacologic, safe, evidence-based therapies including relaxation strategies, biofeedback, and cognitive-behavioral therapy should be the emphasized modalities.[45] For more severe, intractable migraine accompanied by nausea/vomiting and dehydration, medical therapy may be indicated. Although the FDA has phased out the pregnancy risk letter category system for medications and has replaced it with the new pregnancy and lactation labeling rule, the letter system remains a useful hierarchical scheme in the determination of drug safety in pregnant women.

In the first trimester, small doses of caffeine, acetaminophen, and metoclopramide are generally considered safe, but even these agents carry potential risks including the later development of attention deficit hyperactivity disorder in children with antepartum acetaminophen exposure and maternal cardiac conduction changes and extrapyramidal symptoms with metoclopramide exposure.[45] Several nonsteroidal anti-inflammatory drugs are category B in pregnancy and include diclofenac, ibuprofen, ketoprofen, naproxen, and indomethacin; however, these are all category D in the third trimester. Some narcotics, including meperidine and morphine, are category B, except in the third trimester; however, their use is cautioned. Codeine can be used in pregnancy, but has been associated with cardiac, respiratory, and cleft defects. For severe attacks, intravenous fluids and an intravenous antiemetic are often indicated. After the first trimester, antiemetics such as dimenhydrinate and diphenhydramine are classified as category B. In suppository form, prochlorperazine, metoclopramide, and promethazine are generally considered safe. In women who are in status migrainosus and require steroids, prednisone is often preferred to dexamethasone, because the latter crosses the placenta more easily.

In general, triptans (FDA category C), ergots, and aspirin should be avoided; however, under careful consideration and monitoring, these agents may be indicated in specific scenarios. Pregnancy registries have been established to monitor pregnant women who have taken triptans and there remains poor evidence on their specific impact on fetal well-being. Previous studies show that there is no increase in major congenital malformations related to the use of triptans in pregnancy; however, further detailed research was recommended to determine whether there could be a possible link to spontaneous abortions in the triptan-exposed group.[49,50]

Because migraine often improves in pregnancy, prophylactic medication may be unnecessary. When migraine is frequent and disabling, preventative therapy may be required but should be undertaken with the full consent of both the patient and her partner, because no single preventative medication is free of any potential teratogenic effects. Recently, magnesium has come into questions, although further investigation is necessary, because an association between prolonged maternal intravenous magnesium sulfate exposure and low calcium with fetal bone abnormalities (osteopenia and fractures) as well as neonatal hypotonia were reported.[45,51] Medications that may be safe based on limited human and animal studies include pindolol, memantine, and cyproheptadine; for example; however, the data for their use in migraine are limited. Beta-blockers are generally thought to be safe, but may be associated with intrauterine growth restriction.[45]

Interventional therapies including peripheral nerve blocks, trigger point injections and sphenopalatine ganglion blocks using lidocaine (category B) are generally regarded as safe. Potentially, newly approved neuromodulation devices could also provide benefit. These devices include the transcutaneous supraorbital nerve stimulator, a single pulse transcranial magnetic stimulation device, as well as a noninvasive vagus nerve stimulator. Onabotulinum toxin use in pregnancy, at low doses for cosmetic purposes, found fetal loss in 20.9% and major birth defect rate of 2.7%.[52] These authors do not recommend its use in a pregnant migraineur as the PREEMPT doses are much higher.

MIGRAINE DURING LACTATION

Migraine often returns in the postpartum period, presumably related to the rapid decrease in estrogen levels after delivery. Although breastfeeding women have a lower recurrence rate than women who bottle feed, more than one-half of breastfeeding women experience migraine recurrence within 1 month of delivery.[53] Therefore, migraine treatment during lactation may be required, with factors such as drug half-life, protein binding (a highly protein-bound agent will be impeded from entering the milk), and drug bioavailability being important considerations.[54] Acetaminophen, low-dose aspirin (<162 mg/d), ibuprofen, caffeine, metoclopramide, ondansetron, prednisone, lidocaine, bupivacaine, and triptans such as sumatriptan and eletriptan are felt to be relatively safely for acute treatment during breastfeeding.[45]

When prophylactic treatment is required, the patient must be included in the decision-making process as to the benefit and risks of continuing to breast feed while taking a daily medication. Propranolol, timolol, amitriptyline, nortriptyline, verapamil, onabotulinum toxin A, magnesium, riboflavin, escitalopram, paroxetine, and sertraline have been reported to have the best evidence for use by lactating mothers.[45,54]

MIGRAINE IN PERIMENOPAUSE AND MENOPAUSE

Migraine tends to improve with age, specifically in those women who have MRM. Population studies show that on average, women enter into perimenopause in their mid-40s and reach menopause around the age of 50, with most women completing menopause by their mid-50s. Perimenopause marks a period of increased prevalence of migraine in women complicated by other vasomotor symptoms (night sweats, hot flashes) as well as other symptoms including a drop in libido, forgetfulness, difficulty concentrating, fatigue, insomnia and irritability.[44,55]

HRT remains a treatment option for the symptoms of perimenopause; however, few studies have assessed the effect of HRT on migraine and the results are inconsistent.[55] Depending on the duration, type and dose of estrogen, and route of administration, a women's migraine can be exacerbated or alleviated. For those women with migraine who require HRT, a dose reduction, noncycling estrogen, switching from conjugated estrogens to pure estradiol or from synthetic to bioidentical estrogen may be necessary.[56,57] If adjustments in the estrogenic component of the HRT are unsatisfactory and migraine continues to be poorly controlled, the decision should be made as to whether to cease HRT completely versus adjustment of the progesterone component, or adding in agents that may help with the vasomotor symptoms of perimenopause, such as venlafaxine, sertraline, paroxetine, fluoxetine, escitalopram, pregabalin, or gabapentin.[55,58,59]

Once menopause is complete, many women experience a reprieve from their migraines; however, because other factors are still at play such environmental triggers or personal triggers such as poor sleep or stress, migraines may continue but perhaps at a lesser frequency. Some women also experience late life migraine accompaniments, which must of course be differentiated from transient ischemic attacks.

SUMMARY

Migraine is typically a lifelong disorder in women, with fluctuations in their hormonal state leading to worsening or improvement in their migraines. An understanding of these fluctuations and developing an approach to management unique to a woman's particular hormonal status are key to successful management of her migraines throughout her lifetime.

REFERENCES

1. Buse DC, Loder EW, Gorman JA, et al. Sex differences in the prevalence, symptoms, and associated features of migraine, probable migraine and other severe headache: results of the American Migraine Prevalence and Prevention (AMPP) Study. Headache 2013;53(8):1278–99.
2. Delaruelle Z, Ivanova TA, Kahn S, et al. Male and female sex hormones in primary headaches. J Headache Pain 2018;19:117.
3. Maleki N, Kurth T, Field AE. Age at menarche and risk of developing migraine or non-migraine headaches by young adulthood: a prospective cohort study. Cephalalgia 2017;37:1257–63.
4. Lipton RB, Bigal ME, Diamond M, et al. Migraine prevalence, disease burden, and the need for preventive therapy. Neurology 2007;68(5):343–9.
5. Victor T, Hu X, Campbell J, et al. Migraine prevalence by age and sex in the United States: a life-span study. Cephalalgia 2010;30:1065–72.
6. Pavloic JM, Akcali D, Bolay H, et al. Sex-related influences in migraine. J Neurosci Res 2017;95:587.
7. Pinkerman B, Holroyd K. Menstrual and non-menstrual migraines differ in women with menstrually-related migraine. Cephalalgia 2010;30:1187–94.
8. Schroeder RA, Brandes J, Buse D, et al. Sex and gender differences in migraine-evaluating knowledge gaps. J Womens Health 2018;27(8):965–73.
9. Horev A, Wirguin I, Lantsberg L, et al. A high incidence of migraine with aura among morbidly obese women. Headache 2005;45:936–8.
10. Eikermann-Haerter K, Dileköz E, Kudo C, et al. Genetic and hormonal factors modulate spreading depression and transient hemiparesis in mouse models of familial hemiplegic migraine type 1. J Clin Invest 2009;119:99.
11. Eikermann-Haerter K, Baum MJ, Ferrari MD, et al. Androgenic suppression of spreading depression in familial hemiplegic migraine type 1 mutant mice. Ann Neurol 2009;66:564–8.
12. Peres MF, Sanchez Del Rio M, Seabra ML, et al. Hypothalamic involvement in migraine. J Neurol Neurosurg Psychiatry 2001;71:747–51.
13. Ferrini RL, Barrett-Connor E. Sex hormones and age: a cross-sectional study of testosterone and estradiol and their bioavailable fractions in community-dwelling men. Am J Epidemiol 1998;147(8):750–4.
14. Maleki N, Linnman C, Brawn J, et al. Her versus his migraine: multiple sex differences in brain function and structure. Brain 2012;135:2546–59.
15. Martin VT, Behbehani M. Ovarian hormones and migraine headache: understanding mechanisms and pathogenesis -Part I. Headache 2006;46(1):3–23.
16. Martin VT, Behbehani M. Ovarian hormones and migraine headache: understanding mechanisms and pathogenesis-Part 2. Headache 2006;46(1):365–86.
17. Vetvik KG, MacGregor EA. Sex differences in the epidemiology, clinical features, and pathophysiology of migraine. Lancet Neurol 2017;16(1):76–87.

18. Lipton RB, Stewart WF, Diamond S, et al. Prevalence and burden of migraine in the United States: data from the American Migraine Study II. Headache 2001; 41(7):646–57.

19. Gelfand A. Pediatric and adolescent headache. Continuum 2018;24(4, Headache): 1108–36.

20. Headache Classification Committee of the International Headache Society. The international classification of headache disorders 3rd edition. Cephalalgia 2018; 38(1):1–211.

21. Borsook D, Erpelding N, Lebel A, et al. Sex and the migraine brain. Neurobiol Dis 2014;68:200–14.

22. Hershey A, Horn P, Kabbouche M, et al. Genomic expression patterns in menstrual-related migraine in adolescents. Headache 2012;52:68–79.

23. Faber A, Lagman-Bartolome AM, Rajapakse T. Drugs for the acute treatment of migraine in children and adolescents. Paediatr Child Health 2017;22(8):454–8.

24. Lagman-Bartolome AM, Lawler V, Lay C. Headache education active-waiting directive: a program to enhance well-being during long referral wait times. Headache 2018;58:109–17.

25. Richer L, Billing Hurst L, Linsdell MA, et al. Drugs for the acute treatment of migraine in children and adolescents. Cochrane Database Syst Rev 2016;(4):CD005220.

26. Petrovski BE, Vetvik KG, Lundqvist C, et al. Characteristics of menstrual versus non-menstrual migraine during pregnancy: a longitudinal population-based study. J Headache Pain 2018;19:27–33.

27. Calhoun AH. Understanding menstrual migraine. Headache 2018;58(4):626–30.

28. Magos AI, Zilkha KJ, Studd JW. Treatment of menstrual migraine by oestradiol implants. J Neurol Neurosurg Psychiatry 1983;46:1044–6.

29. Murray SC, Muse KN. Effective treatment of severe menstrual migraine headaches with gonadotropin-releasing hormone agonist and "add-back" therapy. Fertil Steril 1997;67:390–3.

30. De Lignieres B, Vincens M, Mauvais-Jarvis P, et al. Prevention of menstrual migraine by percutaneous oestradiol. Br Med J (Clin Res Ed) 1986;293:1540.

31. Allais G, Castagnoli Gabellari I, Mana O, et al. Treatment strategies for menstrually related migraine. Womens Health (Lond) 2012;8(5):529–41.

32. Silberstein SD, Holland F, Freitag F, et al. Evidence-based guideline update: pharmacologic treatment for episodic migraine in adults: reports of the Quality Standards Subcommittee of the American Academy of Neurology and the American Headache Society. Neurology 2012;78:1337–45.

33. Sances G, Martignoni E, Fioroni L, et al. Naproxen sodium in menstrual migraine prophylaxis. Headache 1990;30(11):705–9.

34. Grazzi L, Egeo G, Calhoun AH, et al. Non-invasive vagus nerve stimulation (nan's) as mini-prophylaxis for menstrual/menstrually related migraine: an open-label study. J Headache Pain 2016;17:91–101.

35. Charles A. The migraine aura. Continuum 2018;24(4, Headache):1009–22.

36. Sulak PJ, Scow RD, Preece C, et al. Hormone withdrawal symptoms in oral contraceptive users. Obstet Gynecol 2000;95:261–6.

37. Sacco S, Merki-Feld GS, Aegidus KL, et al. Hormonal contraceptives and risk of ischemic stroke in women with migraine: a consensus statement from the European Headache Federation (EHF) and the European Society of Contraception and Reproductive Health (ESC). J Headache Pain 2017;18:108–28.

38. Warhurst S, Rofe CJ, Brew BJ, et al. Effectiveness of the progestin-only pill for migraine treatment in women: a systematic review and meta-analysis. Cephalalgia 2018;38(4):754–64.
39. Calhoun A. Hormonal contraceptives and migraine with aura-Is there still a risk? Headache 2017;57:184–93.
40. Schurks M, Rist PM, Bigal ME, et al. Migraine and cardiovascular disease: systematic review and meta-analysis. BMJ 2009;339:b3914.
41. Champaloux SW, Tepper NK, Monsour M, et al. Use of combined hormonal contraceptives among women with migraines and risk of ischemic stroke. Am J Obstet Gynecol 2017;216:489e1–7.
42. Tepper NK, Whiteman MK, Zapata LB, et al. Safety of hormonal contraceptives among women with migraine: a systematic review. Contraception 2016;94(6): 630–40.
43. Kurth T, Slomke MA, Kase CS, et al. Migraine, headache, and the risk of stroke in women: a prospective study. Neurology 2005;64:1020–6.
44. Todd C, Lagman-Bartolome AM, Lay C. Women and migraine: role of hormones. Curr Neurol Neurosci Rep 2018;18:42–8.
45. Robbins M. Headache in pregnancy. Continuum 2018;24(4, Headache): 1092–107.
46. Bánhidy F, Acs N, Horvath-Puho E, et al. Pregnancy complications and delivery outcomes in pregnant women with severe migraine. Eur J Obstet Gynecol Reprod Biol 2007;134(2):157–63.
47. Pakalnis A. Migraine and hormones. Semin Pediatr Neurol 2016;23(1):92–4.
48. Grossman TB, Robbins MS, Govindappagari S, et al. Delivery outcomes of patients with acute migraine in pregnancy: a retrospective study. Headache 2017;57:605–11.
49. Ephross SA, Sinclair SM. Final results from the 16-year sumatriptan, naratriptan, and treximent pregnancy registry. Headache 2014;54(7):1158–72.
50. Marchenko A, Etwel F, Olutunfese O, et al. Pregnancy outcome following prenatal exposure to triptan medications: a meta-analysis. Headache 2015;55:490–501.
51. Wells RE, Turner DP, Lee M, et al. Managing migraine during pregnancy and lactation. Curr Neurol Neurosci Rep 2016;14:40–64.
52. Brin MF, Kirby RS, Slavotinek A, et al. Pregnancy outcomes following exposure to onabotulinum toxin A. Pharmacoepidemiol Drug Saf 2016;25(2):179–87.
53. Hoshiyama E, Tatsumoto M, Iwanami H. Postpartum migraines: a long-term prospective study. Intern Med 2012;51(22):3119–23.
54. Riccardo Davanzo JB. Breastfeeding and migraine drugs. Eur J Clin Pharmacol 2014;70:1313–24.
55. MacGregor EA. Migraine, menopause and hormone replacement therapy. Post Reprod Health 2018;24(1):11–8.
56. Lay CL, Broner SW. Adolescent issues in migraine: a focus on menstrual migraine. Curr Pain Headache Rep 2008;12(5):384–7.
57. Martin V, Pavlovic J, Fanning K, et al. Perimenopause and menopause are associated with high frequency headache in women with migraine: results of the American Migraine Prevalence and Prevention Study. Headache 2016;56: 292–305.
58. Shams T, Friwana B, Habib F, et al. SSRIs for hot flashes: a systematic review and meta-analysis of randomized controlled trials. J Gen Intern Med 2013;29(1): 204–13.
59. Santoro N, Epperson CN, Matthews S. Menopausal symptoms and their management. Endocrinol Metab Clin North Am 2015;44(3):497–515.

Trigeminal Autonomic Cephalalgias

Mark J. Burish, MD, PhD[a],*, Todd D. Rozen, MD[b]

KEYWORDS

- Trigeminal autonomic cephalalgia • Cluster headache • Paroxysmal hemicrania
- SUNCT • SUNA • Hemicrania continua

KEY POINTS

- The trigeminal autonomic cephalalgias (TACs) are a group of primary headaches similar in symptoms but different in duration, frequency, and treatment.
- The hypothalamus, trigeminocervical complex, autonomic system, and the vagus nerve all have roles in the pathophysiology of the TACs.
- All patients with paroxysmal hemicrania and hemicrania continua have a dramatic response to indomethacin. In patients suspected of these disorders, a trial of indomethacin up to 75 mg three times daily for up to 2 weeks, with the use of a gastroprotective agent, should be considered.

INTRODUCTION

The trigeminal autonomic cephalalgias (TACs) are a group of 5 primary headache disorders that share features of unilateral pain and ipsilateral cranial autonomic features but differ in frequency, duration, and most importantly treatment (**Table 1**). The new International Classification of Headache Disorders 3 (ICHD3)[1] has brought several changes to the TACs:

1. Hemicrania continua is now classified as a TAC, where it was classified as "other primary headaches" in the ICHD2.[2]
2. The definitions of chronic TACs (not including hemicrania continua) are now remission periods lasting less than 3 months, instead of less than 1 month in the ICHD3-beta.[3]

Disclosure Statement: M.J. Burish has previously received grant funding from the American Headache Society and National Headache Foundation. T.D. Rozen has no disclosures.
[a] Department of Neurosurgery, University of Texas Health Science Center at Houston, Will Erwin Headache Research Center, 6400 Fannin Street, Suite 2010, Houston, TX 77030, USA; [b] Department of Neurology, Mayo Clinic Florida, 4500 San Pablo Road, Jacksonville, FL 32224, USA
* Corresponding author.
E-mail address: Mark.j.burish@uth.tmc.edu

Neurol Clin 37 (2019) 847–869
https://doi.org/10.1016/j.ncl.2019.07.001
0733-8619/19/© 2019 Elsevier Inc. All rights reserved.

neurologic.theclinics.com

Table 1
Features of the trigeminal autonomic cephalalgias

	Cluster Headache	Paroxysmal Hemicrania	SUNCT/SUNA	Hemicrania Continua
ICHD3 criteria				
Severity	Severe or very severe	Severe	Moderate–severe	Baseline any severity, flares moderate-severe
Duration	15–180 min	2–30 min	1–600 s	>3 mo
Frequency	1–8 per d[a]	>5 per d	At least 1 per d	Constant >3 mo with flares
Autonomic features	+	+	+	+
Restlessness or agitation	+	+		+
Indomethacin response		100%		100%
Epidemiology				
Ratio of male to female	3:1	Slightly more women	1.5:1	1:2
Ratio of episodic to chronic	90:10	35:65	10:90	15:85
Associated factors				
Circadian pattern	82%	Rare	Rare	Rare
Triggers				
Alcohol	+	+	–	+
Nitroglycerin	+	+	–	Rare
Neck movements	–	+	+	–
Cutaneous	–	–	+	–
Response to treatment				
Oxygen	70%	–	–	–
Sumatriptan 6 mg subcutaneous	90%	20%	Rare	–

Autonomic features include conjunctival injection, lacrimation, nasal congestion, rhinorrhea, eyelid edema, forehead and facial sweating, miosis, and ptosis.

Abbreviations: ICHD3, International Classification of Headache Disorders 3; SUNA, short-lasting unilateral neuralgiform headache attacks with cranial autonomic symptoms; SUNCT, short-lasting unilateral neuralgiform headache attacks with conjunctival injection and tearing.

[a] Frequency of cluster headache is between 1 every other day and 8 per day.

3. The list of cranial autonomic features have gone through several variations, and the ICHD3 has removed ipsilateral flushing and ipsilateral fullness of the ear.

PATHOPHYSIOLOGY OF THE TRIGEMINAL AUTONOMIC CEPHALALGIAS

The TACs are thought to involve at least 3 brain systems: the trigeminovascular system, the autonomic system, and the hypothalamus (**Fig. 1**). There is emerging evidence that the vagus nerve may also be important. Most research has focused on cluster headache but there is preliminary data for the other TACs as well.

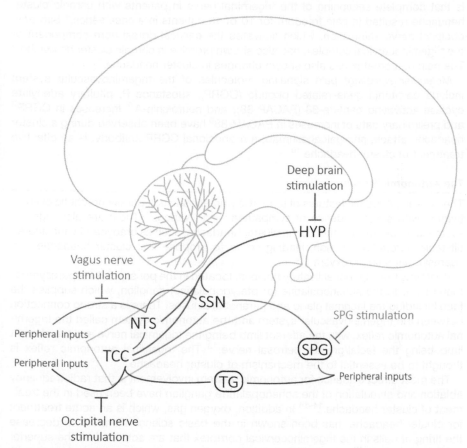

Fig. 1. Pathophysiology of TACs, with most of the data obtained from cluster headache. Several brain systems seem to be important in cluster headache, and neuromodulation of each of these systems can prevent cluster headache as shown. The system responsible for pain is the trigeminal system (*red*) including the trigeminocervical complex (TCC) and trigeminal ganglion (TG). The cranial autonomic system (*green*) includes the superior salivatory nucleus (SSN) and sphenopalatine ganglion (SPG) and connects to the trigeminal system via the trigeminal autonomic reflex. The hypothalamus (HYP, *blue*) connects to be the autonomic and trigeminal systems. Recently the vagus nerve and nucleus tractus solitarius (NTS, *orange*) have been shown in neuromodulation studies to be involved in pain regulation, with connections to the trigeminal system, autonomic system, and the hypothalamus.

The Trigeminovascular System

The trigeminovascular system is a facial pain system.

Anatomy: the ophthalmic branch of the trigeminal nerve receives inputs from the forehead, eye, dura, and large cranial vessels. The trigeminal nerve then connects to the trigeminocervical complex, specifically the most inferior portion of the trigeminal nucleus (the trigeminal nucleus caudalis) and the dorsal horns of the upper cervical spine. From here the system becomes more distributed, but includes connections to the pain neuromatrix, a collection of cortical and subcortical areas involved in pain processing.

Perhaps the most direct evidence for involvement of the trigeminovascular system is that complete sectioning of the trigeminal nerve in patients with chronic cluster headache resulted in pain freedom for 10 of 13 patients in a case series.[4] Similarly, occipital nerve stimulation, which activates the cervical dorsal horn component of the trigeminocervical complex, has also shown promise in chronic cluster headache.[5] The pain neuromatrix has also shown changes in cluster headache.[6]

Molecular signaling: pain signaling molecules of the trigeminovascular system include calcitonin gene–related peptide (CGRP), substance P, pituitary adenylate cyclase-activating peptide-38 (PACAP-38), and neurokinin-A.[7] Increases in CGRP[8] and preliminary data of increases in PACAP-38[9] have been observed during a cluster headache attack, and galcanezumab, a monoclonal CGRP antibody, is an effective treatment of cluster headache.[10]

The Autonomic System

The cranial autonomic features of the TACs primarily include parasympathetic overactivation with some evidence of sympathetic inactivation.[11] There are also signs of systemic autonomic dysfunction in cluster headache, such as bradycardia and altered tilt-table baroreflex function, leading some to propose that cluster headache is a "parasympathetic paroxysm".[12]

Anatomy: the superior salivatory nucleus, located in the pons, provides parasympathetic input to the sphenopalatine (or pterygopalatine) ganglion, which supplies the face including the lacrimal gland and paranasal sinuses. There is a strong connection between the trigeminovascular system and the autonomic system called the trigeminal autonomic reflex, with the afferent limb being the trigeminal nerve and the efferent limb being the facial/greater petrosal nerve.[13] The trigeminal autonomic reflex is thought to be essential to the mechanism of cluster headache.[6]

The most direct evidence for autonomic system involvement is that radiofrequency ablation and stimulation of the sphenopalatine ganglion have been used in the treatment of cluster headache.[14–16] In addition, oxygen gas, which is an acute treatment for cluster headache, has been shown in the basic science literature to decrease the firing of cells in the trigeminocervical complex that are activated by the superior salivatory nucleus.[17]

Molecular signaling: signaling molecules of the autonomic system include vasoactive intestinal peptide (VIP) and PACAP-38. Increases in VIP have been observed during a cluster headache attack.[8]

The Hypothalamus

The hypothalamus is a collection of multiple nuclei that assist in many regulatory behaviors, including endocrine, metabolic, and limbic functions. In cluster headache, researchers have hypothesized that the abnormalities start in the hypothalamus and are then followed by trigeminal and autonomic involvement.[18]

Anatomy: the strongest evidence for hypothalamic involvement comes from functional imaging studies showing activation of the posterior hypothalamus in all TACs during an attack (**Fig. 2**).

Many other areas of the hypothalamus may also be involved. The hypothalamus connects to the autonomic system through the paraventricular nucleus[19] and connects to the trigeminovascular system by an unclear mechanism—orexin, produced by the lateral hypothalamus, modulates neurons in the trigeminal nucleus,[20] and posterior hypothalamic deep brain stimulation activates the trigeminal nucleus.[21] In addition, many cluster headache patients state a predictable daily rhythmicity to their headaches,[22] and the central biological clock is the suprachiasmatic nucleus in the anterior hypothalamus.

Molecular signaling: molecules under direct or indirect hypothalamic control include pituitary hormones, VIP, orexin, corticosteroids, and melatonin. There are data for altered pituitary hormones in cluster headache, including prolactin, growth hormone,

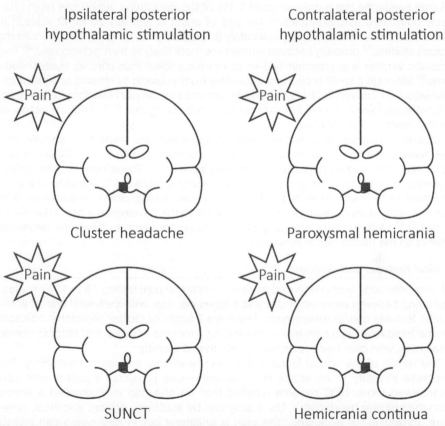

Ipsilateral posterior hypothalamic stimulation

Contralateral posterior hypothalamic stimulation

Cluster headache

Paroxysmal hemicrania

SUNCT

Hemicrania continua

Fig. 2. Functional imaging of the hypothalamus in the trigeminal autonomic cephalalgias. Schematics are shown of coronal sections through the posterior hypothalamus. Activation of the posterior hypothalamus is shown in red and is ipsilateral to the pain in cluster headache and SUNCT and contralateral to the pain in paroxysmal hemicrania and hemicrania continua. Other areas of activation are not shown and include several cortical and subcortical areas, many involved in the pain neuromatrix. Data are based on studies of cluster headache,[125] paroxysmal hemicrania,[126] SUNCT,[127] and hemicrania continua.[128]

thyroid stimulating hormone, and testosterone. VIP, also used by the autonomic system, increases during a cluster attack.[8] Corticosteroids and melatonin, the circadian biomarkers for daytime and nighttime respectively, are decreased in patients with cluster headache.[23–26]

The Vagus Nerve

Noninvasive stimulation of the vagus nerve has recently been shown as an effective treatment of cluster headache[27–29] and possibly for paroxysmal hemicrania and hemicrania continua.[30] Although the exact involvement of the vagus nerve in the TACs is not clear, vagus nerve stimulation can modulate pain in the trigeminal nucleus.[31] And the nucleus tractus solitarius, which receives vagal inputs, connects to both the hypothalamus and the superior salivatory nucleus.[32]

CLUSTER HEADACHE
Epidemiology

Cluster headache has a prevalence of 0.1% of the population, which has been relatively consistent across studies.[33] The age of onset is typically 20 to 40 years.[34] It has a male predominance of approximately 3:1, although this has not been consistent across studies,[33] possibly because women are more likely to be misdiagnosed.[35] The episodic version is approximately 6 times more common than chronic cluster headache[33] although a small proportion will evolve from episodic to chronic or vice versa. Predictors for conversion from episodic to chronic include pain freedom for less than 6 months per year and more frequent cluster headache cycles.[36] The natural history of cluster headache is not clear.

Cluster headache is associated with mood disorders, especially anxiety and depression, and has an alarmingly high rate of suicidal ideation.[22,37–39] Cluster headache may also have an increased risk of sleep apnea.[22,40] The strongest comorbidity, however, may be tobacco use, in particular cigarette smoking.[41] Tobacco use is so common (with many patients smoking before developing cluster headaches) that some investigators have proposed it contributes to the development of cluster headaches.[41,42] Unfortunately, stopping smoking does not seem to have any beneficial effects on the headaches in most patients.

Clinical Features and Diagnosis

Cluster headache is characterized as severe unilateral pain lasting 15 to 180 minutes, occurring between every other day and 8 times per day, with ipsilateral cranial autonomic features and/or restlessness. There are 2 forms of cluster headache: episodic cluster headache, with pain-free cycles lasting 3 months or more, and chronic cluster headache, with pain free cycles lasting less than 3 months.

The details of the clinical features of cluster headache are worth mentioning. The exquisite intensity of an attack is remarkable—one physician scientist who had interviewed more 1000 patients recalled that no one had ever recalled a worse pain than cluster headache.[13] The quality can be stabbing, drilling, electrical, pressure, throbbing, or exploding. The pain is unilateral but in rare cases can switch sides. In these authors' personal experiences, patients with episodic cluster headache who have side-switching often have an entire cycle on one side and the next cycle on the other side; the ipsilateral cranial autonomic features also switch sides. For cranial autonomic features, 70% of patients have lacrimation, conjunctival injection, nasal congestion, rhinnorhea, or ptosis.[43,44] And restlessness is seen in more than 90% of patients.[22]

Although the attacks can last 15 to 180 minutes up to 8 times a day, they usually occur for 45 to 90 minutes and 1 to 3 times per day. Some cluster headache patients will describe a mild interictal discomfort that can be confused for hemicrania continua. For episodic cluster headache, headache cycles usually last 6 to 12 weeks once per year, with no headaches the remainder of the year.[43] The headache cycles often have a "volcano" pattern, gradually becoming more frequent and intense in the middle of the cycle before gradually reducing again.[45]

In addition to the defined cluster headache criteria, there are several other features commonly seen in cluster headache. An attack begins fairly abruptly, with maximal intensity in less than 15 minutes; the attack also ends fairly abruptly. There are several triggers for the headaches, in particular alcohol and nitroglycerin. These triggers generally take effect quickly (less than 2 hours), and in episodic cluster headache they only trigger an attack during a headache cycle (ie, when patients are in the headache-free cycle they can drink alcohol without triggering a headache). Other triggers include increased body temperature (from heat or exercise), strong smells (in particular chemical solvents), nicotine, and possibly sleep.[22,46]

Another feature commonly seen in cluster headache is a daily and yearly rhythmicity to the headaches. As an example from the authors' personal experiences, one patient thought her cluster headaches were a reaction to one of her school classes: the attacks occurred every morning at 10 AM in autumn, coinciding with one specific class. The daily pattern is quite common: a survey of 1134 patients found that 82% of patients have headaches about the same time each day.[22] The most common time is 2 AM based on multiple studies[22,46,47]; these headaches can therefore be misdiagnosed as hypnic headaches. For a yearly pattern, the most common times for headache cycles in episodic cluster headache are spring and autumn.[22] It should be noted that there may also be a yearly pattern to chronic cluster headache, with some patients stating worsening intensity and frequency of the headaches at certain times of year.

The differential diagnosis of cluster headache includes several other types of headaches and facial pain. In a meta-analysis of 15 studies and more than 4000 patients, the most common misdiagnoses were migraine, trigeminal neuralgia, sinusitis, and dental disease.[48] Cluster headache attacks are associated with "migrainous features" (photophobia, phonophobia, nausea, facial allodynia, or aura) in many patients[22,49–53]; the photophobia, however, is often unilateral in cluster headache. Similarly, migraine can be associated with cranial autonomic features, especially lacrimation[50]; however, the cranial autonomic symptoms are often bilateral in migraine. Cluster headache is best differentiated from migraine based on the following:

1. Attack duration: 3 hours or less in cluster headache, 4 hours or more in migraine
2. Attack frequency: more than one per day for cluster headache, one per day for migraine
3. Activity during a headache: cluster headache patients are restless and pace or rock in place, migraine patients often lie still, as movement worsens the headaches
4. Yearly pattern: the episodic form of cluster headache has pain-free cycles lasting several months, whereas patients with migraine generally do not have long periods of remission unless they have the rare cyclic subtype

The differential diagnosis for cluster headache includes other primary headaches such as hemicrania continua and paroxysmal hemicrania; an indomethacin trial thus may be warranted in some patients. Trigeminal neuralgia is similar in pain intensity but shorter in duration, and hypnic headache has a similar onset that is commonly around 2 AM; neither of these disorders have cranial autonomic features. Several nonheadache diseases can also mimic cluster headache, including ocular diseases (acute angle glaucoma), vascular diseases (temporal arteritis), dental diseases (impacted molar), and maxillary sinusitis.[54,55]

Finally, several diseases cause a cluster headache phenotype that has been termed symptomatic cluster headache. Although rare, symptomatic cluster headache has been found with hypothalamic and pituitary tumors, meningiomas (from the cavernous sinus to the upper cervical spine), carotid artery dissections, postcarotid endarterectomy headaches, cavernous malformations and arteriovenous malformations, sinusitis, and obstructive sleep apnea among others.[56–58] Pituitary tumors may be the most common symptomatic lesion, and the headaches may improve with treatment of the underlying endocrine abnormality (with dopamine agonists or surgery). Although surgical treatment of the underlying diseases can lead to resolution of the headaches, it should be noted that many of the diseases listed earlier are commonly incidental and thus it is difficult to predict if treatment will have an effect on the headaches.

Work-up and Treatment

Given the broad differential diagnosis and the list of symptomatic cluster headaches, imaging is recommended for all patients with cluster headache. According to a European Headache Federation consensus, the first recommendation is a brain MRI with dedicated views of the cavernous sinus and pituitary.[59] Should patients not respond to typical preventives, an magnetic resonance angiography (MRA) head and neck could be considered. And in patients refractory to treatment, pituitary laboratory studies and a sleep study (for obstructive sleep apnea) could also be considered. In select patients, an erythrocyte sedimentation rate; indomethacin trial; and referral to ophthalmology, otolaryngology, or dentistry may be considered.

Treatment of cluster headache includes acute, bridge, and preventive treatments (**Table 2**).

Acute treatments

Patients generally do not find relief with acetaminophen, nonsteroidal antiinflammatories, or even opioids. Effective abortive treatments include the following:

Triptans: the recommended triptans are sumatriptan and zolmitriptan. Subcutaneous sumatriptan, in fact, may be the single most effective treatment of cluster headache.[60] Faster routes of delivery are favored: subcutaneous sumatriptan is the most effective, followed by intranasal zolmitriptan and sumatriptan, followed by the oral formulations (which are generally ineffective). However, triptans have several limitations. First, contraindications include cardiovascular and neurovascular disorders such as a history of myocardial infarction or stroke; caution is also recommended with other vascular disorders such as Raynaud's. Second, triptans are not intended to be taken multiple times per day for extended periods of time; thus despite their effectiveness, additional acute medications are often required.

High-flow oxygen: oxygen gas, via a nonrebreather mask at a rate of 6 to 7 L/min or higher, is effective in aborting a cluster attack. Higher rates of oxygen may be more effective, with a recent questionnaire reporting that oxygen at 10 L/min is just as effective as subcutaneous sumatriptan.[61] At doses higher than 10 L/min the oxygen cannister requires the addition of a piece of equipment called a regulator and in some patients this may be necessary: a failure of oxygen is generally only considered if the patient has failed oxygen gas at 15 to 25 L/min for at least 20 minutes. Oxygen can be used multiple times per day with minimal side effects; contraindications include oxygen toxicity in advanced pulmonary diseases such as advanced chronic obstructive pulmonary disease. Oxygen has 2 disadvantages, including portability

Table 2
Recommended treatments of cluster headache from the American Headache Society and the European Federation of Neurologic Societies

Acute	American Recommendation	European Recommendation
Oxygen gas (high-flow)	A	A
Sumatriptan subcutaneous	A	A
Sumatriptan nasal	B	A
Sumatriptan oral	–	–
Zolmitriptan nasal	A	A/B
Zolmitriptan oral	B	B
Octreotide subcutaneous	C	B
Lidocaine nasal	C	B
Noninvasive vagus nerve stimulation	–	–
Transitional		
Greater occipital nerve block	A	–
Oral steroids	U	A
Ergotamine	–	B
Preventive		
Verapamil	C	A
Lithium	C	B
Melatonin	C	C
Topiramate	–	B
Baclofen	–	C
Valproic acid	Unfavorable[a]	C
Noninvasive vagus nerve stimulation	–	–
Galcanezumab	–	–
Refractory		
Sphenopalatine ganglion stimulation	B	–
Occipital nerve stimulation	–	–
Hypothalamic deep brain stimulation	Unfavorable[a]	–

Level A: established effective; level B: probably effective; level C: possibly effective; level U: inadequate data; and "–": no recommendation.
[a] Valproic acid and hypothalamic deep brain stimulation received level B negative ratings (probably ineffective) from the American Headache Society. Monoclonal antibodies to CGRP are currently in trials for cluster headache.

(although smaller cannisters exist) and the fact that some patients find that it delays but does not abort the headaches.

Noninvasive vagus nerve stimulation: 3 studies have shown evidence for a Food and Drug Administration (FDA)–approved noninvasive vagus nerve stimulator in the acute treatment of episodic but not chronic cluster headache.[27–29] The device is more portable than oxygen and, as oxygen, can be used multiple times per day with minimal side effects. It has the advantage of being effective not only as an acute treatment but also possibly as a preventive for both episodic and chronic cluster headaches.[27] The device is not recommended for patients with metal in or near the neck (such as carotid stents or cervical fusion hardware), carotid atherosclerosis, or implanted medical devices (such as pacemakers or hearing aids).

Other acute medications: there is evidence for intranasal lidocaine, between 4% and 10%, sprayed ipsilateral to the pain, which has the advantage of few side effects but has not been found to be as effective as other options[55,60]; there is also evidence for subcutaneous octreotide, especially in patients who have failed other options.[62]

Refractory patients: an implantable sphenopalatine ganglion stimulator has shown evidence in aborting cluster headaches[16]; the device is approved in Europe. The small device is implanted into the sphenopalatine fossa, usually via an intraoral approach and powered wirelessly with a device held over the cheek. Adverse events with implantation were rare but included pain, swelling, and sensory disturbances.

Bridge therapies

Some treatments prevent attacks with quick onset but are generally not recommended for long-term prevention due to side effects or toxicity. Bridge medications are commonly used either (1) when preventive medications are being uptitrated or (2) as the sole preventive in patients with headache cycles that only last several weeks.

Suboccipital steroid injection: greater occipital nerve blocks ipsilateral to the pain, sometimes referred to as suboccipital steroid injections as occipital nerve anesthesia is not required, can reduce headache burden for days to weeks.[63] The dose and type of steroid are unclear; methylprednisolone, triamcinolone, and dexamethasone have been used.

Oral corticosteroids: oral steroid therapy may be the fastest of all the preventives, generally taking effect within 24 hours. Dosing and duration are highly variable, but proposed schedules in the literature include (1) prednisone 1 mg/kg up to 60 mg daily for 5 days, decreasing by 10 mg every 3 days,[18,62] and (2) dexamethasone 4 mg twice daily for 2 weeks then 4 mg daily for 1 week.[55] Generally, courses of approximately 3 weeks, with no more than 2 to 3 steroid cycles per year, are recommended with concern for avascular necrosis of the hip with prolonged steroids.[43] Side effects include insomnia, agitation, hyperglycemia in diabetics, and peptic ulcer disease; adrenal suppression may occur with chronic treatment.

Ergotamines: ergotamine tartrate 2 to 4 mg daily for up to 2 months has been used as a bridge treatment,[55] as has subcutaneous dihydroergotamine 1 mg at bedtime or 1 mg twice daily. The ergotamines have the same contraindications as the triptans, and extreme caution is advised in combining them with triptans.

Refractory patients: intranasal civamide (a synthetic isomer of capsaicin) was shown to be effective in preventing cluster headache over a 7-day period.[64] Civamide is not available in the United States, although some patients have found intranasal capsaicin to the ipsilateral nostril twice daily to be an effective bridge treatment.[55] Although data are limited, daily naratriptan or daily frovatriptan has been suggested as bridge treatments.[65,66] As the ergotamines discussed earlier, caution is advised in combining triptans with ergotamines or other triptans.

Preventive treatments

Preventives are gradually uptitrated during the headache cycle. For episodic cluster headache, patients nearing the end of their headache cycle consider tapering off after 2 weeks of headache freedom. For chronic cluster headache, which can transition to episodic cluster headache, consider tapering after 1 to 2 months of headache freedom.[67]

Verapamil: verapamil is the medication of choice for prevention. Its mechanism is unclear but may involve calcium channel blockade in the hypothalamus.[68] Verapamil is gradually titrated to a typical maintenance dose 240 to 720 mg/d (usually divided into 3 doses), although some patients have required up to 960 mg/d. Although there is little data to support it, the immediate release preparation is often preferred to extended release. Side effects include constipation, lower extremity edema, and rarely gingival hyperplasia. In addition, serial electrocardiogram (EKG) monitoring is recommended because of possible cardiac conduction issues, primarily lengthening of the PR interval leading to heart block or right bundle branch block (RBBB), even on steady dosing. In one study, 19% of patients had EKG abnormalities (usually PR interval lengthening or RBBB), and 4% had complete heart block.[69] Although there is no clear consensus on EKG monitoring, recommendations generally include an EKG before initiating treatment, repeat EKGs every 10 to 14 days after dose increases (especially more than 480 mg/d), and then every 6 months thereafter once on steady state dosing.[11,70]

Lithium: lithium carbonate therapy is still considered a mainstay of cluster prevention, but its narrow therapeutic window and high side-effect profile make it less desirable than newer preventives. Its mechanism in cluster headache is also unclear, but lithium is known to have effects on the hypothalamus, opioid receptors, and the immune system.[71] Lithium is generally titrated to 600 to 900 mg/d, usually for a target lithium level of 0.4 to 0.8 mmol/L measured 12 hours after the last dose.[55] Side effects include weakness, dysarthria, nystagmus, extrapyramidal signs, ataxia, confusion, seizures, and gastrointestinal issues (nausea and diarrhea). In addition, lithium can cause neutrophilia that can be confused for infection. Monitoring is recommended, including a chemistry and liver panel, thyroid stimulating hormone, and lithium level starting 1 week after treatment and periodically thereafter with concern for toxicity, especially thyroid and kidney. Caution in the elderly and caution with diuretics and nonsteroidal antiinflammatories is generally recommended.

Topiramate: the mechanism in cluster headache again is unclear but may involve effects on the posterior hypothalamus.[45] Topiramate is usually uptitrated to a total daily dose of 100 mg or more and generally takes 1 to 4 weeks for effect.[67,72] There can be a paradoxic worsening in some patients if doses are raised too high for that individual. Side effects include paresthesias, word-finding difficulties, weight loss, glaucoma, mood alteration, and kidney stones.

Melatonin: serum melatonin levels are reduced in patients who have cluster headache, particularly during a cluster headache period.[25] A dose of melatonin 10 mg at bedtime seems to be effective in cluster headache.[73] In clinical practice, melatonin is often used as an adjunct along with other preventive medications. Given the minimal side effects, melatonin is a very reasonable option in most patients. Efficacy of melatonin may be brand dependent, thus if a patient fails one brand of melatonin they may want to try another.

Noninvasive vagus nerve stimulation: the device used to abort attacks of episodic cluster headache, as discussed earlier, has also recently been approved for prevention in patients with both episodic and chronic cluster headaches.

Other preventive medications: there is some data for gabapentin between 900 and 3600 mg/d.[74] Valproate was previously used more frequently at 600 to 2000 mg/d; however, recent guidelines from the American Headache Society have given it an unfavorable rating, and thus it is not considered the preferred treatment. Other treatments that have been proposed include baclofen,[72] kudzu,[75] Boswellia serrata,[76] and onabotulinum toxin injections using the PREEMPT protocol.[77]

Galcanezumab: a recent trial of the CGRP antibody galcanezumab showed effectiveness in episodic but not chronic cluster headache, leading to FDA-approval for episodic cluster headache in June 2019. The dose for episodic cluster headache is 300mg monthly during the headache cycle, higher than the migraine dose of 240mg for the first month followed by 120mg per month thereafter.[10] Side effects of galcanezumab in episodic cluster headache were similar to those in migraine, including injection site reactions and nasopharyngitis. It should be noted at another CGRP antibody, fremanezumab, was recently found ineffective in episodic and chronic cluster headache. Given the similar targets of galcanezumab and fremanezumab, the difference in effectiveness is still a matter of debate.

Refractory patients: as many as 20% of patients with chronic cluster headache are refractory to treatment.[78] Although there are no large studies, combinations of preventives are commonly used for patients with refractory cluster headache. There are also several invasive procedures. The sphenopalatine ganglion stimulator, implanted for acute treatment of cluster headache as mentioned earlier, may also have preventive benefits.[79] Occipital nerve stimulation may also have benefit in chronic cluster headache based on open-label studies.[5] Side effects include lead migration or lead erosion and cluster headaches recurring on the side contralateral to the implanted electrodes. Guidelines for occipital nerve stimulation include daily or almost daily attacks for 2 years and failure of preventive medications.[80] Finally, hypothalamic deep brain stimulation has shown benefit, but recent American Headache Society guidelines have given an unfavorable rating based on current studies.[5] Additional research on deep brain stimulation is underway as other targets, such as the ventral tegmental area, subthalamic nucleus, and floor of the third ventricle, are being investigated.[81,82]

A study is currently underway in cluster headache for psilocybin (although currently it cannot be prescribed given its legal status).

PAROXYSMAL HEMICRANIA
Epidemiology

Paroxysmal hemicrania is less common than cluster headache, with a prevalence of 0.5 in 1000 or less.[70] The age of onset is generally between 30 and 40 years.[83] Unlike cluster headache, there is a slight female predominance.[84] Also unlike cluster headache, the chronic version is much more common: approximately 80% of paroxysmal hemicrania is chronic.[85]

Clinical features and diagnosis

Paroxysmal hemicrania is characterized as severe unilateral pain lasting 2 to 30 minutes, occurring more than 5 times a day for at least half the time the disease is active, with ipsilateral cranial autonomic features and/or restlessness. The pain is sharp, stabbing, boring, or throbbing and the exquisite intensity of the pain seems to be similar to cluster headache. The pain is generally located behind or around the eye. In a study of 74 patients, the average attack duration was 26 minutes and the average frequency was 6 per day,[84] although 30 or more attacks per day have been reported.[86] Some patients, however, will have mild interictal pain between attacks. For episodic paroxysmal hemicrania, headache cycles usually last 2 to 20 weeks and remit for 3 to 30 months.[85] Lacrimation is the most common autonomic feature, and restlessness is seen in most patients although not as commonly as in cluster headache.[87]

Paroxysmal hemicrania can be triggered by alcohol and neck movements; there are also reports that it can be triggered with pressure against the occiput or cervical transverse processes, stress, or exercise.[83–87] It typically does not have a predictable circadian pattern. Paroxysmal hemicrania can be associated with "migrainous symptoms" such as photophobia and phonophobia (usually ipsilateral to the pain).[88]

The differential diagnosis for paroxysmal hemicrania is very similar to cluster headache because the 2 diseases overlap in duration and frequency and share the same autonomic and restlessness features. In addition, symptomatic cases of paroxysmal hemicrania also exist. A paroxysmal hemicrania phenotype has been associated with pituitary adenomas, demyelinating lesions, leiomyosarcoma metastatic to the eye, and a gangliocytoma of the sella turcica.[57,58]

Work-up and Treatment

The work-up for all trigeminal autonomic cephalalgias is similar according to the European Headache Federation consensus: a brain MRI with dedicated views of the cavernous sinus and pituitary, followed by an MRA head and neck and pituitary laboratory studies in select patients.[59] In addition, an erythrocyte sedimentation rate may be considered.

Treatment of paroxysmal hemicrania begins with an indomethacin trial. Patients should have a complete or near complete response to an oral indomethacin dose of 225 mg/d or less.[1] A typical trial of indomethacin is 25 mg three times daily for 3 to 7 days, then if ineffective increasing to 50 mg three times daily for 3 to 7 days, then if ineffective increasing to 75 mg three times daily for 2 weeks.[89] A gastroprotectant is generally recommended while taking indomethacin, and sometimes at high doses patients experience a headache different from paroxysmal hemicrania that is throbbing and migrainous in description.[90] Indomethacin is often effective within 24 hours. If the medication is effective, it should slowly be titrated down to find the minimal effective maintenance dose, which may be less than 100 mg/d.[91] If indomethacin is not effective at 225 mg/d for 2 weeks, an alternate diagnosis should be considered.

Indomethacin is commonly associated with side effects. Gastrointestinal side effects seem to be the most common, including nausea, diarrhea, dyspepsia, and rarely gastric ulcers. For these reasons, a gastroprotectant such as a proton pump inhibitor or histamine receptor 2 blocker is often recommended. As other cyclooxygenase inhibitors, indomethacin affects platelet function and has effects on blood pressure, renal function, and liver function; in rare cases indomethacin can cause aseptic meningitis and reversible cerebral vasoconstriction syndrome.[83,92] For all these reasons, periodic downtitrations to find the minimum effective dose are encouraged.

The mechanism of indomethacin in paroxysmal hemicrania is not clear. The cyclooxygenase function is unlikely to be the primary mechanism: other cyclooxygenase inhibitors are typically less effective. Indomethacin is different from other cyclooxygenase inhibitors in several respects. Indomethacin crosses the blood brain barrier at a higher rate than other cyclooxygenase inhibitors[93] and reduces intracranial pressure by reducing cerebral blood flow.[94] Although all cyclooxygenase inhibitors have effects on the trigeminovascular system, indomethacin may also have direct neuronal effects on the hypothalamus or autonomic system.[94] Finally indomethacin has unique effects on the nitric oxide system.[94] None of these proposed mechanisms, however, fully explain why indomethacin is effective for paroxysmal hemicrania and hemicrania continua but not cluster headache, SUNA, or SUNCT. More research is needed.

When indomethacin is effective but is contraindicated or not tolerated, there are several other options. Other cyclooxygenase inhibitors, in particular cyclooxygenase-2 selective inhibitors such as celecoxib, may have benefit.[95] Melatonin is structurally similar to indomethacin and has been used as an adjunct to decrease the amount of indomethacin needed in hemicrania continua; however, there are limited data in paroxysmal hemicrania. Other treatments include those used for cluster headache, such as verapamil, topiramate, greater occipital nerve blocks, sphenopalatine ganglion blocks, and, more recently, noninvasive vagus nerve stimulation.[30,96–99]

SUNCT AND SUNA
Epidemiology

Short-lasting unilateral neuralgiform headache attacks with conjunctival injection and tearing (SUNCT) and short-lasting unilateral neuralgiform headache attacks with cranial autonomic symptoms (SUNA) are similar disorders that differ only in their cranial autonomic features: SUNCT has both conjunctival injection and lacrimation, and SUNA has one or neither. Several investigators have suggested that SUNCT is a subset of SUNA or that the 2 should be considered phenotypes of the same syndrome.[85,100]

SUNCT and SUNA have a prevalence between 1 and 100 in 100,000[101,102]; SUNCT seems to be 5 times more common than SUNA.[103] Typical age of onset is between 40 to 70 years, older than the other TACs.[104] As cluster headache, SUNCT and SUNA are more common in men.

Clinical features and Diagnosis

SUNCT and SUNA are characterized as moderate or severe unilateral pain lasting 1 to 600 seconds, occurring at least once a day, with ipsilateral cranial autonomic features. As mentioned earlier, the presence or absence of conjunctival injection and lacrimation is the only differentiating characteristic. Of note, restlessness, commonly seen in other TACs, is not part of the diagnostic criteria of SUNCT or SUNA. As other TACs there are 2 forms of SUNCT and SUNA: episodic, with pain-free cycles lasting 3 months or more, and chronic, with pain-free cycles lasting less than 3 months.

The pain in SUNCT and SUNA is often burning, stabbing, or electric but is typically not as painful as cluster headache. It generally occurs in the ophthalmic distribution of the trigeminal nerve. It can occur as a single stab, a series of stabs, or a sawtooth pattern (a period of elevated pain punctuated by stabs on top). Attack duration is typically seconds, attack frequency 30 per day (although 100 attacks or more have been seen), and episodic patients usually have 1 to 2 symptomatic periods per year lasting weeks to months.[105] As other TACs, patients can have mild interictal pain. Little is known about the natural history: there seems to be an erratic pattern of symptomatic and silent periods.[104]

SUNCT and SUNA can commonly be triggered by cutaneous stimuli, most commonly touching the face, wind, chewing, or brushing the teeth.[106] Because of the duration, frequency, and cutaneous triggers, SUNCT and SUNA can be misdiagnosed as trigeminal neuralgia. There are several differentiating features:

1. SUNCT and SUNA have cranial autonomic features. Trigeminal neuralgia does not.
2. SUNCT and SUNA generally affect the ophthalmic branch (V1) of the trigeminal nerve. Trigeminal neuralgia generally affects the maxillary and mandibular branches (V2 and V3).
3. SUNCT and SUNA typically do not have refractory periods after trigger zone excitation. Trigeminal neuralgia typically has a refractory period, a few moments after a cutaneous trigger where no more attacks can be triggered.[107]

The differential for SUNCT and SUNA also includes primary stabbing headache, which has a similar duration but can vary in location and lacks cranial autonomic features. Other disorders that can be confused for SUNCT and SUNA include cluster headache and paroxysmal hemicrania (because of the interictal milder pain in SUNCT and SUNA), herpes zoster, and dental issues. Symptomatic cases of SUNCT and SUNA include primarily pituitary tumors and posterior fossa tumors, although vascular malformations, herpes zoster, and compression of the trigeminal nerve by the superior cerebellar artery have also been described.[56–58]

Work-up and Treatment

The work-up according to a European Headache Federation consensus is similar to the other trigeminal autonomic cephalalgias: a brain MRI with dedicated views of the cavernous sinus and pituitary.[59] An MRA of the head may also be considered early in the work-up because SUNCT and SUNA are often difficult to distinguish from trigeminal neuralgia. Should patients not respond to typical preventives, an MRA neck and pituitary laboratory studies could be considered.

The mainstay of treatment is lamotrigine, usually at a dose of 100 to 200 mg/d. A very gradual uptitration is recommended because of the risk of Stevens-Johnson syndrome. More recently the US Food and Drug Administration added a warning to lamotrigine for hemophagocytic lymphohistiocytosis (HLH) based on the identification of 8 cases between 1994 and 2017.[108] Diagnosis of HLH include 5 of the following 8 features: fever/rash, splenomegaly, cytopenia, elevated serum CD25, decreased Natural Killer Cell activity, high triglycerides or low fibrinogen, high ferritin, or biopsy-proven evidence of hemophagocytosis in the bone marrow, spleen, or lymph node.

The most effective treatment of SUNCT and SUNA, however, seems to be intravenous lidocaine at a dose of 1 to 3.5 mg/kg/h for up to 1 week.[102,109] This treatment is generally performed by experienced providers with continuous telemetry given the cardiac conduction effects of lidocaine and is useful for acute SUNCT and SUNA flares. Some patients, however, have received several months of remission after a course of lidocaine.[102]

There are a variety of other medications that have shown effectiveness in SUNCT and SUNA. Several reports have suggested topiramate, gabapentin, duloxetine, or oxcarbazepine as second-line treatments.[110–112] Other treatment options include carbamazepine, pregabalin, greater occipital nerve blocks, and oral steroids.[112,113] For refractory patients research has begun to explore occipital nerve stimulation and microvascular decompression of the trigeminal nerve.[114,115]

HEMICRANIA CONTINUA
Epidemiology

The exact prevalence of hemicrania continua is unknown, but it constitutes about 1% of patients with daily or unilateral headaches, and 1% to 2% of total headache patients in clinic settings.[92,116] The age of onset is typically between 30 and 50 years and may affect women approximately twice as often as men.[92] The unremitting version (continuous pain for 1 year with remission periods <24 hours) seems to be more common.

Clinical Features and Diagnosis

Hemicrania continua is characterized by unilateral pain for at least 3 months, with exacerbations of moderate or severe pain, and with ipsilateral cranial autonomic features and/or restlessness. Instead of chronic and episodic, the 2 versions of hemicrania continua are unremitting (as discussed earlier) and remitting (periods of pain-freedom lasting more than 24 hours).

The pain from hemicrania continua is generally frontal, temporal, or periorbital and remains unilateral; in one review of the literature, a total of 9 cases of side-shifting have been reported.[117] The pain is sharp, throbbing, aching, or stabbing, although patients sometimes describe a foreign body or itchy sensation of the eye. The pain is characterized by a baseline unilateral headache, often of moderate severity with few autonomic features. In addition, there are exacerbations of pain accompanied by ipsilateral autonomic features (most commonly lacrimation) and "migrainous" features such as photophobia, phonophobia, nausea, and vomiting.[118] The autonomic features tend to be less pronounced than other TACs. The duration of the exacerbations is highly variable and has been reported anywhere between seconds and weeks,[117,119] although it most commonly lasts 2 to 3 days. Triggers for exacerbations include those typically associated with migraine, including stress, alcohol, poor sleep quality, bright lights, and skipping meals.[120]

Hemicrania continua is often difficult to distinguish from migraine or cluster headache. Like migraine, flares often have throbbing unilateral pain with photophobia, phonophobia, nausea, and vomiting; auras have rarely been described. Hemicrania continua is best differentiated from migraine by the following:

1. Side-switching: hemicrania continua rarely switches sides; migraine often switches sides or is bilateral
2. Remission: hemicrania continua rarely remits completely; migraine typically has pain-free periods
3. Indomethacin response: hemicrania continua always responds to a therapeutic dose of indomethacin.

Hemicrania continua may also resemble cluster headache, as cluster headache can sometimes have a mild interictal pain.

The differential diagnosis of hemicrania continua includes a much larger list of side-locked unilateral head and facial pains.[121] Some notable diseases include sinus headaches, dental pain, temporomandibular disorder, and temporal arteritis.[92,122] Symptomatic causes of hemicrania continua have also been seen, including several postsurgical and posttraumatic cases, several carotid dissections, and several cortical venous sinus thromboses, as well as cases of cancer (lung cancer metastatic to the brain and nasopharyngeal carcinoma) and orbital pseudotumor.[56,58]

Work-up and Treatment

The work-up is similar to other TACs: a brain MRI with dedicated views of the cavernous sinus and pituitary, followed by an MRA head and neck and pituitary laboratory studies in select patients.[59] In addition, a magnetic resonance venography of the head, neck imaging for cervicogenic headache, and an erythrocyte sedimentation rate may be considered.

The first-line treatment of hemicrania continua is indomethacin. The recommendations for indomethacin in hemicrania continua are identical to those stated earlier for paroxysmal hemicrania, including an uptitration to 225 mg/d for 2 weeks before considering ineffective, the use of gastroprotectants, and the downtitration to find a minimum effective maintenance dose. Periodic titrations of indomethacin should be considered, as the natural history of hemicrania continua is not well understood and some patients may change from the unremitting to the remitting version of the disease.

For patients who cannot tolerate or have contraindications to indomethacin, several other treatments have been proposed. Celecoxib, topiramate, gabapentin, and melatonin have been suggested as second- or third-line medications.[123] Melatonin may be used as an adjunct to reduce the amount of indomethacin needed.[124] Both occipital nerve blocks and onabotulinum toxin using the PREEMPT protocol may also be beneficial. More recently, noninvasive vagus nerve stimulation may have benefit in hemicrania continua.[30] For refractory patients, occipital nerve stimulation as well as radiofrequency of the sphenopalatine ganglion may be beneficial.

SUMMARY

The TACs are primary headache disorders characterized by severe unilateral pain and autonomic symptoms. They differ in their attack duration and frequency. Accurate diagnosis is key because treatment response depends on the condition.

REFERENCES

1. Headache Classification Committee of the International Headache Society (IHS). Headache Classification Committee of the International Headache Society (IHS) The International Classification of Headache Disorders, 3rd edition. Cephalalgia 2018;38(1):1–211.
2. International Headache Society. IHS Classification ICHD-II. 2003. Available at: http://ihs-classification.org/en/. Accessed August 27, 2015.
3. Headache Classification Committee of the International Headache Society (IHS). The International Classification of Headache Disorders, 3rd edition (beta version). Cephalalgia 2013;33(9):629–808.
4. Jarrar RG, Black DF, Dodick DW, et al. Outcome of trigeminal nerve section in the treatment of chronic cluster headache. Headache 2003;17(1):39–40.
5. Robbins MS, Starling AJ, Pringsheim TM, et al. Treatment of cluster headache: The American Headache Society Evidence-Based Guidelines. Headache 2016; 56(7):1093–106.
6. May A, Schwedt TJ, Magis D, et al. Cluster headache. Nat Rev Dis Primers 2018;4:1–17.
7. Goadsby PJ, Holland PR, Martins-oliveira M, et al. Pathophysiology of migraine: a disorder of sensory processing. Physiol Rev 2017;97:553–622.
8. Goadsby PJ, Edvinsson L. Human in vivo evidence for trigeminovascular activation in cluster headache. Neuropeptide changes and effects of acute attacks therapies. Brain 1994;117(Pt 3):427–34.
9. Tuka B, Szabó N, Tóth E, et al. Release of PACAP-38 in episodic cluster headache patients – an exploratory study. J Headache Pain 2016;17(1):69.
10. Goadsby PJ, Dodick DW, Leone M, et al. Trial of Galcanezumab in Prevention of Episodic Cluster Headache. N Engl J Med 2019;381(2):132–41.
11. Alstadhaug KB, Ofte HK. Cluster headache. Tidsskr Nor Laegeforen 2015; 135(15):1361–4.
12. Barloese MCJ. The pathophysiology of the trigeminal autonomic cephalalgias, with clinical implications. Clin Auton Res 2018;28(3):315–24.
13. Goadsby PJ. Pathophysiology of cluster headache: a trigeminal autonomic cephalgia. Lancet Neurol 2002;1(4):251–7.
14. Robbins MS, Robertson CE, Kaplan E, et al. The sphenopalatine ganglion: anatomy, pathophysiology, and therapeutic targeting in headache. Headache 2016; 56(2):240–58.
15. Sanders M, Zuurmond WWA. Efficacy of sphenopalatine ganglion blockade in 66 patients suffering from cluster headache: a 12- to 70-month follow-up evaluation. J Neurosurg 1997;87(6):876–80.
16. Schoenen J, Jensen RH, Lantéri-Minet M, et al. Stimulation of the sphenopalatine ganglion (SPG) for cluster headache treatment. Pathway CH-1: a randomized, sham-controlled study. Cephalalgia 2013;33(10):816–30.
17. Akerman S, Holland PR, Lasalandra MP, et al. Oxygen inhibits neuronal activation in the trigeminocervical complex after stimulation of trigeminal autonomic reflex, but not during direct dural activation of trigeminal afferents: Harold g. wolff lecture award winner. Headache 2009;49(8):1131–43.

18. Matharu M, Goadsby P. Cluster headache. Pract Neurol 2001;1:42–9.
19. Holland PR, Goadsby PJ. Cluster headache, hypothalamus, and orexin. Curr Pain Headache Rep 2009;13(2):147–54.
20. Bartsch T, Levy MJ, Knight YE, et al. Differential modulation of nociceptive dural input to [hypocretin] orexin A and B receptor activation in the posterior hypothalamic area. Pain 2004;109(3):367–78.
21. May A, Leone M, Boecker H, et al. Hypothalamic deep brain stimulation in positron emission tomography. J Neurosci 2006;26(13):3589–93.
22. Rozen TD, Fishman RS. Cluster headache in the United States of America: demographics, clinical characteristics, triggers, suicidality, and personal burden. Headache 2012;52(1):99–113.
23. Chazot G, Claustrat B, Brun J, et al. A chronobiological study of melatonin, cortisol growth hormone and prolactin secretion in cluster headache. Cephalalgia 1984;4(4):213–20.
24. Waldenlind E, Gustafsson SA, Ekbom K, et al. Circadian secretion of cortisol and melatonin in cluster headache during active cluster periods and remission. J Neurol Neurosurg Psychiatry 1987;50(2):207–13.
25. Bruera O, Sances G, Leston J, et al. Plasma melatonin pattern in chronic and episodic headaches. Evaluation during sleep and waking. Funct Neurol 2008; 23(2):77–81.
26. Leone M, Lucini V, D'Amico D, et al. Twenty-four-hour melatonin and cortisol plasma levels in relation to timing of cluster headache. Cephalalgia 1995; 15(3):224–9.
27. Gaul C, Diener H-C, Silver N, et al. Non-invasive vagus nerve stimulation for PREVention and Acute treatment of chronic cluster headache (PREVA): a randomised controlled study. Cephalalgia 2016;36(6):534–46.
28. Silberstein SD, Mechtler LL, Kudrow DB, et al. Non-Invasive Vagus Nerve Stimulation for the ACute Treatment of Cluster Headache: Findings From the Randomized, Double-Blind, Sham-Controlled ACT1 Study. Headache 2016; 56(8):1317–32.
29. Goadsby PJ, de Coo IF, Silver N, et al. Non-invasive vagus nerve stimulation for the acute treatment of episodic and chronic cluster headache: a randomized, double-blind, sham-controlled ACT2 study. Cephalalgia 2018;38(5):959–69.
30. Tso AR, Marin J, Goadsby PJ. Noninvasive vagus nerve stimulation for treatment of indomethacin-sensitive headaches. JAMA Neurol 2017;74(10):1266–7.
31. Akerman S, Simon B, Romero-Reyes M. Vagus nerve stimulation suppresses acute noxious activation of trigeminocervical neurons in animal models of primary headache. Neurobiol Dis 2017;102:96–104.
32. Moeller M, Schroeder CF, May A. Vagus nerve stimulation modulates the cranial trigeminal autonomic reflex. Ann Neurol 2018;84(6):886–92.
33. Fischera M, Marziniak M, Gralow I, et al. The incidence and prevalence of cluster headache: a meta-analysis of population-based studies. Cephalalgia 2008; 28(6):614–8.
34. Manzoni GC, Taga A, Russo M, et al. Age of onset of episodic and chronic cluster headache – a review of a large case series from a single headache centre. J Headache Pain 2016;17(1):44.
35. Lund N, Barloese M, Petersen A, et al. Chronobiology differs between men and women with cluster headache, clinical phenotype does not. Neurology 2017; 88(11):1069–76.
36. Torelli P, Cologno D, Cademartiri C, et al. Possible predictive factors in the evolution of episodic to chronic cluster headache. Headache 2000;40(10):798–808.

37. Louter MA, Wilbrink LA, Haan J, et al. Cluster headache and depression. Neurology 2016;87(18):1899–906.

38. Liang J-F, Chen Y-T, Fuh J-L, et al. Cluster headache is associated with an increased risk of depression: a nationwide population-based cohort study. Cephalalgia 2013;33(3):182–9.

39. Trejo-Gabriel-Galan JM, Aicua-Rapún I, Cubo-Delgado E, et al. Suicide in primary headaches in 48 countries: a physician-survey based study. Cephalalgia 2018;38(4):798–803.

40. Graff-Radford SB, Newman A. Obstructive sleep apnea and cluster headache. Headache 2004;44(6):607–10.

41. Govare A, Leroux E. Licit and illicit drug use in cluster headache. Curr Pain Headache Rep 2014;18(5):413.

42. Rozen TD. Linking cigarette smoking/tobacco exposure and cluster headache: a pathogenesis theory. Headache 2018;58(7):1096–112.

43. Bahra A, May A, Goadsby PJ. Cluster headache: a prospective clinical study with diagnostic implications. Neurology 2002;58(3):354–61.

44. Donnet A, Lanteri-Minet M, Guegan-Massardier E, et al. Chronic cluster headache: a French clinical descriptive study. J Neurol Neurosurg Psychiatry 2007; 78(12):1354–8.

45. Leone M, Bussone G. Pathophysiology of trigeminal autonomic cephalalgias. Lancet Neurol 2009;8(8):755–64.

46. Barloese M, Lund N, Petersen A, et al. Sleep and chronobiology in cluster headache. Cephalalgia 2015;35(11):969–78.

47. Steinberg A, Fourier C, Ran C, et al. Cluster headache – clinical pattern and a new severity scale in a Swedish cohort. Cephalalgia 2017;38(7):1286–95.

48. Buture A, Ahmed F, Dikomitis L, et al. Systematic literature review on the delays in the diagnosis and misdiagnosis of cluster headache. Neurol Sci 2018;40(1): 25–39.

49. Schürks M, Kurth T, De Jesus J, et al. Cluster headache: Clinical presentation, lifestyle features, and medical treatment. Headache 2006;46(8):1246–54.

50. Uluduz D, Ayta S, Ozge A, et al. Cranial autonomic features in migraine and migrainous features in cluster headache. Noro Psikiyatr Ars 2016;55(3):220–4.

51. Ashkenazi A, Young WB. Dynamic mechanical (brush) allodynia in cluster headache. Headache 2004;44(10):1010–2.

52. Silberstein SD, Niknam R, Rozen TD, et al. Cluster headache with aura. Neurology 2000;54(1):219–22.

53. Wilbrink LA, Louter MA, Teernstra OP, et al. Allodynia in cluster headache. Pain 2017;158(6):1113–7.

54. Goadsby PJ. Trigeminal autonomic cephalalgias. Continuum (Minneap Minn) 2012;18(4):883–95.

55. Dodick DW. Trigeminal autonomic cephalgias. In: Lipton RB, Bigal ME, editors. Migraine and other headache disorders. New York: Taylor & Francis Group; 2006. p. 471–93.

56. de Coo IF, Wilbrink LA, Haan J. Symptomatic trigeminal autonomic cephalalgias. Curr Pain Headache Rep 2015;19(8):305–12.

57. Cittadini E, Matharu MS. Symptomatic trigeminal autonomic cephalalgias. Neurologist 2009;15(6):305–12.

58. Chowdhury D. Secondary (symptomatic) trigeminal autonomic cephalalgia. Ann Indian Acad Neurol 2018;21(Suppl 1):S57–69.

59. Mitsikostas DD, Ashina M, Craven A, et al. European headache federation consensus on technical investigation for primary headache disorders. J Headache Pain 2015;17(1):5.
60. Lademann V, Jansen J-P, Evers S, et al. Evaluation of guideline-adherent treatment in cluster headache. Cephalalgia 2015;36(8):760–4.
61. Schindler EAD, Wright DA, Weil MJ, et al. Survey analysis of the use, effectiveness, and patient-reported tolerability of inhaled oxygen compared with injectable sumatriptan for the acute treatment of cluster headache. Headache 2018;58(10):1568–78.
62. Goadsby PJ, Cohen AS, Matharu MS. Trigeminal autonomic cephalalgias: diagnosis and treatment. Curr Neurol Neurosci Rep 2007;7(2):117–25. Available at: http://www.ncbi.nlm.nih.gov/pubmed/17355838. Accessed July 9, 2017.
63. Leroux E, Ducros A. Occipital injections for trigemino-autonomic cephalalgias: evidence and uncertainties. Curr Pain Headache Rep 2013;17(4):325.
64. Saper JR, Klapper J, Mathew NT, et al. Intranasal civamide for the treatment of episodic cluster headaches. Arch Neurol 2002;59(6):990–4.
65. Ito Y, Mitsufuji T, Asano Y, et al. Naratriptan in the prophylactic treatment of cluster headache. Intern Med 2017;56(19):2579–82.
66. Pageler L, Katsarava Z, Lampl C, et al. Frovatriptan for prophylactic treatment of cluster headache: lessons for future trial design. Headache 2011;51(1):129–34.
67. Leone M, Franzini A, Cecchini AP, et al. Cluster headache: pharmacological treatment and neurostimulation. Nat Clin Pract Neurol 2009;5(3):153–62.
68. Tfelt-hansen P, Tfelt-hansen J. Verapamil for cluster headache. clinical pharmacology and possible mode of action. Headache 2009;49:117–25.
69. Cohen AS, Matharu MS, Goadsby PJ. Electrocardiographic abnormalities in patients with cluster headache on verapamil therapy. Neurology 2007;69(7):668–75.
70. Eller M, Goadsby P. Trigeminal autonomic cephalalgias. Oral Dis 2014;22(1):1–8.
71. Abdel-Maksoud MB, Nasr A, Abdul-Aziz A. Lithium treatment in cluster headache: review of literature. Eur J Psychiatry 2009;23(1):53–60.
72. May A, Leone M, Afra J, et al. EFNS guidelines on the treatment of cluster headache and other trigeminal-autonomic cephalalgias. Eur J Neurol 2006;13(10):1066–77.
73. Leone M, D'Amico D, Moschiano F, et al. Melatonin versus placebo in the prophylaxis of cluster headache: a double-blind pilot study with parallel groups. Cephalalgia 1996;16(7):494–6.
74. Schuh-Hofer S, Israel H, Neeb L, et al. The use of gabapentin in chronic cluster headache patients refractory to first-line therapy. Eur J Neurol 2007;14(6):694–6.
75. Sewell RA. Response of cluster headache to Kudzu. Headache 2009;49(1):98–105.
76. Lampl C, Haider B, Schweiger C. Long-term efficacy of Boswellia serrata in four patients with chronic cluster headache. Cephalalgia 2012;32(9):719–22.
77. Lampl C, Rudolph M, Bräutigam E. OnabotulinumtoxinA in the treatment of refractory chronic cluster headache. J Headache Pain 2018;19(1):45.
78. Newman LC. Trigeminal autonomic cephalalgias. Continuum (Minneap Minn) 2015;21(4 Headache):1041–57.
79. Barloese M, Petersen A, Stude P, et al. Sphenopalatine ganglion stimulation for cluster headache, results from a large, open-label European registry. J Headache Pain 2018;19(1):6.
80. Leone M, Franzini A, Cecchini AP, et al. Stimulation of occipital nerve for drug-resistant chronic cluster headache. Lancet Neurol 2007;6(4):289–91.

81. Vyas DB, Ho AL, Dadey DY, et al. Deep brain stimulation for chronic cluster headache: a review. Neuromodulation 2019;22(4):388–97.
82. Huotarinen A, Reich M, Volkmann J, et al. STN DBS for advanced parkinson disease simultaneously alleviates cluster headache. Case Rep Neurol 2017; 9(3):289–92.
83. Osman C, Bahra A. Paroxysmal hemicrania. Ann Indian Acad Neurol 2018; 21(Suppl 1):S16–22.
84. Boes CJ, Dodick DW. Refining the clinical spectrum of chronic paroxysmal hemicrania: a review of 74 patients. Headache 2002;42(8):699–708.
85. Cohen AS, Matharu MS, Goadsby PJ. Trigeminal autonomic cephalalgias: current and future treatments. Headache 2007;47(6):969–80.
86. Benoliel R, Sharav Y. Paroxysmal hemicrania. Case studies and review of the literature. Oral Surg Oral Med Oral Pathol Oral Radiol Endod 1998;85(3):285–92.
87. Cittadini E, Matharu MS, Goadsby PJ. Paroxysmal hemicrania: a prospective clinical study of 31 cases. Brain 2008;131(Pt 4):1142–55.
88. Irimia P, Cittadini E, Paemeleire K, et al. Unilateral photophobia or phonophobia in migraine compared with trigeminal autonomic cephalalgias. Cephalalgia 2008;28(6):626–30.
89. Cittadini E, Goadsby PJ. Update on hemicrania continua. Curr Pain Headache Rep 2011;15(1):51–6.
90. Jürgens TP, Schulte LH, May A. Indomethacin-induced de novo headache in hemicrania continua—fighting fire with fire? Cephalalgia 2013;33(14):1203–5.
91. Pareja J, Caminero A, Franco E, et al. Dose, efficacy and tolerability of long-term indomethacin treatment of chronic paroxysmal hemicrania and hemicrania continua. Cephalalgia 2001;21(9):906–10.
92. Charlson RW, Robbins MS. Hemicrania Continua. Curr Neurol Neurosci Rep 2014;14(3):436.
93. Summ O, Evers S. Mechanism of action of indomethacin in indomethacin-responsive headaches. Curr Pain Headache Rep 2013;17(4):327.
94. Lucas S. The pharmacology of indomethacin. Headache 2016;56(2):436–46.
95. Siow H. Seasonal episodic paroxysmal hemicrania responding to cyclooxygenase-2 inhibitors. Cephalalgia 2004;24(5):414–5.
96. Rossi P, Di Lorenzo G, Faroni J, et al. Seasonal, extratrigeminal, episodic paroxysmal hemicrania successfully treated with single suboccipital steroid injections. Eur J Neurol 2005;12(11):903–6.
97. Morelli N, Mancuso M, Felisati G, et al. Does sphenopalatine endoscopic ganglion block have an effect in paroxysmal hemicrania? A case report. Cephalalgia 2010;30(3):365–7.
98. Boes C. Differentiating paroxysmal hemicrania from cluster headache. Cephalalgia 2005;25(4):241–3.
99. Zhu S, Mcgeeney B. When indomethacin fails : additional treatment options for b indomethacin responsive headaches. Curr Pain Headache Rep 2015;19(3):7.
100. Favoni V, Grimaldi D, Pierangeli G, et al. SUNCT/SUNA and neurovascular compression: New cases and critical literature review. Cephalalgia 2013; 33(16):1337–48.
101. Williams MH, Broadley SA. SUNCT and SUNA: clinical features and medical treatment. J Clin Neurosci 2008;15(5):526–34.
102. Cohen A. SUN: short-lasting unilateral neuralgiform headache attacks. Headache 2017;57(6):1010–20.
103. Pareja JA, Álvarez M, Montojo T. SUNCT and SUNA: recognition and treatment. Curr Treat Options Neurol 2013;15(1):28–39.

104. Pareja JA, Caminero AB, Sjaastad O. SUNCT syndrome: diagnosis and treatment. CNS Drugs 2002;16(6):373–83.

105. Alore PL, Jay WM, Macken MP. SUNCT syndrome: short-lasting unilateral neuralgiform headache with conjunctival injection and tearing. Semin Ophthalmol 2006;21(1):9–13.

106. Benoliel R, Sharav Y, Haviv Y, et al. Tic, triggering, and tearing: from CTN to SUNHA. Headache 2017;57(6):997–1009.

107. Weng H-Y, Cohen AS, Schankin C, et al. Phenotypic and treatment outcome data on SUNCT and SUNA, including a randomised placebo-controlled trial. Cephalalgia 2018;38(9):1554–63.

108. Lamictal (lamotrigine): Drug Safety Communication - Serious Immune System Reaction. 2018. Available at: https://www.fda.gov/safety/medwatch/safetyinformation/safetyalertsforhumanmedicalproducts/ucm605628.htm. Accessed December 20, 2018.

109. Pareja JA, Álvarez M. The usual treatment of trigeminal autonomic cephalalgias. Headache 2013;53(9):1401–14.

110. Goadsby PJ, Cittadini E, Burns B, et al. Trigeminal autonomic cephalalgias: diagnostic and therapeutic developments. Curr Opin Neurol 2008;21(3):323–30.

111. Matharu MS, Cohen AS, Boes CJ, et al. Short-lasting unilateral neuralgiform headache with conjunctival injection and tearing syndrome: a review. Curr Pain Headache Rep 2003;7(4):308–18.

112. Lambru G, Matharu MS. SUNCT and SUNA: medical and surgical treatments. Neurol Sci 2013;34(S1):75–81.

113. Baraldi C, Pellesi L, Guerzoni S, et al. Therapeutical approaches to paroxysmal hemicrania, hemicrania continua and short lasting unilateral neuralgiform headache attacks: a critical appraisal. J Headache Pain 2017;18(1):71.

114. Lambru G, Shanahan P, Watkins L, et al. Occipital nerve stimulation in the treatment of medically intractable SUNCT and SUNA. Pain Physician 2014;17(1):29–41.

115. Sebastian S, Schweitzer D, Tan L, et al. Role of trigeminal microvascular decompression in the treatment of SUNCT and SUNA. Curr Pain Headache Rep 2013;17(5):332.

116. Prakash S, Patel P. Hemicrania continua: clinical review, diagnosis and management. J Pain Res 2017;10:1493–509.

117. Prakash S, Adroja B. Hemicrania continua. Ann Indian Acad Neurol 2018;21(Suppl 1):S23–30.

118. Peres MF, Silberstein SD, Nahmias S, et al. Hemicrania continua is not that rare. Neurology 2001;57(6):948–51.

119. Cortijo E, Guerrero ÁL, Herrero S, et al. Hemicrania continua in a headache clinic: referral source and diagnostic delay in a series of 22 patients. J Headache Pain 2012;13(7):567–9.

120. Cittadini E, Goadsby PJ. Hemicrania continua: a clinical study of 39 patients with diagnostic implications. Brain 2010;133(Pt 7):1973–86.

121. Prakash S, Rathore C, Makwana P, et al. A cross-sectional clinic-based study in patients with side-locked unilateral headache and facial pain. Headache 2016;56(7):1183–93.

122. Rossi P, Faroni J, Tassorelli C, et al. Diagnostic delay and suboptimal management in a referral population with hemicrania continua. Headache 2009;49(2):227–34.

123. Rossi P, Tassorelli C, Allena M, et al. Focus on therapy: hemicrania continua and new daily persistent headache. J Headache Pain 2010;11(3):259–65.

124. Rozen TD. How effective is melatonin as a preventive treatment for hemicrania continua? A clinic-based study. Headache 2015;55(3):430–6.
125. May A, Bahra A, Büchel C, et al. Hypothalamic activation in cluster headache attacks. Lancet 1998;352(9124):275–8.
126. Matharu MS, Cohen AS, Frackowiak RSJ, et al. Posterior hypothalamic activation in paroxysmal hemicrania. Ann Neurol 2006;59(3):535–45.
127. May A, Bahra A, Büchel C, et al. Functional magnetic resonance imaging in spontaneous attacks of SUNCT: short-lasting neuralgiform headache with conjunctival injection and tearing. Ann Neurol 1999;46(5):791–4.
128. Matharu MS, Cohen AS, McGonigle DJ, et al. Posterior hypothalamic and brainstem activation in hemicrania continua. Headache 2004;44(8):747–61.

Other Primary Headaches
An Update

Vicente González-Quintanilla, MD, PhD, Julio Pascual, MD, PhD*

KEYWORDS

- Cough headache • Epicranea fugax • Exercise headache • Hypnic headache
- New daily-persistent headache • Nummular headache • Stabbing headache
- Thunderclap headache

KEY POINTS

- Within the umbrella of "Other Primary Headaches," ICHD-3 includes activity-related headaches, headaches due to direct physical stimuli, epicranial headaches, and a miscellanea with hypnic headache and new daily-persistent headache.
- These entities are a challenging diagnostic problem, as they can be primary or secondary and their etiologies differ depending on the headache type.
- Activity-related headaches can be brought on by Valsalva maneuvers ("cough headache") or prolonged exercise ("exercise and sexual headaches").
- Cough headache is primary in almost half of the cases. Chiari type I malformation is the most frequent etiology in secondary cases. Contrary to cough headache, only 20% of exertional/sexual headaches are secondary, sentinel subarachnoid bleeding being the most frequent etiology.

The classification of the International Headache Society (IHS) includes 4 sections within the primary headaches: "Migraine," "Tension-Type Headache," "Trigeminal Autonomic Cephalalgias," and "Other Primary Headaches." Within the umbrella of "other primary headaches," the classification defines a variety of clinically heterogeneous headaches phenotypes (**Box 1**). They are grouped into 4 categories and coded in the recently published third version of the International Classification of Headache Disorders (ICHD-3) accordingly: 1. Headaches associated with physical exertion, including Primary cough headache, Primary exercise headache, Primary headache associated with sexual activity and Primary thunderclap headache. 2. Headaches attributed to direct physical stimuli (considered to be primary headache disorders because they are brought on by physiologic [non-damaging] stimuli), including Cold-stimulus headache and External-pressure headache. 3. Epicranial headaches,

Disclosure Statement: The authors have nothing to disclose.
Service of Neurology, University Hospital Marqués de Valdecilla, IDIVAL, Av. Valdecilla s/n, Santander 39008, Spain
* Corresponding author.
E-mail address: juliopascual@telefonica.net

Neurol Clin 37 (2019) 871–891
https://doi.org/10.1016/j.ncl.2019.07.010
0733-8619/19/© 2019 Elsevier Inc. All rights reserved.

neurologic.theclinics.com

Box 1
Other primary headache disorders

4.1 Primary cough headache
    4.1.1 Probable primary cough headache

4.2 Primary exercise headache
    4.2.1 Probable primary exercise headache

4.3 Primary headache associated with sexual activity
    4.3.1 Probable primary headache associated with sexual activity

4.4 Primary thunderclap headache

4.5 Cold-stimulus headache
    4.5.1 Headache attributed to external application of a cold stimulus
    4.5.2 Headache attributed to ingestion or inhalation of a cold stimulus
    4.5.3 Probable cold-stimulus headache
        4.5.3.1 Headache probably attributed to external application of a cold stimulus
        4.5.3.2 Headache probably attributed to ingestion or inhalation of a cold stimulus

4.6 External-pressure headache
    4.6.1 External-compression headache
    4.6.2 External-traction headache
    4.6.3 Probable external-pressure headache
        4.6.3.1 Probable external-compression headache
        4.6.3.2 Probable external-traction headache

4.7 Primary stabbing headache
    4.7.1 Probable primary stabbing headache

4.8 Nummular headache
    4.8.1 Probable nummular headache

4.9 Hypnic headache
    4.9.1 Probable hypnic headache

4.10 New daily-persistent headache (NDPH)
    4.10.1 Probable new daily-persistent headache

From Headache Classification Committee of the International Headache Society (IHS). The International Classification of Headache Disorders. 3rd edition. Cephalalgia 2018; 38: 1-211; with permission.

---

including Primary stabbing headache and Nummular headache (as well as Epicrania fugax in the Appendix). 4. Other miscellaneous primary headache disorders including Hypnic headache and New daily-persistent headache.[1] This review focuses on all of them. The pathogenesis of these headaches is poorly understood, and their treatments are based on uncontrolled trials or anecdotal reports. One important issue in confronting these headaches is that they also can be symptomatic of structural lesions or other disorders; therefore, when they appear, evaluation by neuroimaging or other appropriate tests is usually needed.

PRIMARY COUGH HEADACHE

Primary cough headache, previously also known as benign cough headache or Valsalva-maneuver headache, is a headache precipitated by coughing or straining, but not by prolonged physical exercise. This diagnosis requires the absence of any other intracranial disorder. Primary cough headache is considered a rare entity. Rasmussen and Olesen[2] have shown that the lifetime prevalence of cough headache is

1% (95% confidence interval 0%–2%). In our series, of the 6412 patients attending our Neurology Department due to headache, 68 (1.1%) consulted because of cough headache.[3]

Current ICHD-3 diagnostic criteria for primary cough headache appear in **Box 2**. Cough headache may occur either as a primary headache or as a headache secondary to potentially serious processes, so careful evaluation for underlying causes is mandatory. Before computed tomography (CT) and MRI availability, series concluded that only approximately 20% of patients with cough headache had structural lesions, most of them a Chiari type I deformity (**Fig. 1**). In the MRI era, the proportion of patients who have an underlying structural cause has varied between 11% and 59% in different studies.[3–7] In consequence, structural lesions should be ruled out before making the diagnosis of primary cough headache.[1,8] The most common causes are, after Chiari type I malformation, miscellaneous posterior fossa lesions[3,9] (**Fig. 2**), acquired tonsillar descent due to low intracranial pressure[10] (**Fig. 3**), carotid or vertebrobasilar diseases, and causes of thunderclap headache, including reversible cerebral vasoconstriction syndrome. In summary, it can be concluded that approximately one-half and two-thirds of patients with cough headache will show no demonstrable etiology, whereas the remaining cases will be secondary to a structural lesion, mostly at the foramen magnum level.[3,4,11]

The clinical picture of primary cough headache is very characteristic, which allows differentiation from secondary cases.[3,9,12] Primary cough headache most often affects people older than 40 (range 44–81 years) and is more common in women.[3] Cough headaches are sudden in onset, bilateral in distribution, and usually last from seconds to a few minutes, although some patients may have headache for up to 2 hours.[13] Precipitants include cough, sneezing, blowing the nose, laughing, crying, singing, lifting (including weightlifting), straining at stool, and stooping. Sustained physical exercise is not a precipitating factor for primary cough headache. These headaches are not associated with nausea, vomiting, light or sound sensitivity, conjunctival injection, rhinorrhea, or lacrimation, and respond to indomethacin.[3,9,11,12]

The pathophysiology of secondary cough headache is reasonably well understood. The headache seems to be to a temporary impaction of the cerebellar tonsils below the foramen magnum.[14–18] In 2 patients with cough headache and tonsillar herniation, Williams demonstrated a pressure difference between the ventricle and the lumbar subarachnoid space during coughing.[14,18] The pressure difference, named craniospinal pressure dissociation, displaced the cerebellar tonsils into the foramen

---

Box 2
International Classification of Headache Disorders, Third Version (ICHD-3) diagnostic criteria for primary cough headache

A. At least 2 headache episodes fulfilling criteria B to D.

B. Brought on by and occurring only in association with coughing, straining, and/or other Valsalva maneuver.

C. Sudden onset.

D. Lasting between 1 second and 2 hours.

E. Not better accounted for by another ICHD-3 diagnosis.

From Headache Classification Committee of the International Headache Society (IHS). The International Classification of Headache Disorders. 3rd edition. Cephalalgia 2018; 38: 1-211; with permission.

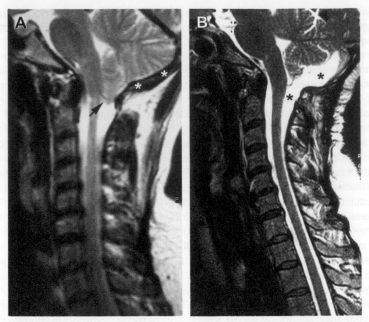

Fig. 1. Preoperative (*A*) and postoperative (*B*) T2-weighted sagittal MRI of a 36-year-old woman with cough headache. Note the presence of tonsillar descent (*arrow*) and flattening of posterior fossa (*asterisks*) and the absence of cisterna magna. (*B*) After posterior fossa reconstruction, notice the appearance of cisterna magna with restitution of CSF transit (*asterisks*) with upward migration of the tonsils. (*From* Pascual J. Activity-related headache. In: Roos R., editor-in-chief. MedLink Neurology. San Diego: MedLink Corporation. Available at http://www.medlink.com/article/activity-related_headache. Republished by permission.)

Posterior fossa occupying lesions presenting as cough headache

arachnoid cyst   dermoid tumor   meningioma

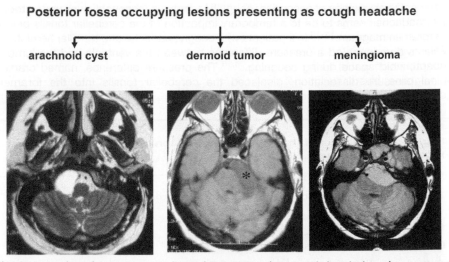

Fig. 2. Examples of patients consulting due to secondary cough headache who were not diagnosed with Chiari type I malformation. Notice the identical location of the 3 tumors. *Location of the dermoid tumor in a patient presenting with cough headache. (*Adapted from* Pascual J, Iglesias F, Oterino A, et al. Cough, exertional, and sexual headaches: an analysis of 72 benign and symptomatic cases. Neurology 1996; 46: 1520-4; with permission.)

magnum. Williams also observed that the headache disappeared after decompressive craniectomy.[15] Subsequently, Nightingale and Williams[16] described 4 more patients who had headache due to episodic impaction of the cerebellar tonsils in the foramen magnum after abrupt Valsalva maneuvers. In our series, not only it was demonstrated that tonsillar descent is the actual cause of cough headache, but it was shown that the presence of cough headache in patients with Chiari type I only correlated with the degree of tonsillar descent.[9] Pujol and colleagues,[19] using cine phase-contrast MRI, were able to detect this abnormal pulsatile motion of the cerebellar tonsils in patients with Chiari type I and not in controls. This movement produced a selective obstruction of the cerebrospinal fluid (CSF) flow from the cranial cavity to the spine (see **Fig. 3**). The amplitude of the tonsillar pulsation and the severity of the arachnoid space reduction were associated with cough headache. All these data confirm that symptomatic cough headache is secondary to Chiari type I deformity and that this pain is due to compression or traction of the causally displaced cerebellar tonsils on pain-sensitive dura and other anchoring structures around the foramen magnum innervated by the first cervical roots.

The pathophysiology of primary cough headache is poorly understood, and several hypotheses have been proposed, including the possibility that coughing induces sudden increases in intra-abdominal and intrathoracic pressures that are transmitted through the venous system into the intracranial venous sinuses, causing activation of intradural or perivascular nociceptive neurons.[20] However, coughs in daily life are usually insufficient to activate intracranial nociceptive fibers, suggesting that other factors that decrease activation thresholds and result in recurrent depolarization of the nociceptive fibers may play a role in headache onset. There should be other contributing factors, such as a hypersensitivity of some receptors, sensitivity to pressure.[21] One of the potential etiologies for this transient receptor sensitization could be a hidden or previous infection.[17] Finally, Chen and colleagues[22] found that patients with primary cough headache are associated with a more crowded posterior cranial fossa, which may be a further contributing factor to the pathogenesis of this headache syndrome. Other investigators reported that some patients have incompetent or absent internal jugular venous valves and might be more prone to transient elevation of central venous pressure and intracranial pressure. Wang and colleagues[20] postulated that CSF hypervolemia could lead to a transient increase in intracranial pressure during cough, which would be a potential cause of the headache.

Migraine, cluster headache, post-lumbar puncture headache and idiopathic intracranial hypertension can be aggravated, but not elicited, by cough. Given the differential diagnosis outlined previously, every patient with cough headache should have an

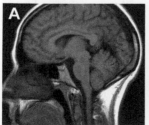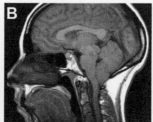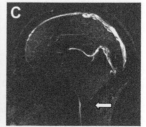

Fig. 3. (A) MRI of a 33-year-old woman with pseudotumor cerebri with no tonsillar descent. (B) MRI after lumboperitoneal shunt when she consulted due to cough headache, showing acquired tonsillar descent. (C) Cine phase-contrast MRI showing difficulties in CSF circulation in the foramen magnum region (*arrow*).

MRI of the brain to rule out a posterior fossa lesion. In spite of scattered reports, there is not enough scientific background to support unruptured aneurysms,[23] carotid stenosis, or vertebrobasilar disease as specific causes for cough headache. Therefore, a magnetic resonance angiogram (MRA) study is not mandatory in these patients (**Fig. 4**).

The prognosis for spontaneous recovery is limited. In a reported series of 21 cases, only 9 had spontaneous recovery within 18 months to 12 years.[4] Acute treatment is impractical because of the short duration and multiplicity of cough headaches. However, because symptoms can be quite debilitating, a preventive treatment strategy should be considered.

Primary cough headache responds to indomethacin, given prophylactically at doses usually ranging from 25 to 150 mg daily.[24,25] Indomethacin decreases intracranial pressure,[26] and this would explain the benefits seen with lumbar puncture or acetazolamide, both known to decrease intracranial pressure in patients with primary cough headache.[20,27,28] No consensus exists on indomethacin treatment duration. Besides indomethacin, beneficial effects of topiramate, methysergide, propranolol, naproxen and intravenous metoclopramide have been reported in small case series.[29–32] For some patients with primary cough headache, stopping cough-inducing antihypertensives can be enough.

Patients with symptomatic cough headache do not consistently respond to any known pharmacologic treatment, including indomethacin, and may need specific surgical treatment. In experienced hands, suboccipital craniectomy combined with a C1-C3 laminectomy, relieves cough headache in most patients with a Chiari malformation type I.[3,9]

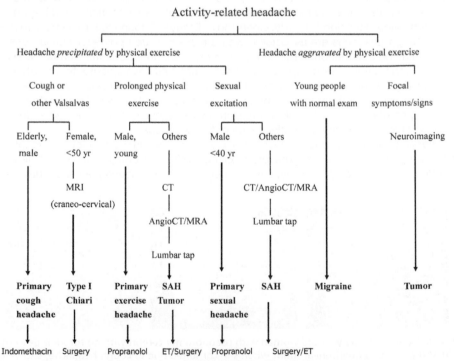

Fig. 4. Differential diagnosis and management of activity-related headaches. ET, endovascular treatment; SAH, subarachnoid hemorrhage.

PRIMARY EXERCISE HEADACHE

This entity, previously known as exertional headache, is a headache precipitated by any form of exercise in the absence of any intracranial disorder.[1] Current diagnostic criteria for primary exercise headache (**Box 3**) require sustained strenuous physical activity, which distinguishes this entity from other short-duration precipitated factors, such as cough or Valsalva maneuver. Also, as specified in the diagnostic criteria, it is mandatory to exclude symptomatic causes of exercise headache, including arterial dissection, reversible cerebral vasoconstriction syndrome, and subarachnoid hemorrhage.

Contrary to primary cough headache, primary exercise headache is typical of young people (range 10–48 years in our series), and its prevalence has been estimated between 1% and 26%.[2,3] Our prospective series found that 11 of 6412 patients with headache met the criteria for primary exercise headache.[3] Gender estimates vary; first series identified a higher prevalence in men, but recent studies found a higher prevalence in women than men at a ratio of 1.38 in adults and 1.49 in adolescents.[33,34]

In terms of consultation, exercise headache is less common than cough headache. Most cases occur in patients who have a personal and/or family history of migraine.[3,9,11] This headache may be triggered by any kind of prolonged physical exercise,[28,35] at least exercise sufficient to double the resting pulse for more than 10 seconds, but ordinarily for minutes or even hours. Headache usually occurs at the peak of the exercise and subsides when the activity ceases, even though in some occasions headache can last up to 2 days. Most patients present with a bilateral, pulsating headache, which begins within 30 minutes of the onset of exercise in more than half of patients.[33] However, the average duration may be shorter in adolescents.[36]

Exercise headache is described as aching, pounding, or throbbing and has many migraine characteristics, with associated nausea, vomiting, and photophobia and some phonophobia. It may be bilateral (approximately 60% of the cases) or unilateral.[3,9,11]

Even in the presence of a typical clinical picture, the diagnosis of primary exercise headache can be made only after an extensive investigation. Contrary to cough headache, however, more than 80% of patients consulting due to exertional headache are primary cases (see **Fig. 4**). Patients with exercise-induced headache should have neuroimaging, preferably brain MRI, and MRA to rule out vascular abnormalities or other structural causes. Such investigations are especially needed when headaches appear de novo after the age of 40, are prolonged, or are accompanied by vomiting or focal neurologic symptoms. It is mandatory to exclude any kind of intracranial space-occupying lesion and sentinel hemorrhage due to vascular malformations.[3,9,11]

Box 3
ICHD-3 diagnostic criteria for primary exercise headache

A. At least 2 headache episodes fulfilling criteria B and C.

B. Brought on by and occurring only during or after strenuous physical exercise.

C. Lasting less than 48 hours.

D. Not better accounted for by another ICHD-3 diagnosis.

From Headache Classification Committee of the International Headache Society (IHS). The International Classification of Headache Disorders. 3rd edition. Cephalalgia 2018; 38: 1-211; with permission.

Other possible entities to be investigated include pheochromocytoma,[37] carcinoid syndrome, intracranial pressure disorders, and cerebral venous sinus thrombosis. Cardiac cephalalgia is another important mimic of primary exercise headache,[38] especially in patients with multiple vascular risk factors.[39] Older patients (typically older than 50 years), patients with vascular risk factors, and those with unusual associated symptoms, such as chest pain or sweating, should have a cardiac assessment, including electrocardiogram, echocardiography, and consideration of referral to a cardiologist.

The etiology of benign exercise headache is presumed to be related to cerebral vasodilation, both extracranial and intracranial in nature. In these patients, cerebral blood flow velocity increases and the pulsatility index decreases as compared with controls. In this respect, exertional headache may resemble the headaches associated with high altitude and fever. The finding of a higher prevalence of internal jugular venous valve incompetence in patients with exercise headache could indicate that in some cases the pathophysiological mechanism could be an intracranial venous congestion.[40]

Treatment of exercise headache is usually prophylactic or preventive when exercise is predictable. For non-incapacitating cases or for those with a low exercise frequency, the first, and sometimes the only, recommendation should be transient exercise moderation or abstinence. From a pharmacologic perspective, antimigraine preventive medications show some benefit. For most patients, beta-blockers at the usual antimigraine doses seem to be useful.[3,9,11] There are well-documented cases with exertional headache that did not improve or could not tolerate beta-blockers. Small studies have suggested a role for indomethacin.[24,41] The therapeutic dose may range from 25 to 150 mg per day, although higher doses may be necessary. Indomethacin can be used daily, but administering it 30 to 60 minutes before activity or exercise may be more effective The mechanism of indomethacin's benefit in these syndromes is not known, although an effect on CSF pressure has been suggested.[26]

There is no consensus on the treatment duration in these cases. Primary exertional headache is usually a transient clinical issue and is typically thought to resolve spontaneously in most patients. Therefore, we recommend stopping the preventive treatment after 3 to 6 months to check for headache reappearance.

Acute therapy could theoretically be a good alternative for some patients. Simple analgesics and nonsteroidal anti-inflammatory drugs do not seem to prevent the development of exertional headaches. Ergotamine seems to be useful. Triptans could theoretically be an alternative treatment to ergotamine, but, again, there is no definite scientific evidence as to the possible value of triptans in the acute treatment of exertional headache.

PRIMARY HEADACHE ASSOCIATED WITH SEXUAL ACTIVITY

Headache associated with sexual activity has been referred to as sexual headache, benign vascular sexual headache, coital cephalalgia, coital headache, intercourse headache, (pre)orgasmic cephalalgia, and (pre)orgasmic headache. It is a relatively uncommon headache. This entity describes headaches precipitated by sexual activity, usually starting as a dull bilateral ache as sexual excitement increases and suddenly becoming intense at orgasm, in the absence of any intracranial disorder.[1]

Headaches may occur during sexual activities associated with intercourse or independent of intercourse (eg, masturbation) or orgasm. Two subtypes (*preorgasmic headache* and *orgasmic headache*) were included in previous International

Classifications of Headache (ICHD-1 and ICHD-2), but clinical studies have been unable to distinguish these; therefore, it is now regarded as a single entity with variable presentation.[1,42]

Headache associated with sexual activity is bilateral in approximately two-thirds of patients and unilateral in one-third, with predominance in the occipital area.[1] Pain is variable in terms of onset (sudden or gradual), quality (pressurelike or throbbing), peak intensity (mild to severe), and duration (minutes to hours). The most common is the explosive type. These patients often suffer from exertional headaches as well, and rarely also from cough headache.[3,9,43,44] As occurs in exertional headache, there is a bidirectional comorbidity between sexual headache and migraine.[45] These coincidences seem logical, as sexual intercourse combines prolonged physical exercise and the Valsalva maneuver.

Primary headache associated with sexual activity is rare in terms of consultation, but its exact prevalence and incidence remain unclear. A population-based study found a lifetime prevalence of sexual headache of 1%.[2] This headache occurs typically in young to middle-aged people (average in our series 40 years) and is most common in men (ratios range from 1.2:1–3:1). The prognosis is generally good,[42] although recent studies have shown that up to 40% of all cases run a chronic course over more than a year. Current diagnostic criteria for orgasmic headache appear in **Box 4**.

The pathophysiology of orgasmic headache is unknown, although sudden hemodynamic changes have been proposed as an explanation.[43,44] The etiologies for secondary cases comprise subarachnoid bleeding, intracranial and extracranial arterial dissection, reversible cerebral vasoconstriction syndrome, and, more rarely, intracranial masses.[3,9] Therefore, diagnostic investigation in these headaches must begin first with a neuroimaging study (CT or MRI). Conventional angiography and/or lumbar puncture would be indicated only in those cases with a high suspicion of bleeding despite a negative angioMRI, but not as routine (see **Fig. 4**). Multiple explosive headaches during sexual activities should be considered as headache attributed to reversible cerebral vasoconstriction syndrome until proven otherwise by angiographic studies.

Management is identical to that of prolonged exertional headache. Treatment principles include education and reassurance of the benign, self-limiting natural history of the headache. Indomethacin or triptans 30 minutes before sexual activity can be effective.[46] For longer periods, beta-blockers provide an alternative.[3]

Box 4
ICHD-3 diagnostic criteria for primary headache associated with sexual activity

A. At least 2 episodes of pain in the head and/or neck fulfilling criteria B to D.

B. Brought on by and occurring only during sexual activity.

C. Either or both of the following:
   1. Increasing in intensity with increasing sexual excitement.
   2. Abrupt explosive intensity just before or with orgasm.

D. Lasting from 1 minute to 24 hours with severe intensity and/or up to 72 hours with mild intensity.

E. Not better accounted for by another ICHD-3 diagnosis.

From Headache Classification Committee of the International Headache Society (IHS). The International Classification of Headache Disorders. 3rd edition. Cephalalgia 2018; 38: 1-211; with permission.

PRIMARY THUNDERCLAP HEADACHE

This is a high-intensity headache of abrupt onset mimicking that seen in the case of a ruptured cerebral aneurysm in the absence of any intracranial pathology. The diagnostic criteria for primary thunderclap headache appear in **Box 5**. The recognition that thunderclap headache can be a primary headache disorder has only recently been considered, and evidence of its existence is poor.[1] This syndrome predominantly affects individuals between 20 and 50 years of age, with a female predominance,[11] but its real prevalence is not known.

Thunderclap headache may occur as a benign and recurring headache disorder in the absence of structural intracranial lesions. The clinical picture is very characteristic. Headache appears suddenly and reaches its maximum intensity within 1 minute or less of onset. Headache can be diffuse and may present either in isolation or accompanied by additional symptoms such as nausea or vomiting. In approximately two-thirds of patients, the headache repeats over a period of 2 weeks, whereas the remaining patients may even experience headache attacks over several years. A thunderclap headache is typically described as a relevant event, one clearly different from other types of headaches the patient may have previously experienced. Headache may appear spontaneously or may be triggered by exercise, bathing in hot water, hyperventilation, or by sexual intercourse. By definition, there are no focal symptoms/signs and neuroimaging (CT and MRI) and the cerebrospinal test must be normal.[11,47–49]

The pathophysiology of primary thunderclap headache is unclear, but hypersensitivity of cranial autonomic system has been proposed as an explanation. An excessive sympathetic activity, an abnormal vascular response to circulating catecholamines, or an aberrant central sympathetic neurogenic reflex could explain the occurrence of thunderclap headache in patients with pheochromocytoma, with acute hypertensive crisis, or in patients who take amphetamine or cocaine or foods containing tyramine while concurrently using monoaminoxidase inhibitors.[11]

Thunderclap headache is a medical emergency that requires urgent evaluation, as it is frequently associated with secondary causes. Furthermore, the search for an underlying cause should be quick and exhaustive. The clinician must initially presume that the patient presenting with a thunderclap headache has a secondary cause. Only after exclusion of underlying causes should the diagnosis of primary headache be considered. Differential diagnosis must include serious vascular intracranial disorders, particularly subarachnoid hemorrhage, but also intracerebral hemorrhage, cerebral venous thrombosis, unruptured vascular malformations, arterial dissection (intracranial and extracranial), pheochromocytoma, central nervous system angeitis, colloid cyst of the third ventricle, cerebrospinal hypotension, acute

---

Box 5
ICHD-3 diagnostic criteria for primary thunderclap headache

A. Severe head pain fulfilling criteria B and C.

B. Abrupt onset, reaching maximum intensity in less than 1 minute.

C. Lasting for ≥5 minutes.

D. Not better accounted for by another ICHD-3 diagnosis.

From Headache Classification Committee of the International Headache Society (IHS). The International Classification of Headache Disorders. 3rd edition. Cephalalgia 2018; 38: 1-211; with permission.

sinusitis with barotrauma, and consumption of sympathomimetic drugs, especially amphetamines or cocaine.

It is possible that many patients diagnosed with primary thunderclap headache suffer from the syndrome of reversible cerebral vasculitis/vasoconstriction of unknown etiology.[47–49] This syndrome includes a group of conditions that show reversible multifocal narrowing of the cerebral arteries with clinical manifestations that include thunderclap headache and focal neurologic deficits related to brain edema, stroke, or seizure. Over the past years, these syndromes have been described using variable terminology, including the Call-Fleming syndrome, thunderclap headache with reversible vasospasm, benign angiopathy of the central nervous system, postpartum angiopathy, migrainous vasospasm or migraine angeitis, and drug-induced cerebral arteritis or angiopathy. In a few patients, this condition is complicated by reversible posterior leukoencephalopathy syndrome. There is no confirmatory test for the diagnosis of the syndrome of reversible cerebral vasoconstriction. In patients presenting with thunderclap headache, the usual presenting symptoms mandate CT and MRI, as well as laboratory tests, including vasculitis and toxicologic screening. Transcranial Doppler can show diffusely elevated blood velocities, which typically normalize over a period of days to weeks. The characteristic angiographic pattern of multifocal narrowing and dilation of the intracerebral arteries is best seen by conventional angiography or with less invasive tests like MRA. This technique is particularly useful for documenting reversal of the vasoconstriction.[11,47–50]

If secondary causes have been ruled out, treatment for a primary thunderclap headache can be challenging. Patients generally do not respond well to typical headache pain relievers and there is no established treatment. A short course of steroids can be justified to cover for cerebral vasculitis while awaiting results of serial angiography. Nimodipine has been demonstrated to prevent further attacks of thunderclap headaches in most patients and should be recommended for 2 to 3 months.[49,51] It is also important to avoid vasoconstrictors, such as triptans, ergot derivatives, cocaine, or similar drugs.[11,47–51]

COLD-STIMULUS HEADACHE

This headache, also known as ice-cream headache or brain-freeze headache, is triggered by exposure of the unprotected head to a cold environment, such as diving into cold water or receiving cryotherapy.[1] In addition, cold-stimulus headache can be triggered by passing solid, liquid, or gaseous cold materials over the palate and posterior pharynx. Common examples include eating ice cream or crushed ice.

Typically, headache begins seconds after the stimulus and lasts from seconds (most episodes last <30 seconds) to 5 minutes in some patients.[52,53] Headache is localized commonly in frontal or temporal areas, and frequently is bilateral. There must be at least 2 episodes of headache brought on by a cold stimulus and that are not better accounted for by another ICHD-3 diagnosis to meet the diagnostic criteria.

Epidemiologic studies of cold-stimulus headache are limited. Prevalence varies, ranging from 7.6% to 93.0%,[54,55] and it is more common in people who suffer from migraine.[56] Its pathophysiology is not completely understood, but theoretically a cold stimulus may act as a trigeminal trigger followed by possible reflex vasoconstriction. Rapid constriction and dilation of vessels thus activates the nociceptors in the vessel wall and, in an example of referred pain, cold stimulation of the palate or posterior pharyngeal wall results in frontal or temporal head pain.

Because headache is generally short-lived, cold-stimulus headache does not require a specific treatment aside from trigger avoidance.

EXTERNAL-PRESSURE HEADACHE

External-pressure headache has been moved to this group of headaches from Group 13 of the ICHD-2. This headache is caused by sustained compression of or traction on pericranial soft tissues without damage to the scalp. The inclusion of this headache in the primary headaches is because compression and traction are considered too subtle to cause damage to the scalp. In other words, they are physiologic stimuli.

Several causative factors have been attributed to the wearing of bands around the head, specifically goggles (such as those worn for swimming), tight hats, or even professional helmets.[57] On the other hand, external-traction headache occurs only during traction on the scalp. In both cases, headache relief needs pressure removal. The duration of headache varies with the severity and duration of the external pressure.[1]

Clinical features include a headache moderate in intensity, frequently constant, non-pulsating, and maximal at the site of traction but often extending to other areas of the head. Like other headaches in this section, headache from external pressure is more frequent in patients who also have migraine, and is more usual in women, although men are the most frequent users of the professional helmet. The diagnostic criteria appear in **Box 6**.

The pathophysiological mechanisms are still unclear. It has been suggested that headache is triggered by the compression of nerve endings or branches of the trigeminal and occipital nerves.[58] Treatment is based on the recommendation that the patient removes the stimulus that is causing the headache. Subsequent treatment with drugs is rarely needed.

PRIMARY STABBING HEADACHE

This headache, previously known as ice-pick pain, jabs and jolts, or ophthalmodynia periodica, consists of transient and localized stabs of pain in the head that occur spontaneously in the absence of organic disease of underlying structures or of the cranial nerves.[1] The IHS diagnostic criteria for stabbing headache appear in **Box 7**.[1,11]

Box 6
ICHD-3 diagnostic criteria for external-pressure headache

External-compression headache
A. At least 2 episodes of headache fulfilling criteria B to D.
B. Brought on by and occurring within 1 hour during sustained external compression of the forehead or scalp.
C. Maximal at the site of external compression.
D. Resolving within 1 hour after external compression is relieved.
E. Not better accounted for by another ICHD-3 diagnosis.

External-traction headache
A. At least 2 episodes of headache fulfilling criteria B to D.
B. Brought on by and occurring only during sustained external traction on the scalp.
C. Maximal at the traction site.
D. Resolving within 1 hour after traction is relieved.
E. Not better accounted for by another ICHD-3 diagnosis.

From Headache Classification Committee of the International Headache Society (IHS). The International Classification of Headache Disorders. 3rd edition. Cephalalgia 2018; 38: 1-211; with permission.

> **Box 7**
> **ICHD-3 diagnostic criteria for primary stabbing headache**
>
> A. Head pain occurring spontaneously as a single stab or series of stabs and fulfilling criteria B and C.
>
> B. Each stab lasts for up to a few seconds.
>
> C. Stabs recur with irregular frequency, from 1 to many per day.
>
> D. No cranial autonomic symptoms.
>
> E. Not better accounted for by another ICHD-3 diagnosis.
>
> *From* Headache Classification Committee of the International Headache Society (IHS). The International Classification of Headache Disorders. 3rd edition. Cephalalgia 2018; 38: 1-211; with permission.

Primary stabbing headache is likely to be common. Prevalence is difficult to estimate, as many individuals only suffer from very few stabs throughout their lives, such stabs being easily forgotten. In various studies, prevalence has ranged from 1% to 35% of the general population.[11,59] Interestingly, stabbing headache is more frequent in migraineurs (approximately 40%), in which stabs tend to be localized to the site habitually affected by migraine headaches, and to patients with cluster headache (approximately 30%).[60] Stabbing headache is more frequent in women (3:1) and usually occurs after adolescence.[59]

Primary stabbing headache is characterized by transient, sharp, jabbing pains that occur either as single episodes or as brief repeated volleys. The pains occur anywhere in the head, involve extratrigeminal regions in 70% of cases, and frequently cause the patient to wince. It may move from one area to another, in either the same or the opposite hemicranium: and only one-third of patients have a fixed location. To meet ICHD-3 diagnostic criteria, no cranial autonomic symptoms are associated. Also, these episodes are not triggered by stimuli, such as eating, talking, or touch.[1]

Stabbing headaches have the shortest duration of all known headaches, lasting 1 to 2 seconds in more than two-thirds of cases; only rarely is pain prolonged by up to 10 seconds. The episodes occur at an irregular frequency, from a single stab to more than 50 episodes per day. The pathophysiology is not understood, the clinical picture suggests a trigeminal nerve hyperexcitability, but the mechanisms remain unknown.[11,60]

The differential diagnosis of primary headache includes disorders presenting with short-lived pains such as trigeminal neuralgia, short-lasting unilateral neuralgiform headache attacks with conjunctival injection and tearing (SUNCT), short-lasting unilateral neuralgiform headache attacks with cranial autonomic symptoms, and chronic paroxysmal hemicrania. Trigeminal neuralgia involving the first division of the trigeminal nerve is a possible differential diagnosis. The existence of trigger points and the response to carbamazepine in trigeminal neuralgia are important clues. The ultrashort duration and the lack of autonomic features distinguish stabbing headache from SUNCT syndrome and also from chronic paroxysmal hemicrania.[11,60]

Adult patients with new-onset primary stabbing headache should undergo a diagnostic evaluation to exclude secondary causes, although most cases are idiopathic. Neuroimaging may be indicated depending on headache red flags. Short stabs of pain have been described with intracranial lesions, such as pituitary tumors or meningioma, at the onset of cerebrovascular disease or herpes zoster, with ocular or cranial trauma and with acute glaucoma.[11–61]

Primary stabbing headache is benign and typically does not require pharmacologic treatment. No therapies have been evaluated in controlled trials. For patients with frequent attacks, indomethacin is the medication of choice.[1,11,60,62,63] Duration of treatment must be individualized. Melatonin, gabapentin and celecoxib have been useful in a few cases and can be given in patients who are intolerant or show a partial response to indomethacin.

NUMMULAR HEADACHE

Also called coin-shaped headache, nummular headache is an unusual headache disorder characterized by pain in a small circumscribed area of the scalp in the absence of any underlying structural lesion.[1] Diagnostic criteria appear in **Box 8**.

The true prevalence of nummular headache is unknown. Although it is considered an uncommon headache, one hospital series estimated an incidence of 6.4 per 100,000 per year.[64] As with other primary headaches, nummular headaches are more common in women with a mean age of onset at 45 years. Interestingly, although approximately 13% of patients report prior head trauma, limited correlation exists between the site of trauma and the location of the pain. A preexisting headache diagnosis has been described in approximately 50% of patients, the most common migraine.

Nummular headache clinical features are characterized by small circumscribed areas of continuous pain on any area of the head.[1,65] Generally, it is considered to be of mild to moderate intensity and confined to a round or elliptical unchanging area from 2 to 6 cm in diameter, the pain being continuous or intermittent. Superimposed on the continuous pain, lancinating pain may occur. The pain remains focal and well circumscribed and characteristically never radiates. The affected area may also suffer sensory dysfunction (allodynia, paresthesia, or hyperesthesia) with the parietal region being the area of scalp most often affected.[66] Typically, nummular headache is not accompanied by photophobia, nausea, vomiting, or autonomic symptoms.

The differential diagnosis includes such secondary headaches or underlying structural lesions as cranial bone lesions caused by metastatic cancer, multiple myeloma, Paget disease, or osteomyelitis.[65] Among primary headaches must be considered the primary stabbing headache, which tends to be multifocal and variable in location,

---

Box 8
ICHD-3 diagnostic criteria for primary nummular headache

A. Continuous or intermittent head pain fulfilling criterion B.

B. Felt exclusively in an area of the scalp, with all of the following 4 characteristics:
1. Sharply-contoured.
2. Fixed in size and shape.
3. Round or elliptical.
4. 1 to 6 cm in diameter.

C. Not better accounted for by another ICHD-3 diagnosis.

From Headache Classification Committee of the International Headache Society (IHS). The International Classification of Headache Disorders. 3rd edition. Cephalalgia 2018; 38: 1-211; with permission.

epicrania fugax (in motion rather than a single focal coin-shaped area), and other cranial neuralgias.

The mechanism for nummular headache is unclear. Nummular headache may be a focal form of complex regional pain syndrome,[67] whereas other investigators have suggested a possible relationship between autoimmunity and nummular headache.[68]

Little evidence exists for nummular headache treatment. Approximately 60% of patients respond to analgesics and nonsteroidal anti-inflammatory drugs. For patients with more severe, refractory, or continuous pain, preventive treatment should be offered. Gabapentin and tricyclic antidepressants have been reported to be effective. Other options include indomethacin, and even transcutaneous electrical nerve stimulation. New approaches include the use of local onabotulinumtoxinA, which in different series has achieved pain relief in patients with nummular headache.[69] However, nummular headache often becomes refractory to prophylactic and analgesic therapies.

HYPNIC HEADACHE

Hypnic headache is characterized by recurring headache attacks developing only during sleep. First described by Raskin in 1988,[21] it was adopted by the second edition of the ICHD and confirmed in the third one. Its epidemiology is unknown, but in terms of clinical practice, hypnic headache is rare. Among patients consulting tertiary headache centers, the overall proportion of patients with hypnic headache ranged from 0.07% to 0.35%.[70] Hypnic headache is more frequent in women, the onset typically occurs after the age of 50 years (mean approximately 60) but may occur in younger people. Diagnostic criteria appear in **Box 9**.

By definition, attacks occur at night during sleep (or during a nap in 10% of cases), waking the patient at constant time intervals ("alarm clock headache"). When awaking with headache, most patients do not stay in bed, but instead display motor activity and engage in elaborate activities. Headache is usually mild-moderate in intensity, being severe in 34% of the cases, and lasts from 15 to 240 minutes after waking, but longer attacks of up to 10 hours also have been described.[71] To meet ICHD-3 diagnostic criteria, patients must have recurrent headache attacks and occur on 10 or more days per month for more than 3 months.[1]

Pain location is not characteristic, being bilateral in approximately two-thirds of cases. Regarding frequency, half of the patients have daily attacks (ranging from

---

Box 9
ICHD-3 diagnostic criteria for hypnic headache

A. Recurrent headache attacks fulfilling criteria B to E.

B. Developing only during sleep, and causing wakening.

C. Occurring on ≥10 days per month for more than 3 months.

D. Lasting from 15 minutes up to 4 hours after waking.

E. No cranial autonomic symptoms or restlessness.

F. Not better accounted for by another ICHD-3 diagnosis.

From Headache Classification Committee of the International Headache Society (IHS). The International Classification of Headache Disorders. 3rd edition. Cephalalgia 2018; 38: 1-211; with permission.

1 per week to 6 per night). Triggers or autonomic phenomena are not part of the clinical picture of hypnic headache. Contrary to stabbing headache, a history of the most common primary headaches is not associated with the development of hypnic headache.[71–76]

Pathophysiological mechanisms of hypnic headache are speculative. It has been hypothesized that hypnic headache is the result of dysfunction within the suprachiasmatic nucleus in the hypothalamus, which is considered the brain pacemaker. Supporting this hypothesis, one study found a significant gray matter volume loss within the posterior hypothalamus in patients with hypnic headache compared with age and gender-matched healthy controls.[77] Melatonin is secreted by the pineal gland and is also a marker of circadian rhythms. A decrease in nocturnal secretion of melatonin has also been suggested as a potential mechanism for hypnic headache. Finally, although early reports suggested a rapid eye movement (REM) sleep disorder, later studies showed that most hypnic headaches attacks arise from non-REM sleep stages, mainly sleep stage N2.[78,79]

Secondary causes of headache must be ruled out before the diagnosis of hypnic headache. The differential diagnosis for nocturnal headaches includes nocturnal hypertension, increased intracranial pressure (mass lesion or idiopathic intracranial hypertension), trigeminal autonomic cephalalgias (specifically cluster headache), medication-overuse (rebound) headache, and sleep apnea headache. In our personal experience, the most common confounding diagnoses for patients consulting because of a suspicion of hypnic headache are (1) nocturnal peaks of arterial hypertension, frequently in hypertensive patients who receive treatment early in the morning; and (2) rebound phenomenon in migraineurs with overuse.

There are no controlled trials for the treatment of hypnic headache, so treatment recommendations are based on case reports or small open case series. Main treatment options include caffeine, lithium, indomethacin, and melatonin. Lithium interacts with the pain-modulating systems possibly involved in this syndrome, and also indirectly increases nocturnal production of melatonin, and remains the most popular treatment for hypnic headache.[80] Lithium carbonate can be initiated at 300 mg at night and increased to 600 mg after 1 or 2 weeks if necessary. Poor tolerability to lithium is not rare, mainly in elderly patients. Melatonin has been shown to be useful in some cases, as well as nocturnal caffeine, which appears to be a well-tolerated option to consider before initiating a higher toxicity option such as lithium. Indomethacin outcome seems to be mixed, with half of patients responding to therapy.[77] There are scattered case reports documenting the usefulness of topiramate, amitriptyline, verapamil, prednisone, acetazolamide, gabapentin, and pizotifen.[76]

NEW DAILY-PERSISTENT HEADACHE

New daily-persistent headache (NDPH) was recognized by the second edition of the IHS classification as a separate entity from chronic tension-type headache and remains in the new classification.[1] NDPH is a daily and unremitting from, or almost from, the moment of onset (within 24 hours at most), typically in individuals without a prior history of headache. As stated by the IHS, NDPH may take either of 2 subforms: a self-limiting subtype that typically resolves within several months without therapy, and a refractory subtype that is resistant to aggressive treatment regimens, but both subforms are not separately coded.[1]

The incidence and prevalence of NDPH are unknown, studies from headache centers suggest that NDPH is more frequent in women than in men and affects children

> **Box 10**
> **ICHD-3 diagnostic criteria for new daily-persistent headache (NDPH)**
>
> A. Persistent headache fulfilling criteria B and C.
>
> B. Distinct and clearly remembered onset, with pain becoming continuous and unremitting within 24 hours.
>
> C. Present for more than 3 months.
>
> D. Not better accounted for by another ICHD-3 diagnosis.
>
> *From* Headache Classification Committee of the International Headache Society (IHS). The International Classification of Headache Disorders. 3rd edition. Cephalalgia 2018; 38: 1-211; with permission.

more often than adults. Diagnosed at all ages, NDPH usually begins in the second and third decade in women and in the fifth decade in men.[81] Typically, patients can pinpoint the exact date their headache started. In at least half of the cases, headache begins in relation to an infection or flulike illness or a stressful life event.

NDPH clinical features include mild to severe intensity, variable pain location, and potentially associated migrainous features that include nausea, vomiting, photophobia, and phonophobia. Current diagnostic criteria for NDPH appear in **Box 10**.[81–83]

The exact pathogenic mechanism is unknown, but there are several proposed etiologies. After a viral infection or stressful event, such as surgery, a persistent central nervous system inflammation has been proposed, secondary to glial activation and increased tumor necrosis factor alpha levels in the CSF.[81,84] Another theory suggests cervical spine joint hypermobility as a predisposing factor for the development of NDPH. Joint hypermobility in the cervical spine can theoretically lead to persistent daily headache, as there is convergence of trigeminal and cervical afferents in the trigeminal nucleus caudalis.[85]

Diagnosis of NDPH is one of exclusion. Secondary causes of NDPH appear in **Box 11**. Low CSF headache due to spontaneous CSF leak, or cerebral vein thrombosis, as well as headache attributed to infection (particularly viral) and medication-overuse headache can all mimic NDPH presentation and should always be carefully ruled out with appropriate investigations.

At present no specific treatment strategy can be suggested based on clinical evidence. NDPH is difficult to manage. In general, it is recommended to classify the

> **Box 11**
> **Secondary causes of new daily-persistent headache**
>
> Cerebral vein thrombosis
>
> Low cerebrospinal fluid pressure headache
>
> High cerebrospinal fluid pressure headache
>
> Medication-overuse headache
>
> Carotid or vertebral artery dissection
>
> Giant cell arteritis
>
> Meningitis
>
> Sphenoid sinusitis
>
> Cervical facet syndrome
>
> Posttraumatic headache

dominant headache phenotype (migraine or tension-type headache) and treat with preventives accordingly.[81–84] Even with aggressive treatment, many patients do not improve and become treatment refractory. Consequently, other possible and heterogeneous alternatives, such as doxycycline, a tumor necrosis factor alpha inhibitor,[86] mexiletine,[87] endovenous corticosteroids, or nerve blockade have been desperately tried in these patients.

REFERENCES

1. Headache Classification Committee of the International Headache Society (IHS) The International Classification of Headache Disorders. Cephalalgia 2018;38: 1–211.

2. Rasmussen BK, Olesen J. Symptomatic and nonsymptomatic headaches in a general population. Neurology 1992;42:1225–31.

3. Pascual J, González-Mandly A, Martín R, et al. Headaches precipitated by cough, prolonged exercise or sexual activity: a prospective etiological and clinical study. J Headache Pain 2008;9:259–66.

4. Symonds C. Cough headache. Brain 1956;79:557–68.

5. Nick J. La céphalée d'effort. A propos d'une série de 43 cas. Sem Hop 1980;56: 525–31.

6. Rooke ED. Benign exertional headache. Med Clin North Am 1968;52:801–8.

7. Sands GH, Newman L, Lipton R. Cough, exertional and other miscellaneous headaches. Med Clin North Am 1991;75:733–47.

8. Cordenier A, De Hertogh W, De Keyser J, et al. Headache associated with cough: a review. J Headache Pain 2013;14:42.

9. Pascual J, Iglesias F, Oterino A, et al. Cough, exertional, and sexual headaches: an analysis of 72 benign and symptomatic cases. Neurology 1996;46:1520–4.

10. Ramón C, Gónzalez-Mandly A, Pascual J. What differences exist in the appropriate treatment of congenital versus acquired adult Chiari type I malformation? Curr Pain Headache Rep 2011;15:157–63.

11. Dodick D, Pascual J. Primary stabbing, cough, exertional, and thunderclap headaches. In: Olesen J, Goadsby PJ, Ramadan NM, et al, editors. The headaches. 3rd edition. Philadelphia: Lippincott Williams & Wilkins; 2006. p. 831–9.

12. Pascual J. Activity-related headache. In: Gilman S, editor. MedLink neurology. San Diego (CA): MedLink Corporation. Available at: www.medlink.com. Accessed January 2, 2019.

13. Diamond S. Prolonged benign exertional headache: its clinical characteristics and response to indomethacin. Headache 1982;22:96–8.

14. Williams B. Cerebrospinal fluid pressure changes in response to coughing. Brain 1976;99:331–46.

15. Williams B. Cough headache due to craniospinal pressure dissociation. Arch Neurol 1980;37:226–30.

16. Nightingale S, Williams B. Hindbrain hernia headache. Lancet 1987;1:731–4.

17. Sansur CA, Heiss JD, DeVroom HL, et al. Pathophysiology of headache associated with cough in patients with Chiari I malformation. J Neurosurg 2003;98: 453–8.

18. Williams B. Simultaneous cerebral and spinal fluid pressure recordings. 2. Cerebrospinal dissociation with lesions at the foramen magnum. Acta Neurochir (Wien) 1981;59(1-2):123–42.

19. Pujol J, Roig C, Capdevilla A, et al. Motion of the cerebellar tonsils in Chiari type I malformation studied by cine-phase constrast MRI. Neurology 1995;45:1746–53.

20. Wang SJ, Fuh JL, Lu SR. Benign cough headache is responsive to acetazolamide. Neurology 2000;55:149–50.
21. Raskin NH. Short-lived head pains. Neurol Clin 1997;15:143–52.
22. Chen YY, Lirng JF, Fuh JL, et al. Primary cough headache is associated with posterior fossa crowdedness: a morphometric MRI study. Cephalalgia 2004;24: 694–9.
23. Smith WS, Messing RO. Cerebral aneurysm presenting as cough headache. Headache 1993;33:203–4.
24. Diamond S, Medina JL. Benign exertional headache: successful treatment with indomethacin. Headache 1979;19:249.
25. Mathew NT. Indomethacin-responsive headache syndromes. Headache 1981;21: 147–50.
26. Slavik RS, Rhoney DH. Indomethacin: a review of its cerebral blood flow effects and potential use for controlling intracranial pressure in traumatic brain injury patients. Neurol Res 1999;21:491–9.
27. Chalaupka FD. Therapeutic effectiveness of acetazolamide in hindbrain hernia headache. Neurol Sci 2000;21:117–9.
28. Dalessio DJ. Effort migraine. Headache 1974;14:53.
29. Medrano V, Mallada J, Sempere AP, et al. Primary cough headache responsive to topiramate. Cephalalgia 2005;25:627–8.
30. Bahra A, Goadsby PJ. Cough headache responsive to methysergide. Cephalalgia 1998;18:495–6.
31. Calandre L, Hernandez-Lain A, Lopez-Valdes E. Benign Valsalva's maneuver-related headache: an MRI study of six cases. Headache 1996;36:251–3.
32. Gupta VK. Metoclopramide aborts cough-induced headache and ameliorates cough–a pilot study. Int J Clin Pract 2007;61:345–8.
33. Chen SP, Fuh JL, Lu SR, et al. Exertional headache-a survey of 1963 adolescents. Cephalalgia 2008;29:401–7.
34. Sjaastad O, Bakketeig LS. Exertional headache. I. Vågå study of headache epidemiology. Cephalalgia 2002;22:784–90.
35. Indo T, Takahashi A. Swimmer's headache. Headache 1990;30:485–7.
36. Tofangchiha S, Rabiee B, Mehrabi F. A study of exertional headache's prevalence and characteristics among conscripts. Asian J Sports Med 2016;7:e30720.
37. Paulson GW, Zipf RE, Beekman JF. Pheochromocytoma causing exercise-related headache and pulmonary edema. Ann Neurol 1979;5:96–9.
38. Wei JH, Wang HF. Cardiac cephalalgia: case reports and review. Cephalalgia 2008;28:892–6.
39. Wang M, Wang L, Liu C, et al. Cardiac cephalalgia: one case with cortical hypoperfusion in headaches and literature review. J Headache Pain 2017;8:1–8.
40. Doepp F, Valdueza JM, Schreiber SJ. Incompetence of internal jugular valve in patients with primary exertional headache: a risk factor? Cephalalgia 2008;28: 182–5.
41. Halker R, Vargas B. Primary exertional headache: updates in the literature. Curr Pain Headache Rep 2013;17:337.
42. Frese A, Eikermann A, Frese K, et al. Headache associated with sexual activity: demography, clinical features, and comorbidity. Neurology 2003;61:796–800.
43. Evers S, Lance JW. Primary headache attributed to sexual activity. In: Olesen J, Goadsby PJ, Ramadan NM, et al, editors. The headaches. 3rd edition. Philadelphia: Lippincott Williams & Wilkins; 2006. p. 841–5.

44. Silbert PL, Edis RH, Stewart-Wynne EG, et al. Benign vascular sexual headache and exertional headache: interrelationships and long-term prognosis. J Neurol Neurosurg Psychiatry 1991;54:417–21.

45. Biehl K, Evers S, Frese A. Comorbidity of migraine and headache associated with sexual activity. Cephalalgia 2007;27:1271–3.

46. Evans RW, Pascual J. Expert opinion: orgasmic headaches: clinical features, diagnosis, and management. Headache 2000;40:491–4.

47. Calabrese LH, Dodick DW, Schwedt TJ, et al. Narrative review: reversible cerebral vasoconstriction syndromes. Ann Intern Med 2007;146:34–44.

48. Dodick DW, Brown RD Jr, Britton JW, et al. Non-aneurysmal thunderclap headache with diffuse, multifocal, segmental and reversible vasospasm. Cephalalgia 1999;19:118–23.

49. Chen SP, Fuh JL, Lirng JF, et al. Recurrent primary thunderclap headache and benign CNS angiopathy: spectra of the same disorder? Neurology 2006;67: 2164–9.

50. Singhal AB, Topcuoglu MA, Fok JW, et al. Reversible cerebral vasoconstriction syndromes and primary angiitis of the central nervous system: clinical, imaging, and angiographic comparison. Ann Neurol 2016;79:882.

51. Lu SR, Liao YC, Fuh JL, et al. Nimodipine for treatment of primary thunderclap headache. Neurology 2004;62:1414–6.

52. Boes CJ, Copobianco DJ, Cutrer FM, et al. Headache and other craniofacial pain. In: Bradley WG, Daroff RB, Fenichel GM, et al, editors. Neurology in clinical practice. Philadelphia: Butterworth Heinemann; 2004. p. 2055.

53. Cheshire WP Jr, Ott MC. Headache in divers. Headache 2001;41:235–47.

54. Fuh JL, Wang SJ, Lu SR, et al. Ice-cream headache—a large survey of 8359 adolescents. Cephalalgia 2003;23:977–81.

55. Starling AJ. Unusual headache disorders. Continuum (Minneap Minn) 2018;24: 1192–208.

56. Raskin NH, Knittle SC. Ice cream headache and orthostatic symptoms in patients with migraine. Headache 1976;16:222–5.

57. Krymchantowski AV. Headaches due to external compression. Curr Pain Headache Rep 2010;14:321–4.

58. Lance J, Goadsby PJ. Miscellaneous headaches unassociated with a structural lesion. In: Olesen J, Tfelt-Hansen P, Welch KM, editors. The headaches. 2nd edition. Philadelphia: Lippincott Williams & Wilkins; 2000. p. 752–3.

59. Sjaastad O, Pettersen H, Bakketeig LS. The Vaga study; epidemiology of headache I: the prevalence of ultrashort paroxysms. Cephalalgia 2001;21:207–15.

60. Pareja JA, Ruiz J, de Isla C, et al. Idiopathic stabbing headache (jabs and jolts syndrome). Cephalalgia 1996;16:93.

61. Mascellino AM, Lay CL, Newman LC. Stabbing headache as the presenting manifestation of intracranial meningioma: a report of two patients. Headache 2001;41:599–601.

62. Dodick D. Indomethacin responsive headache syndromes. Curr Pain Headache Rep 2004;8:19–28.

63. VanderPluym J. Indomethacin-responsive headaches. Curr Neurol Neurosci Rep 2015;15:516.

64. Pareja JA, Pareja J, Barriga FJ, et al. Nummular headache: a prospective series of 14 new cases. Headache 2004;44:611.

65. Pareja JA, Caminero AB, Serra J, et al. Nummular headache: a coin-shaped cephalgia. Neurology 2002;58:1678.

66. Schwartz DP, Robbins MS, Grosberg BM. Nummular headache update. Curr Pain Headache Rep 2013;17:340.
67. Grosberg BM, Solomon S, Lipton RB. Nummular headache. Curr Pain Headache Rep 2007;11:310–2.
68. Chen WH, Chen YT, Lin CS, et al. A high prevalence of autoimmune indices and disorders in primary nummular headache. J Neurol Sci 2012;320:127–30.
69. Linde M, Hagen K, Stovner LJ. Botulinum toxin treatment of secondary headaches and cranial neuralgias: a review of evidence. Acta Neurol Scand (Suppl) 2011;109:50–5.
70. Lanteri-Minet M, Donnet A. Hypnic headache. Curr Pain Headache Rep 2010;14:309–15.
71. Liang JF, Wang SJ. Hypnic headache: a review of clinical features, therapeutic options and outcomes. Cephalalgia 2014;34:795–805.
72. Rains JC, Poceta JS. Sleep-related headache syndromes. Semin Neurol 2005;25:69–80.
73. Dodick DW, Eross EJ, Parish JM, et al. Clinical, anatomical, and physiologic relationship between sleep and headache. Headache 2003;43:282–92.
74. Evans RW, Dodick DW, Schwedt TJ. The headaches that awake us. Headache 2006;46:678–81.
75. Newman LC, Mosek A. Hypnic headaches. In: Olesen J, Goadsby PJ, Ramadan NM, et al, editors. The headaches. 3rd edition. Philadelphia: Lippincott Williams & Wilkins; 2006. p. 847–9.
76. Lanteri-Minet M. Hypnic headache. Headache 2014;54:1556–9.
77. Holle D, Naegelk S, Krebs S, et al. Hypothalamic gray matter volume loss in hypnic headache. Ann Neurol 2011;69:533–9.
78. Holle D, Naegel S, Obermann M. Hypnic headache. Cephalalgia 2013;33:1349–57.
79. Holle D, Naegel S, Obermann M. Pathophysiology of hypnic headache. Cephalalgia 2014;34:806–12.
80. Tarig N, Estemalik E, Vij B, et al. Long-term outcomes and clinical characteristics of Hypnic Headache Syndrome: 40 patients series from a Tertiary Referral Center. Headache 2016;56:717–24.
81. Li D, Rozen TD. The clinical characteristics of new daily persistent headache. Cephalalgia 2002;22:66–9.
82. Evans RW, Rozen TD. Etiology and treatment of new daily persistent headache. Headache 2001;4:830–2.
83. Rozen TD, Jensen R. New daily persistent headache. In: Olesen J, Goadsby PJ, Ramadan NM, et al, editors. The headaches. 3rd edition. Philadelphia: Lippincott Williams & Wilkins; 2006. p. 855–7.
84. Rozen T. New daily persistent headache: an update. Curr Pain Headache Rep 2014;18:431–6.
85. Piovesan EJ, Kowacs PA, Oshinsky ML. Convergence of cervical and trigeminal sensory afferents. Curr Pain Headache Rep 2003;2:155–61.
86. Rozen TD. Doxycycline for treatment resistant new daily persistent headache. Neurology 2008;70(Suppl 1):A348.
87. Marmura MJ, Passero FC, Young WB. Mexiletine for refractory chronic daily headache: a report of 9 cases. Headache 2008;48:1506–10.

Moving?

Make sure your subscription moves with you!

To notify us of your new address, find your **Clinics Account Number** (located on your mailing label above your name), and contact customer service at:

Email: journalscustomerservice-usa@elsevier.com

800-654-2452 (subscribers in the U.S. & Canada)
314-447-8871 (subscribers outside of the U.S. & Canada)

Fax number: 314-447-8029

Elsevier Health Sciences Division
Subscription Customer Service
3251 Riverport Lane
Maryland Heights, MO 63043

*To ensure uninterrupted delivery of your subscription, please notify us at least 4 weeks in advance of move.

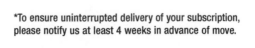

Printed and bound by CPI Group (UK) Ltd, Croydon, CR0 4YY

03/10/2024

01040484-0011